T0256601

Pediatric Otorhinolaryngology:
Diagnosis and Treatment

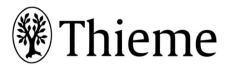

Pediatric Otorhinolaryngology: Diagnosis and Treatment

Greg R. Licameli, M.D., M.H.C.M., F.A.C.S.
Assistant Professor of Otology and Laryngology
Harvard Medical School
Boston, Massachusetts

Attending Surgeon
Department of Otolaryngology and Communication Enhancement
Children's Hospital Boston
Boston, Massachusetts

David E. Tunkel, M.D., F.A.A.P, F.A.C.S.
Director
Department of Pediatric Otolaryngology

Associate Professor of Otolaryngology – Head and Neck Surgery
Pediatrics, and Anesthesiology – Critical Care Medicine
Johns Hopkins University School of Medicine
Baltimore, Maryland

Thieme Medical and Scientific Publishers Private Limited
A-12, Second Floor, Sector - 2
Noida, Uttar Pradesh - 201 301, India
Email: customerservice@thieme.in
www.thieme.com

Thieme
Delhi • Stuttgart • New York

Thieme Medical and Scientific Publishers Private Limited
A-12, Second Floor, Sector - 2
Noida, Uttar Pradesh - 201 301, India

Managing Editor: Sangeeta P.C.
Assistant Manager - Publishing: Kumar Kunal
National Sales and Marketing Manager: Harish Singh Bora
Chief Executive Officer: Ajit Kohli

Pediatric Otorhinolaryngology: Diagnosis and Treatment / [edited by] Greg R. Licameli, David E. Tunkel.

Includes bibliographical references and index.

ISBN 978-93-82076-04-9

Licameli, Greg R. II. Tunkel, David E.

Copyright © 2013 by Thieme Medical and Scientific Publishers Private Limited. This book, including all parts thereof, is legally protected by copyright. Any use, exploitation, or commercialization outside the narrow limits set by copyright legislation without the publisher's consent is illegal and liable to prosecution. This applies in particular to photostat reproduction, copying, mimeographing or duplication of any kind, translating, preparing of microfilms, and electronic data processing and storage.

Important note: Medical knowledge is ever changing. As new research and clinical experience broaden our knowledge, changes in treatment and drug therapy may be required. The authors and editors of the material herein have consulted sources believed to be reliable in their efforts to provide information that is complete and in accord with the standards accepted at the time of publication. However, in view of the possibility human error by the authors, editors, or publishers of the work herein or changes in medical knowledge, neither the authors, editors, nor publishers, nor any other party who has been involved in the preparation of this work, warrants that the information contained herein is in every respect accurate or complete, and they are not responsible for any errors or omissions or for the results obtained from use of such information. Readers are encouraged to confirm the information contained herein with other sources. For example, readers are advice to check the product information sheet included in the package of each drug they plan to administer to be certain that the information contained in this publication is accurate and that changes have not been made in the recommended dose or in the contraindications for administration. This recommendation is of particular importance in connection with new or infrequently used drugs. Some of the product names, patents, and registered designs referred to in this book are in fact registered trademarks or proprietary names even though specific reference to this fact is not always made in the text. Therefore, the appearance of a name without designation as proprietary is not to be construed as a representation by the publishers that it is in the public domain.

5 4 3 2 1

ISBN: 978-93-82076-04-9
eISBN: 978-93-82076-10-0

Pediatric Otorhinolaryngology: Diagnosis and Treatment
Published by Thieme Medical and Scientific Publishers Private Limited
A-12, Second Floor, Sector - 2, Noida, Uttar Pradesh - 201 301, India
Email: customerservice@thieme.in
www.thieme.com
Printer: Gopsons Papers Limited, Noida

Pediatric Otorhinolaryngology: Diagnosis and Treatment

Table of Contents

Foreword

Pediatric otorhinolaryngology is indeed a young subspecialty, yet we continue to see remarkable advances in the diagnostic and therapeutic approaches to ear, nose, and throat disease in young children. We recognize that the care of children with such disorders starts with the primary care provider, usually the pediatrician, and may involve otolaryngologists or subspecialty-trained pediatric otolaryngologists. With this volume on pediatric otorhinolaryngology, we aim to provide up-to-date information useful to all who provide care for children with otolaryngologic disease. For example, the chapters on otitis media, tonsillar infections, and sinusitis will be valuable to both generalists and specialists, while chapters on tracheostomy, laryngotracheal reconstruction, and cochlear implantation may prove most valuable to specialists or specialists-in-training.

While the breadth of pediatric otorhinolaryngology, is daunting, we have provided information about the common ailments as well as those topics that have changed rapidly over the past decade. We thank Prof. M.V. Kirtane and Dr. Chris de Souza, the series editors, for involving us in this endeavor. We applaud the many authors in this volume, whose efforts have provided concise, expert, and fully-researched chapters. Of course, we recognize the readers of this text, who will apply the information provided within to improve the health and quality of lives of children.

Greg R. Licameli, M.D., M.H.C.M., F.A.C.S.
David E. Tunkel, M.D., F.A.A.P, F.A.C.S.

Acknowledgment

It is a daunting task to single out any one individual who contributed to my development as a pediatric otolaryngologist, as so many have influenced my career. As a resident, John Stram, M.D. and Greg Grillone, M.D. at Boston University taught me how to operate under pressure in the shadow of the old City Hospital; as my fellowship director at Johns Hopkins, David Tunkel, M.D. could create an unparalleled differential diagnosis from his encyclopedic knowledge of our field and is a role model to trainees and colleagues alike. I have been fortunate to find myself currently in the company of very talented surgeons; all to whom I have turned to for advice; particularly Margaret Kenna M.D., whose passion for the advancement of pediatric otolaryngology is inspiring and whose door is always open. Finally, to my wife Megan and our two children—your support along every step of the way during this process has been invaluable.

Greg R. Licameli, M.D., M.H.C.M., F.A.C.S.

I have been a practitioner and a student of pediatric otolaryngology for over 20 years, and have experienced many rewards and challenges. As this volume came to completion, I fondly think of both my mentors and my students in pediatric otolaryngology. As a young resident and again as a slightly older faculty member, I had the pleasure of learning from two masters of the pediatric airway, Bernard R. Marsh, M.D.—simply the best endoscopist I have ever seen, and Haskins K. Kashima, M.D.—a true innovator and clinician-researcher. While Dr. Marsh is retired and Dr. Kashima has passed away, I am guided by their lessons almost daily. I also had the good fortune to receive fellowship training, now two decades ago, under the direction of Kenneth M. Grundfast, M.D. Dr. Grundfast's humble expertise, availability, and insightful analysis have helped me in the past and the present, and I am sure will do so in the future. Finally, I thank my wife Theda and my daughter Alexandra, who have encouraged me at every point from conception to editing to publication of this volume.

David E. Tunkel, M.D., F.A.A.P, F.A.C.S.

Contributors

Manali Shailesh Amin, M.D., F.A.C.S.
Department of Otolaryngology
DuPage Medical Group
Glen Ellyn and Naperville, Illinois

Max M. April, M.D., F.A.A.P., F.A.C.S.
Division of Pediatric Otolaryngology
Department of Otolaryngology – Head and Neck Surgery
Weill Cornell Medical College
New York, New York

Fuad M. Baroody, M.D.
Section of Otolaryngology – Head and Neck Surgery
Departments of Surgery and Pediatrics
The Comer Children's Hospital
The University of Chicago Medical Center
Chicago, Illinois

Emily F. Boss, M.D., M.P.H.
Department of Otolaryngology – Head and Neck Surgery
Johns Hopkins University School of Medicine
Baltimore, Maryland

Farrel Joel Buchinsky, M.B.Ch.B.
Department of Otolaryngology – Head and Neck Surgery
Drexel University College of Medicine
Allegheny General Hospital
Pittsburgh, Pennsylvania

David H. Chi, M.D., F.A.C.S.
Department of Otolaryngology
Children's Hospital of Pittsburgh of UPMC
University of Pittsburgh School of Medicine
Pittsburgh, Pennsylvania

Aliza P. Cohen, M.A.
Division of Pediatric Otolaryngology – Head and Neck Surgery
Cincinnati Children's Hospital Medical Center
Cincinnati, Ohio

Michael J. Cunningham, M.D.
Department of Otolaryngology and Communication Enhancement
Children's Hospital Boston
Boston, Massachusetts

Department of Otology and Laryngology
Harvard Medical School
Boston, Massachusetts

David H. Darrow, M.D., D.D.S.
Departments of Otolaryngology and Pediatrics
Eastern Virginia Medical School
Norfolk, Virginia

Department of Otolaryngology
Children's Hospital of The King's Daughters
Norfolk, Virginia

Yaniv Ebner, M.D.
Division of Pediatric Otolaryngology
Department of Otolaryngology – Head and Neck Surgery
Weill Cornell Medical College
New York, New York

Stacey L. Ishman, M.D.
Department of Otolaryngology – Head and Neck Surgery
Center for Snoring and Sleep Surgery
Johns Hopkins School of Medicine
Baltimore, Maryland

Ian N. Jacobs, M.D.
The Center for Pediatric Airway Disorders
The Children's Hospital of Philadelphia
Philadelphia, Pennsylvania

Department of Otolaryngology – Head and Neck Surgery
University of Pennsylvania Perelman School of Medicine
Philadelphia, Pennsylvania

Dennis J. Kitsko, D.O., F.A.C.S.
Department of Otolaryngology
Children's Hospital of Pittsburgh of UPMC
University of Pittsburgh School of Medicine
Pittsburgh, Pennsylvania

Tali Lando, M.D.
Department of Otolaryngology
New York Medical College
Vallhala, New York

Gi Soo Lee, M.D., Ed.M.
Department of Otolaryngology and Communication Enhancement
Boston Children's Hospital
Boston, Massachusetts

Greg R. Licameli, M.D., M.H.C.M., F.A.C.S.
Departments of Otology and Laryngology
Harvard Medical School
Boston, Massachusetts

Children's Hospital Boston
Department of Otolaryngology and Communication Enhancement
Boston, Massachusetts

Myriam Loyo, M.D.
Department of Otolaryngology – Head and Neck Surgery
The Johns Hopkins Hospital
Baltimore, Maryland

David L. Mandell, M.D., F.A.A.P., F.A.C.S.
Department of Otolaryngology
Miller School of Medicine
University of Miami
Miami, Florida

Charles E. Schmidt College of Biomedical Sciences
Florida Atlantic University
Boca Raton, Florida

Division of Otolaryngology
NOVA Southeastern University College of Osteopathic Medicine
Ft. Lauderdale, Florida

Center for Pediatric ENT
Bethesda Health City
Boynton Beach, Florida

Timothy B. McDonald, M.D., J.D.
Departments of Anesthesiology and Pediatrics
University of Illinois College of Medicine
Chicago, Illinois

Deepak Mehta, M.D., F.R.C.S.
Department of Otolaryngology
Children's Hospital of Pittsburgh
University of Pittsburgh
Pittsburgh, Pennsylvania

Andrea Ellen Nath, M.D.
Section of Otolaryngology – Head and Neck Surgery
Department of Surgery
The University of Chicago Medicine
Chicago, Illinois

Roger C. Nuss, M.D.
Department of Otolaryngology and Communication Enhancement
Children's Hospital Boston
Boston, Massachusetts

Kara K. Prickett, M.D.
Department of Otolaryngology – Head and Neck Surgery
Emory University
Atlanta, Georgia

Roy Rajan, M.D.
Department of Otolaryngology – Head and Neck Surgery
Emory Univesity
Atlanta, Georgia

Christopher R. Roxbury, M.D.
Department of Otolaryngology – Head and Neck Surgery
The Johns Hopkins Hospital
Baltimore, Maryland

Michael J. Rutter, M.B.Ch.B., F.R.A.C.S.
Division of Pediatric Otolaryngology – Head and Neck Surgery
Cincinnati Children's Hospital Medical Center
Cincinnati, Ohio

Department of Pediatric Otolaryngology – Head and Neck Surgery
University of Cincinnati College of Medicine
Cincinnati, Ohio

Eliot Shearer, B.Sc.
Departments of Molecular Physiology and Biophysics
Department of Otolaryngology – Head and Neck Surgery, Molecular Otolaryngology and Renal Research Laboratories
University of Iowa
Iowa City, Iowa

Jonathan M. Sherman, M.D.
Section of Otolaryngology – Head and Neck Surgery
Department of Surgery
University of Chicago Medical Center
Chicago, Illinois

Margaret L. Skinner, M.D.
Division of Pediatric Otolaryngology – Head and Neck Surgery
Pediatric Aerodigestive Center
Johns Hopkins Medical Institutions
Baltimore, Maryland

Richard J.H. Smith, M.D.
Departments of Otolaryngology – Head and Neck Surgery, Molecular Otolaryngology and Renal Research Laboratories
University of Iowa
Iowa City, Iowa

Nicholas Smith, M.D.
Pediatric ENT Associates
Children's of Alabama
Division of Otolaryngology, UAB School of Medicine
Birmingham, Alabama

Steven E. Sobol, M.D., M.Sc.
Division of Otolaryngology
Center for Pediatric Airway Disorders
The Children's Hospital of Philadelphia
Philadelphia, Pennsylvania

Department of Otolaryngology – Head and Neck Surgery,
Perelman School of Medicine
University of Pennsylvania
Philadelphia, Pennsylvania

Rose Stavinoha, M.D.
Pediatric Ear, Nose, and Throat Institute
San Antonio, Texas

Dana Suskind, M.D.
Section of Otolaryngology – Head and Neck Surgery
Department of Surgery
University of Chicago Medical Center
Chicago, Illinois

Rosalie F. Tassone, M.D., M.P.H.
Department of Anesthesiology
University of Illinois College of Medicine
Chicago, Illinois

David E. Tunkel, M.D.
Department of Otolaryngology – Head and Neck Surgery Otolaryngology
Johns Hopkins University School of Medicine
Baltimore, Maryland

Frank W. Virgin, M.D.
Division of Pediatric Otolaryngology
Department of Otolaryngology – Head and Neck Surgery
Vanderbilt University Nashville
Nashville, Tennessee

Kenneth R. Whittemore Jr., M.D., M.S.
Department of Otolaryngology and Communication Enhancement
Children's Hospital Boston
Boston, Massachusetts

Department of Otology and Laryngology
Harvard Medical School
Boston, Massachusetts

J. Paul Willging, M.D.
Pediatric Otolaryngology
University of Cincinnati College of Medicine
Cincinnati Children's Hospital Medical Center
Cincinnati, Ohio

SECTION I: Otology

1 Otitis Media

David H. Chi and Dennis J. Kitsko

Otitis media (OM) is one of the most common infectious diseases in children, particularly in infants and toddlers. Approximately 30 to 35% of all visits for acute illness in the primary care setting in the first 5 years of life are for middle ear disease. Up to 40% of total office visits at 4 to 5 years of age will result in the diagnosis of some middle ear problem. This includes approximately 10% of children who present at well-child visits and are without any subjective complaint.[1] Nearly half of all antibiotics prescribed in children less than 10 years old was for OM.[2] The financial burden for medical and surgical intervention for OM is estimated at $5 billion yearly in the United States alone.[3] But perhaps the impact on the day-to-day lives of families is far greater than any monetary figure. It can be associated with speech, language, and balance difficulties, which can contribute to further learning problems. The parental burden of dealing with a fussy, irritable child who sleeps poorly can be very frustrating. Also, parents may be forced to miss multiple days of work as daycare settings frequently forbid children with high fevers to attend; this is in addition to the time missed from work for physician visits.

For the sake of clarity, the following terms and their definitions will be used in this chapter. *Otitis media* will refer to nonspecific inflammation within the middle ear space. *Acute otitis media* (AOM) will refer to acute infection of fluid within the middle ear space, with associated otalgia and an erythematous or bulging tympanic membrane. *Otitis media with effusion* (OME) will be defined as fluid collection in the middle ear space in the absence of signs of acute infection mentioned above. Finally, *middle ear effusion* (MEE) will refer generally to fluid in the middle ear space, whether this fluid is associated with acute infection or not.

Epidemiology

AOM

The vast majority of children will have at least one episode of AOM in childhood. Approximately 62% of infants will have AOM by 12 months of age, with this number rising to 84% at 3 years of age, and 95% by age 7. After age 7, children are much less likely to develop AOM.[1] Many children will have recurrent episodes of AOM as well. Up to 20% of infants will have three episodes by their first birthday, and by age 7, 75% of children will have had at least three episodes.

OME

Determining the incidence of OME is much more difficult because many children will present without any complaints. Furthermore, many episodes of AOM will "become" OME as ear pain and tympanic membrane erythema and bulging resolve, but MEE remains. Identifying the onset and interval to resolution of OME is challenging, as it requires very short observation intervals. This is particularly true given that approximately 65% of OME episodes will resolve in 1 month.[4] Casselbrant et al found a 53 to 61% incidence of OME in 2- to 6-year-old daycare children followed monthly with pneumatic otoscopy and tympanometry. This number dropped to 22% in 5- to 12-year-old schoolchildren.[4,5] Lous and Fiellau-Nikolajsen reported a similar 26% incidence in 7-year-old children who they followed-up for 1 year.[6]

Multiple studies in various countries have looked at the point prevalence of MEE, which includes both AOM and OME, with a great variety of ranges from 1 to 40%. Given the variability in race, sample sizes, age ranges, number of screenings, and screening tools, it is difficult to generalize these incidence data in a meaningful way. What is clear, though, is that almost all children developed MEE at some point during the first 3 years of life.[7,8]

Anatomy and Pathophysiology

The anatomic structures involved in regulating the middle ear system include the mastoid cavity, the middle ear cavity, the eustachian tube (ET), and the nose/nasopharynx and palate. The ET is perhaps the most important of these structures, particularly as it relates to the development of AOM and OME. The ET serves three important functions physiologically: (1) pressure regulation/ventilation and equilibration to atmospheric pressure, (2) protection of the middle ear from pathogens ascending from the nasopharynx via a gas cushion, and (3) clearance of secretions from the middle ear. The origin of middle ear disease is poor ET function and inability to regulate pressure. In infants, the ET is shorter and more horizontal than in an adult, and this is one anatomic factor that leads to poor pressure regulation.

ET dysfunction may occur spontaneously, particularly in infants, but is more commonly associated with antecedent events that cause either anatomic or, more commonly, functional obstruction. Anatomic causes include enlarged adenoids, nasal polyposis, foreign body, or tumor. Functional obstruction is associated with inflammation within the nasal cavity and nasopharynx, most commonly from a viral upper respiratory illness (URI) in children. Other causes include allergic rhinitis and gastroesophageal reflux disease (GERD). This inflammation leads to edema around the ET orifice, which is located in the nasopharynx, and subsequent inability of the ET to open in its usual passive fashion to regulate pressure. As negative pressure builds, secretions and pathogens can be aspirated from the nasopharynx into the middle ear space, creating MEE. This fluid may persist and not become infected, resulting in OME. If, however, the fluid becomes infected, either with viruses or more commonly bacteria, an AOM develops.

Certain populations have a much higher incidence of ET dysfunction and, subsequently, OM. Anatomically, those children with craniofacial abnormalities, Down syndrome, and cleft palate may have persistent ET dysfunction and difficulties with OM throughout their lives. Immunocompromised children are also at increased risk—this includes those with primary ciliary dyskinesia, immunoglobulin deficiencies, T- or B-cell defects, chemotherapy, or human immunodeficiency virus infections.

Microbiology
Bacteriology

The most common bacteria isolated in AOM are *Haemophilus influenzae* (35 to 50%) and *Streptococcus pneumoniae* (25 to 40%). It was hoped that the introduction of the pneumococcal conjugate vaccine—PCV7—in 2000 would dramatically decrease the number of episodes of AOM, but the decrease has been reported at a modest 7.8%, with an increase in the number of infections from nonvaccine serotypes and *Haemophilus* infections.[9–11] *Moraxella catarrhalis* is the third most common bacteria (3 to 20%) isolated, followed by group A *Streptococcus* and *Staphylococcus aureus* (1 to 10%). Also, although neonates and infants usually have the same bacteriologic pattern as older children, gram-negative bacteria such as *Escherichia coli*, *Klebsiella*, and *Pseudomonas* are seen with a higher frequency. Anaerobic bacteria such as *Peptostreptococcus*, *Fusobacterium*, and *Bacteroides* are more commonly seen in chronic suppurative OM (persistent drainage via a tympanostomy tube or perforation) and in cases of cholesteatoma. A myriad of other bacteria have been recovered from the middle ear in rare cases, including *Mycoplasma*, *Mycobacterium tuberculosis*, group B *Streptococcus* species, and *Neisseria* and *Chlamydia* species.

Cultures in OME more commonly do not grow bacteria, and this "sterile" culture occurs in one-third of cases. Another one-third of the cultures will grow the three most common AOM bacteria (*S. pneumoniae*, *H. influenzae*, and *M. catarrhalis*), with *Haemophilus* being the most common.

The final one-third is composed of nonpathogenic bacteria such as the normal skin bacterium *S. epidermidis*, as well as viruses.[12]

More recently, the role of bacterial biofilms in the pathogenesis of OM has been debated. A biofilm occurs when a community of bacteria interact together to surround themselves with a polysaccharide matrix, which protects them from a host's immune response. Because of its low metabolic rate, it is also resistant to antimicrobial therapy. Initially, it was thought that biofilms only existed on hard surfaces such as teeth and tympanostomy tubes. But research has shown that biofilms can also be found in the middle ear.[13] These biofilms were identified in 48% of patients undergoing tympanostomy tube insertion even in the face of negative middle ear fluid cultures. Biofilms have also been found in the nasopharynx of children with OM. This suggests that these biofilms may act as a bacterial reservoir for repeated OM via the ET, and may help explain why adenoidectomy benefits some patients with OM. At this point, the existence of biofilms cannot be disputed. Their exact role in the pathogenesis of OM, particularly as it relates to treatment strategies, has yet to be clearly defined.

Virology

Before the advent of polymerase chain reaction, the incidence of viral AOM was unknown and largely underestimated, because isolating viruses in culture was technically challenging. Currently, it is thought that viruses alone account for approximately 20% of episodes of AOM and are present in approximately 20 to 30% of fluid in OME. Rhinovirus and respiratory syncytial virus are the most common, but influenza, parainfluenza, and adenovirus are also seen.[14] The role of viruses in OM extends beyond their role in the middle ear directly. Viral URIs are often precursor events to episodes of OM. In one study, 70% of episodes of OM were associated with a viral URI, and viruses were isolated from MEE in 77% of these cases.[15] This suggests that mixed bacterial and viral OM is common and perhaps viruses "set up" the middle ear space for bacterial infection, similar to the pathogenesis of sinusitis.

Diagnosis
History

The most recent guidelines released by the American Academy of Pediatrics/American Academy of Family Physicians outline three components in diagnosing AOM: (1) history of acute onset, (2) confirmed presence of MEE, and (3) presence of signs and symptoms of acute inflammation.[16] Common symptoms of AOM include ear pulling, poor sleep, fever, and irritability, although some children may have no symptoms. OME, as previously mentioned, is the presence of fluid in the middle ear without acute inflammation.

This can be more challenging to diagnose and is often not accompanied by any symptoms, particularly in young children. If symptoms are present, the most common ones include hearing loss, fullness, otalgia (especially at night), and imbalance.

Physical Examination

Physical examination findings of acute inflammation in AOM include a bulging tympanic membrane (TM), erythema of the TM, or otorrhea associated with spontaneous perforation. The TM may be thickened and dull, and purulence may be visualized through the TM. However, caution must be taken when assessing redness of the eardrum. One study showed the predictive value of redness of the TM alone to be only 7%, and hyperemia of the TM alone is a common normal finding, particularly in a crying child.[17] OME usually is seen as opacification of the TM with abnormal color, typically pink, yellow, amber, or blue. Bubbles or air–fluid interfaces may be visible, and the TM may be in a neutral or retracted position. Pneumatic otoscopy is a critical part of the otoscopic examination, particularly when determining whether MEE is present. This involves the application of positive and negative pressure to the TM. To properly perform pneumatic otoscopy, the largest speculum that adequately fits in the ear canal should be used and an airtight seal must be created within the cartilaginous ear canal. Decreased or absent mobility of the TM is suggestive of fluid and may be used to confirm MEE and OME. Other sources of poor mobility include scarring (myringosclerosis) or thickening of the TM, and obviously a perforation or tympanostomy tube will prohibit mobility. Myringosclerosis is seen as white plaques within the TM, and commonly occurs in a horseshoe pattern centrally around the pars tensa portion of the TM. This occurs with long-standing ear disease, either with or without the previous presence of a tympanostomy tube. Retraction, or atelectasis, of the TM is another common otoscopic finding, and may be associated with OME. In severe cases, hearing loss associated with ossicular chain erosion or cholesteatoma formation can occur. If available, binocular microscopy can also be a valuable tool in examining the TM and assessing for the presence of MEE. One study showed an 88% sensitivity and 89% specificity for binocular microscopy in identifying MEE, compared with 68 and 81%, respectively, for pneumatic otoscopy.[18] Obviously, binocular microscopy will not be available in all diagnostic settings and may not be practical in every patient, particularly young children, therefore, pneumatic otoscopy remains the gold standard for identifying MEE.

Ancillary Testing

Immittance testing, or tympanometry, is an audiologic tool that can also be useful in diagnosing MEE. It is particularly useful in young children, those with small ear canals, and those patients in whom an airtight seal cannot be obtained for pneumatic otoscopy. Tympanometry involves placing a probe in the ear canal with an airtight seal. The probe emits a tone, and a curve is obtained by plotting the immittance of the middle ear as a function of pressure in the ear canal. A normal (or type A) tympanogram will have a sharp peak, which usually will occur near 0 daPa. A flat (or type B) tympanogram is classically associated with MEE, as compliance of the drum is poor. Other sources of flat tympanograms, however, include presence of a tympanostomy tube, or a false-positive result if a seal is not created with the probe. A type C tympanogram occurs when a peak is obtained, but this peak occurs at a pressure of 150 daPa or greater. This suggests high negative pressure, or a vacuum type effect, in the middle ear, and is much less specific in diagnosing MEE. Tympanometry is highly sensitive, with ranges around 80 to 90% reported in multiple studies, but its specificity is much lower, reportedly as low as 47%.[18] It is particularly poor in children less than 1 year of age, and this may be due to the increased compliance of the ear canal in infants. This can be overcome to some degree by using a 1000 Hz probe tone instead of the usual 226 Hz tone. The role of other supplementary testing, including acoustic reflectometry and ultrasound, is less well defined and not readily available in most physicians' offices.

Medical Treatment of AOM and OME

AOM

There has been controversy for quite some time about the need for antibiotic therapy in all cases of AOM. It has been shown that only a 12% increase in resolution rate was observed in children who received antibiotics versus clinical observation at 2 to 7 days.[19] Furthermore, the incidence of meningitis, mastoiditis, and other suppurative complications are similar in those treated with antibiotics versus observation (0.17 vs. 0.59%, respectively). In fact, routine antibiotic usage may select out for more invasive, resistant bacteria. A scientific review of the best available studies was performed and new guidelines from the American Academy of Pediatrics (AAP) and American Academy of Family Physicians (AAFP) were introduced in 2004.[16] This was the first set of guidelines from these academies that included observation as initial management in certain cases of AOM. The factors used to determine initial treatment include age, certainty of diagnosis, and severity of illness, and reliability of the caregiver/follow-up were the factors used to create this recommendation (**Table 1.1**). Certain diagnosis meets the three criteria mentioned previously in this chapter. Severe illness was defined as severe otalgia or fever greater than 39°C (102.2°F).

Observation

By definition, the "observation option" refers to observation for a period of 48 to 72 hours, and limiting management to symptomatic relief. This includes particularly the management of pain, another recommendation from the committee. The most important initial factor in determining

Table 1.1 Criteria for Initial Antibacterial Agent Treatment or Observation in Children with AOM

Age	Certain Diagnosis	Uncertain Diagnosis
<6 mo	Antibacterial therapy	Antibacterial therapy
6 mo to 2 y	Antibacterial therapy	Antibacterial therapy if severe illness; observation option[a] if nonsevere illness
≥2 y	Antibacterial therapy if severe illness; observation option[a] if nonsevere illness	Observation option[a]

[a]Observation is an appropriate option only when follow-up can be ensured and antibacterial agents started if symptoms persist or worsen. Nonsevere illness is mild otalgia and fever <39°C in the past 24 hours. Severe illness is moderate to severe otalgia or fever ≥39°C. A certain diagnosis of AOM meets all three criteria: (1) rapid onset, (2) signs of middle ear effusion and (3) signs and symptoms of middle ear inflammation.

Adapted from: American Academy of Pediatrics/American Academy of Family Physicians Subcommittee Guidelines on Management of Acute Otitis Media.

AOM, acute otitis media; mo, months; y, years.

whether observation is even an option in a child is the reliability of the caregiver. This not only relates to assurance of follow-up, but also their ability to recognize worsening severity of illness and to be able to provide them with prompt access to medical care if necessary. If there are serious concerns with any of these factors, then a physician may choose to initially treat a child with antibiotics empirically. When observation is chosen, a strategy should be in place to ensure that some follow-up occurs. This may include a scheduled clinic or phone follow-up, a parent-initiated visit if there is no improvement in 48 to 72 hours, or a safety-net antibiotic prescription given to parents to fill if there is no improvement in 48 to 72 hours. Other exclusion criteria for the observation option include immunodeficiency, genetic abnormalities, craniofacial anomalies, underlying persistent OME, and AOM in the past 30 days.

All children under the age of 6 months should receive initial antibiotic therapy for AOM, regardless of certainty of diagnosis or severity of illness. The reason for this is the concern for serious infection in this very young age group and the diagnostic challenge in assessing worsening symptoms or signs of progression to suppurative complications. In the age of 6 months to 2 years, initial antibiotic therapy should be instituted if there is a certain diagnosis, or if there is an uncertain diagnosis in the presence of severe illness. If the diagnosis is uncertain and there is nonsevere illness, then observation is an option. In children older than age 2, observation is an option even in the presence of a certain diagnosis of AOM, as long as the patient has nonsevere illness. Initial antibiotic therapy should be instituted in the presence of severe illness (**Table 1.1**).

Although these guidelines are widely accepted, further research may give us a clearer picture of which patients should be treated initially and which can be observed. There have been problems cited with the studies that were used to show high spontaneous resolution rates in AOM. The definition of AOM may have included criteria that allowed inclusion of patients with OME, the antibiotics may have been inappropriate or at an insufficient dosage, and the sickest children and those less than 2 years of age may have been excluded/underrepresented.[20] All these factors would make antibiotic therapy appear less efficacious. Another challenge is of getting parents to agree to observation, which can be difficult particularly given the empiric historic use in AOM. Practitioners have also not universally accepted this into their practice, and one study showed that although 83% of physicians felt observation was a reasonable practice, it was used in only a median of 15% of practices.[21]

Initial Antibiotic Therapy

The initial antibiotic for an uncomplicated, nonrecurring AOM is amoxicillin (**Table 1.2**). Amoxicillin has been shown to be effective against the most common AOM organisms, particularly *S. pneumoniae* and nonbeta lactamase-producing *H. influenzae*. The dosage recommendation is 80 to 90 mg/kg/d versus the standard 40 mg/kg/d. This higher dose has been shown to be more effective, particularly against the increasing intermediate and highly resistant strains of *S. pneumoniae* that have emerged. In addition, amoxicillin is cost-effective and easy to take, with a low incidence of side effects. In patients with severe illness (severe otalgia or temperature >39°C), the recommendation is high-dose amoxicillin (90 mg/kg/d)/clavulanate (6.4 mg/kg/d). The challenge in determining appropriate initial antibiotic therapy is the changing landscape of the bacteriology of AOM. Nearly 50% of *H. influenzae* and 100% of *M. catarrhalis* are beta-lactamase–producing, and therefore resistant to amoxicillin alone. But there is also evidence to suggest that AOM caused by these bacteria are more likely to resolve spontaneously, and the combination of *S. pneumoniae* and amoxicillin-sensitive *H. influenzae* still represent the majority of AOM pathogens.

In penicillin-allergic patients without type I hypersensitivity, cefdinir, cefpodoxime, or cefuroxime can be used. Azithromycin or clarithromycin are alternatives in those patients with type I hypersensitivity, although studies

Table 1.2   AAP/AAFP Therapy Options for AOM in Varying Clinical Circumstances

At diagnosis when observation is not an option
Recommended: amoxicillin 80–90 mg/kg/d
Alternative for penicillin allergy: nontype I: cefdinir, cefuroxime, cefpodoxime; type I: azithromycin, clarithromycin
Clinically defined failure of observation option after 48 to 72 h
Recommended: amoxicillin 80–90 mg/kg/d
Alternative for penicillin allergy: nontype I: cefdinir, cefuroxime, cefpodoxime; type I: azithromycin, clarithromycin
Clinically defined failure of initial antibiotic treatment after 48 to 72 h
Recommended: amoxicillin/clavulanate (90 mg/kg/d of amoxicillin component, with 6.4 mg/kg/d of clavulanate)
Alternative for penicillin allergy: nontype I: ceftriaxone—3 d; type I: clindamycin
At diagnosis when observation is not an option
Recommended: amoxicillin/clavulanate (90 mg/kg/d of amoxicillin with 6.4 mg/kg/d of clavulanate
Alternative for penicillin allergy: ceftriaxone—1 or 3 d
Clinically defined failure of observation option after 48 to 72 h
Recommended: amoxicillin/clavulanate (90 mg/kg/d of amoxicillin with 6.4 mg/kg/d of clavulanate)
Alternative for penicillin allergy: ceftriaxone 1 or 3 d
Clinically defined failure of initial antibiotic treatment after 48 to 72 h
Recommended: ceftriaxone 3 d
Alternative for penicillin allergy: tympanocentesis, clindamycin

Adapted from: Pichichero ME, Casey JR. Acute otitis media: making sense of recent guidelines on antimicrobial treatment. *J Fam Pract* 2005;54(4): 313–322.
AAP, American Academy of Pediatrics; AAFP, American Academy of Family Physicians; AOM, acute otitis media; d, day(s); h, hour(s).

suggest increasing resistance rates to these macrolide antibiotics. Other possibilities include erythromycin/sulfisoxazole or trimethoprim/sulfamethoxazole. Clindamycin is also effective if the pathogen is resistant *S. pneumoniae*. In the case of severe illness or the inability of the patient to tolerate oral medication, intramuscular ceftriaxone is also an option. The above protocols are designed not only for patients who are treated initially, but also for those in whom the observation option has failed after 72 hours. **Table 1.3** outlines antibiotic guidelines from a combination of the AAP/AAFP and Centers for Disease Control and Prevention guidelines.

The optimal duration of therapy for AOM is not completely certain. Evidence suggests fewer treatment failures in younger children with a standard 10-day course, and the current recommendation is 10 days in children younger than 6 years. A 5- to 7-day course may be appropriate in children older than 6 years of age without severe disease.

Table 1.3   Consistency of Guidelines for AOM

All recommend as first-line therapy	Amoxicillin, mostly at 80–90 mg/kg/d
All recommend as second-line therapy	Amoxicillin/clavulanate, mostly "ES" 80–90 mg/kg/d
Some recommend as second-line therapy	Cefdinir 14 mg/kg/d Cefprozil 30 mg/kg/d Cefuroxime axetil 30 mg/kg/d Cefpodoxime 10 mg/kg/d Ceftriaxone 50 mg/kg/d
Not recommended by any guideline Unless pathogen known to be sensitive; patient had severe allergic reaction to penicillin or amoxicillin; or combined with another antibiotic that is effective against additional organisms	Azithromycin Clarithromycin Trimethoprim/sulfamethoxazole Erythromycin/sulfisoxazole Cefaclor Loracarbef Cefixime Ceftibuten Clindamycin

Adapted from: Pichichero ME, Casey JR. Acute otitis media: making sense of recent guidelines on antimicrobial treatment. *J Fam Pract* 2005;54(4): 313–322.
AOM, acute otitis media; d, day(s); ES, extra strength.

Specific antibiotics have been approved for shorter courses even in younger children. Cefdinir and cefpodoxime have been approved for 5-day courses, and azithromycin has been approved for 1-, 3-, and 5-day courses.

Antibiotics for Treatment Failures

When initial antibiotic therapy fails, the patient should be started on high-dose amoxicillin/clavulanate if there is no allergy. If they have failed this therapy already, alternatives such as cefdinir, cefpodoxime, and cefuroxime can be considered. A 3-day course of intramuscular ceftriaxone can also be considered. In type I penicillin hypersensitivity patients, clindamycin is also an option because of its high (up to 95%) success against highly resistant *S. pneumoniae*.[22] Finally, in the severely ill patient, tympanocentesis can be performed to make a bacteriologic diagnosis for culture-directed therapy.

Nonantibiotic Therapies

Analgesics

Symptomatic management of pain with analgesics is important in patients with AOM, regardless of whether or not they receive antibiotic therapy. Multiple options exist, with acetaminophen and ibuprofen being the most common and highly effective. Topical analgesia with benzocaine has also shown to be effective, though the benefits are short-lasting.[23] Narcotic analgesics such as codeine and its derivatives can also be used, but must be used cautiously, particularly in younger children. Lethargy from the narcotic may mask the worsening symptoms of suppurative complications, and respiratory depression is also a side effect that needs to be monitored.

Corticosteroids

Although some small studies have shown short-term benefit with oral or intranasal steroid, the benefits have been marginal. A large study showed no benefit with oral steroid over antibiotic alone, and steroids are not routinely recommended in AOM.[24]

Antihistamines and Decongestants

Both large individual studies and meta-analysis of studies have shown no benefit in terms of early cure, symptom resolution, duration of effusion, or prevention of complication or surgery with antihistamines or decongestants.[24] These are not routinely recommended in AOM.

Alternative Therapies

Homeopathy, acupuncture, chiropractic treatment, and nutritional supplements have all been used for AOM, but there are no data suggesting a beneficial effect of these therapies. These alternative therapies are not currently recommended for AOM.

OME

Observation

OME is common in children both with URIs and after AOM, and fluid may persist up to 1 month after an acute episode of AOM in 50% of cases. In a child without speech, language, or learning delays, observation of fluid is recommended for up to 3 months. If a child is at risk or OME persists beyond 3 months, audiologic evaluation should be done. If the child's hearing is normal (<20 dB), continued watchful waiting is recommended. If there is a moderate or worse conductive hearing loss (>40 dB) then surgical intervention is recommended. When the hearing falls in the mild conductive hearing loss range (21 to 39 dB), the duration and particularly the severity of symptoms related to the hearing loss must be addressed. If there is parental or teacher concern about the child's hearing, surgical intervention may be considered. Otherwise, observation at 3- to 6-month intervals is recommended until the fluid resolves, language delays occur, or structural abnormalities of the eardrum are observed. These recommendations are from the AAP/AAFP clinical practice guidelines for OME, also published in 2004.[25]

Medical Therapy

Little evidence exists to support the use of any medical therapy to shorten the duration of OME. The 2004 guidelines conclude that antihistamines and decongestants are ineffective in treating OME and they do not recommend their use, particularly from a risk–benefit standpoint. Antibiotics and corticosteroids are also not recommended. Although there may be short-term benefit of both antibiotics and steroids, these benefits become nonsignificant within several weeks of stopping them. In addition, their side effect profiles are led to a less than optimal risk–benefit ratio. Autoinflation of the eustachian tube, described by Politzer, has been shown to have limited short-term benefit in very small studies, but adherence to the procedure can be difficult in children.[26] No definitive recommendation has been made regarding autoinflation.

Surgical Treatment of AOM and OME

Myringotomy/Tympanocentesis

Myringotomy, or an incision in the eardrum, may temporarily relieve pressure associated with an AOM and allow culture for bacteriology, but has not been shown to be as effective as antibiotic therapy, does not decrease duration of effusion, and does not prevent recurrent AOM. It also has been shown to be ineffective in the long-term management of chronic OME. Therefore, there is little role for myringotomy alone in OM.

Myringotomy with pressure equalization tube (PET)

placement is the first-line surgical therapy for recurrent AOM, complicated AOM, as well as chronic OME.[25] Children are in general considered candidates for PET placement if they have three to four episodes of AOM in 6 months or have four to six episodes in 1 year. Studies show that PETs reduce the frequency of AOM episodes by 56% and decrease the duration of OM.[26,27] Although OM can still occur with a PET in place in the form of otorrhea, many of these episodes are not accompanied by any symptoms and can be treated with ototopical antibiotic drops without oral antibiotics. PET placement is also considered in a complicated AOM episode, such as AOM with mastoiditis, labyrinthitis, facial nerve paralysis, or other complications.

PET placement is also the most common initial surgical intervention in chronic OME. Indications for intervention, however, are somewhat more controversial. As mentioned previously, hearing loss, particularly as it relates to speech, language, or learning delays is usually the primary factor in determining whether PET placement is necessary. In a child with speech or language delays, particularly those at-risk patients with genetic abnormalities or other developmental delays, prompt PET placement is indicated. Otherwise, OME is observed for 3 months for spontaneous resolution. If the fluid persists and audiologic evaluation reveals moderate hearing loss (>40 dB) or speech or language delays develop, then PET placement is indicated at this time. With a normal audiogram, observation is recommended at 3- to 6-month intervals until resolution occurs, significant hearing loss develops, or structural damage of the TM is identified—if any of this occurs, PET placement should be considered. With mild (21 to 40 dB) hearing loss, a discussion with parents is necessary and either (1) a PET can be placed or (2) close observation at 3-month intervals can be continued.

The average length of time a PET stays in place is between 1 and 2 years with minor variations related to the type and model of tube inserted. An episode of tube otorrhea is not uncommon during this time and is often associated with a URI or exposure to water. Younger children (<2 to 3 years of age) have otorrhea more commonly associated with URIs, and the typical sinonasal bacteria (*S. pneumoniae, H. influenzae,* and *M. catarrhalis*) are usually cultured. In older children, (>3 years of age) otorrhea is more likely to occur with exposure to water, particularly when swimming, and the most common bacterial pathogens are *Pseudomonas* and *S. aureus.* Topical antibiotic therapy has been shown to be at least as effective as and perhaps more effective than oral antibiotics. Oral antibiotics are usually reserved for those patients with severe systemic symptomatology or those who have failed initial topical therapy. Aural toilet (i.e., suctioning) can also help clear the ear canal and allow the eardrops easier access to the middle ear space. This is even more important in those patients with acutely inflamed, edematous and narrow ear canals. Chronic or recurrent otorrhea is a rarer problem that can be more difficult to manage. If a patient has failed both topical and oral antibiotic culture-directed therapy in the presence of repeated aural toilet, consideration can be given

to a variety of adjuvant therapies. This could include tube replacement, adenoidectomy, tube removal, intravenous (IV) antibiotic therapy, and mastoidectomy. Particularly in those patients with long-standing chronic otorrhea, a computed tomography (CT) scan can also be considered to evaluate for the presence of cholesteatoma.

There are other less frequently seen sequelae of PET placement. Early extrusion may occur, usually in the setting of an acute otorrhea episode. A tube may become blocked with cerumen, dried blood, or dried mucus which can often be cleared either with ototopical drops or manually in the office setting. Persistent perforation may occur after PET extrusion, with myringoplasty or tympanoplasty necessary to close the hole. A PET may not extrude spontaneously and be retained in the TM which may eventually need to be removed in the operative setting. Myringosclerosis (scarring of the TM), atrophy of the TM at the prior PET site, and retraction pockets can also occur after tube extrusion. Although these TM abnormalities can also occur without prior PET placement, they have been shown to be more common after PET placement.

Adenoidectomy

Twenty-five percent of children who have had PETs will have a relapse of OM when the tubes extrude or become obstructed.[28] In those instances where repeated PET placement is indicated, there is a role for adenoidectomy, as it decreases by 50% the need for further surgeries (i.e., a third set of PETs). The groups that benefit the most from adenoidectomy are those with chronic OME who are older than age 4 and those with recurrent AOM older than age 2 with a history of extruded PETs.[29] Interestingly, the benefit from adenoid removal is independent of the size of the adenoid tissue, suggesting that not only adenoid size, but chronic inflammation, contributes to OM. Adenoidectomy with myringotomy alone was equivalent to PET placement alone in older children, but this is not recommended routinely because it is more invasive than PET placement alone. Adenoidectomy is not recommended routinely with a first set of PETs unless an indication such as chronic adenoiditis or chronic sinusitis coexists.[25] Tonsillectomy is not recommended in the treatment of either AOM or OME, as it has shown limited evidence of benefit and poses significantly higher risks.

Complications of AOM

Extracranial

Acute Mastoiditis

Acute mastoiditis describes acute infection and inflammation within the mastoid cavity with bony destruction of the architecture of the air cells, or "coalescence." Clinically, the child would have postauricular edema, erythema, and tenderness in the setting of an AOM. There is commonly protrusion of the pinna as well. A CT scan can confirm the presence of coalescence. Management is controversial, but IV antibiotic therapy alone is often the initial choice. If the child shows no improvement within 48 hours, the surgical options include myringotomy +/– PET placement and/or simple mastoidectomy. Another management strategy that is commonly employed is to perform a myringotomy and PET insertion initially in conjunction with IV antibiotics, with mastoidectomy performed if there is no improvement in 48 hours.

Subperiosteal and Bezold Abscesses

These occur when an acute mastoiditis erodes through the cortical bone either adjacent to the lateral surface of the mastoid cortex (subperiosteal) or through the mastoid tip into the neck (Bezold). This can most commonly be via direct bony erosion but may also occur hematogenously through mastoid emissary vessels. Purulence collects in these areas, with resultant fluctuance and erythema. Again, a CT scan can confirm the presence of an abscess and its precise location (**Fig. 1.1**). Management in these cases includes myringotomy +/– PET placement with incision and drainage of the abscess alone or in combination with simple mastoidectomy.

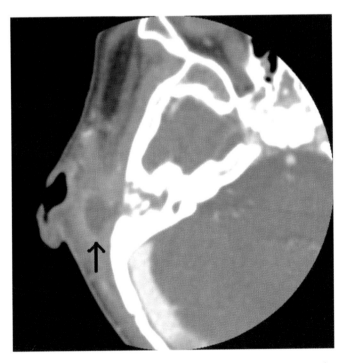

Figure 1.1 Axial computed tomography scan showing acute right mastoiditis with cortical bony erosion and subperiosteal abscess (arrow).

Petrous Apicitis (Gradenigo Syndrome)

Petrous apicitis occurs when infection spreads from the middle ear and mastoid medially to the petrous portion of the temporal bone, either directly or hematogenously via vascular channels. The classic triad in petrous apicitis is otitis/otorrhea, retrobulbar pain/headache, and abducens nerve (cranial nerve VI) palsy. A CT scan or a magnetic resonance imaging (MRI) examination can usually confirm the diagnosis, and initial management with IV antibiotic therapy alone is often successful.[30] Petrous apicectomy, typically via a transmastoid approach, is usually reserved for antibiotic failures or infections with complications.

Labyrinthitis

This occurs when inflammation in the middle ear spreads to the labyrinth, which includes the cochlea and semicircular canals. This may be via direct bacterial spread (suppurative labyrinthitis), but is also commonly caused by inflammatory mediators in the absence of the organisms themselves (serous labyrinthitis). Transmission can occur at the oval or round windows, or via microscopic bony labyrinthine defects. The diagnosis is made clinically with acute debilitating vertigo and sensorineural hearing loss (SNHL) in the setting of an AOM. An MRI examination, although not necessary, will also show labyrinthine involvement. IV antibiotics are recommended initially to both treat the infection and to try prevent meningitis. Conversely, labyrinthitis can also be a complication of meningitis; this is in part due to a normal communication channel between the extracranial labyrinth and intracranial meninges through the cochlear aqueduct. Myringotomy +/– PET placement drains the fluid and allows for culture-directed therapy, and vertiginous symptoms are managed in the usual fashion. Serous and suppurative labyrinthitis are treated similarly from a medical standpoint and it is rather difficult to distinguish them acutely. In general, however, serous labyrinthitis presents with milder vestibulocochlear symptoms than suppurative labyrinthitis and labyrinthine function is more likely to return in serous labyrinthitis.

Facial Nerve Paresis/Paralysis

The horizontal portion of the facial nerve runs through the middle ear space, and when AOM affects the facial nerve, either through the tiny vascular channels in the normal bony canal or directly secondary to dehiscence of the nerve, facial palsy can occur. This can be a partial weakness (paresis) or complete weakness (paralysis), with the former event more common. Management includes IV antibiotic therapy and wide-field myringotomy versus myringotomy with PET, with culture-directed therapy. A CT scan may be considered to rule out other intracranial or other extracranial involvement. More aggressive intervention is rarely indicated.

Intracranial

Meningitis/Otitic Hydrocephalus

Bacterial meningitis is the most common intracranial complication of AOM. Transmission of disease from the middle ear can be due to hematogenous spread or directly, via the oval and round windows, cochlear aqueduct, or other bony defects. Symptoms include high fever, altered level of consciousness, vomiting, and neck stiffness. There may be papilledema, Kernig and Brudzinski signs, bulging fontanelles, or cranial neuropathies on physical examination. Lumbar puncture is performed to confirm the diagnosis. A CT scan or an MRI examination is usually performed upfront to exclude tumor and mass effect, but they may also be used to look for other complications. Broad-spectrum antibiotic therapy with myringotomy +/– PET for culture is the treatment. Audiologic evaluation of these patients is recommended when neurologic status improves, as SNHL is very common, particularly with pneumococcal meningitis.

Although hydrocephalus is a common finding in bacterial meningitis, another entity has been described, known as otitic hydrocephalus. Lumbar puncture demonstrates high cerebrospinal fluid opening pressure with normal cytology, thereby excluding meningitis. The pathophysiology is thought to be due to nonobstructing thrombus of the transverse sinus, and MRI is useful to demonstrate the presence of a thrombus. Management includes antibiotic treatment of the underlying AOM and supportive measures to decrease intracranial pressure.

Sigmoid Sinus Thrombosis

This occurs when a septic thrombus occurs in the sigmoid dural sinus, usually as a result of direct extension of infection from the mastoid cavity. Clinically, it may present with "picket-fence" spiking fevers, headache, and photophobia. Abducens palsy, as well as swelling and tenderness over the mastoid process (Griesinger sign) have also been described. Either CT with contrast or MRI +/– venography can make the diagnosis (**Fig. 1.2**). Management includes IV antibiotic therapy and PET placement +/– mastoidectomy. If the choice to perform mastoidectomy is made, the bone directly

over the sigmoid sinus should be decompressed. Surgical thrombectomy and anticoagulation are both controversial without strong evidence to support their benefit. This, combined with literature suggesting that recanalization usually occurs spontaneously in 4 to 6 weeks, suggests that a more conservative approach may be appropriate.[31]

Intracranial Abscesses (Epidural, Subdural, and Brain Abscesses)

Intracranial abscesses are defined by the space they occupy within the cranium. An epidural abscess is located between the bone and the dura mater, a subdural abscess is located between the dura and arachnoid maters, and a brain abscess is located intraparenchymally. The mortality associated with subdural and particularly brain abscess is much higher than that with epidural abscess. MRI is the imaging study of choice for these abscesses, but most can also be detected with contrast-enhanced CT.

Many epidural abscesses can be managed with IV antibiotic alone, close clinical observation, and interval imaging studies (CT or MRI) for comparison. When an epidural abscess is present in continuity with mastoiditis or sigmoid sinus thrombosis (**Fig. 1.3**), it may be decompressed via a transmastoid approach. If there is no improvement with antibiotic therapy, or if neurologic status deteriorates, surgical drainage either via craniotomy or burr holes should be performed.

Subdural abscesses tend to spread rapidly through the subdural space, partially contributing to their more aggressive clinical picture. Symptoms include fever, altered mental status, and headache. Neurosurgical drainage is

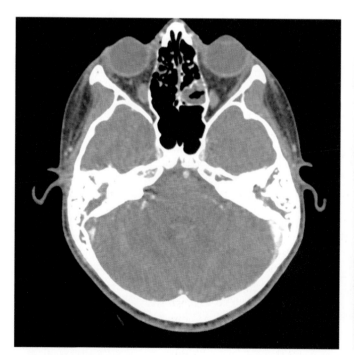

Figure 1.2 Axial computed tomography scan showing thrombosis of the right sigmoid sinus. Comparison can be made to the normally enhancing left sigmoid sinus.

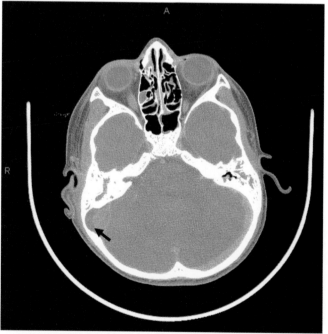

Figure 1.3 Axial computed tomography scan showing epidural abscess adjacent to a thrombosed right sigmoid sinus.

always indicated, while otolaryngologic intervention should be performed if the patient is stable and deferred if the patient is unstable. Other measures to decrease cerebral edema should also be undertaken, as well as seizure prophylaxis.

Brain abscess is a catastrophic complication of AOM, with a reported mortality of as high as 50%.[32] Signs and symptoms may include fever, altered mental status, seizure, and focal neurologic deficits. These focal deficits depend on the location of the abscess within the brain parenchyma. The disease can have an indolent course, making diagnosis all the more difficult. Management is similar to that of subdural abscess.

References

1. Teele DW, Klein JO, Rosner B, et al. Middle ear disease and the practice of pediatrics. Burden during the first five years of life. JAMA 1983;249(8):1026–1029

2. Nelson WL, Kuritsky JN, Kennedy DL, et al. Outpatient pediatric antibiotic use in the US: trends and therapy for acute otitis media, 1977–1986. In: Program and Abstracts of the 27th Interscience Conference on Antimicrobial Agents and Chemotherapy. Washington, D.C.: American Society for Microbiology; 1987

3. Gates GA. Cost-effectiveness considerations in otitis media treatment. Otolaryngol Head Neck Surg 1996;114(4):525–530

4. Casselbrant ML, Brostoff LM, Cantekin EI, et al. Otitis media with effusion in preschool children. Laryngoscope 1985;95(4):428–436

5. Casselbrant ML, Brostoff LM, Cantekin EI, et al. Otitis media in children in the United States. Acute and secretory otitis media. Proceedings of the International Conference on Acute and Secretory Otitis Media, Part I. Amsterdam: Kugler Publications; 1996:161

6. Lous J, Fiellau-Nikolajsen M. Epidemiology and middle ear effusion and tubal dysfunction. A one-year prospective study comprising monthly tympanometry in 387 non-selected 7-year-old children. Int J Pediatr Otorhinolaryngol 1981;3(4):303–317

7. Owen MJ, Baldwin CD, Luttman D, et al. Otitis media with effusion detected by tympanometry on frequent home visits in Galveston, Texas. In: Lim DJ, Bluestone CD, Klein JO, Melson JD, eds. Recent Advances in Otitis Media. Proceedings of the Fifth International Symposium. Hamilton, Ontario: Decker Periodicals; 1993:17.

8. Zeisel SA, Roberts JE, Gunn EB, et al. Prospective surveillance for otitis media with effusion among black infants in group child care. J Pediatr 1995;127(6):875–880

9. Pichichero ME, Casey JR. Acute otitis media: making sense of recent guidelines on antimicrobial treatment. J Fam Pract 2005;54(4):313–322

10. McEllistrem MC, Adams JM, Patel K, et al. Acute otitis media due to penicillin-nonsusceptible *Streptococcus pneumoniae* before and after the introduction of the pneumococcal conjugate vaccine. Clin Infect Dis 2005;40(12):1738–1744

11. Black S, Shinefield H, Fireman B, et al; Northern California Kaiser Permanente Vaccine Study Center Group. Efficacy, safety and immunogenicity of heptavalent pneumococcal conjugate vaccine in children. Pediatr Infect Dis J 2000;19(3):187–195

12. Bluestone CD, Stephenson JS, Martin LM. Ten-year review of otitis media pathogens. Pediatr Infect Dis J 1992;11(8, Suppl):S7–S11

13. Post JC, Preston RA, Aul JJ, et al. Molecular analysis of bacterial pathogens in otitis media with effusion. JAMA 1995;273(20):1598–1604

14. Heikkinen T, Thint M, Chonmaitree T. Prevalence of various respiratory viruses in the middle ear during acute otitis media. N Engl J Med 1999;340(4):260–264

15. Winther B, Alper CM, Mandel EM, Doyle WJ, Hendley JO. Temporal relationships between colds, upper respiratory viruses detected by polymerase chain reaction, and otitis media in young children followed through a typical cold season. Pediatrics 2007;119(6):1069–1075

16. American Academy of Pediatrics Subcommittee on Management of Acute Otitis Media. Diagnosis and management of acute otitis media. Pediatrics 2004;113(5):1451–1465

17. Pelton SI. Otoscopy for the diagnosis of otitis media. Pediatr Infect Dis J 1998;17(6):540–543, discussion 580

18. Rogers DJ, Boseley ME, Adams MT, Makowski RL, Hohman MH. Prospective comparison of handheld pneumatic otoscopy, binocular microscopy, and tympanometry in identifying middle ear effusions in children. Int J Pediatr Otorhinolaryngol 2010;74(10):1140–1143

19. Marcy M, Takata G, Chan LS, et al. Management of Acute Otitis Media. Evidence Report / Technology Assessment No. 15. AHRQ Publication No. 01–E010. Rockville, MD: Agency for Healthcare Research and Quality; 2001

20. Wald ER. Acute otitis media: more trouble with the evidence. Pediatr Infect Dis J 2003;22(2):103–104

21. Vernacchio L, Vezina RM, Mitchell AA. Knowledge and practices relating to the 2004 acute otitis media clinical practice guideline: a survey of practicing physicians. Pediatr Infect Dis J 2006;25(5):385–389

22. Marchetti F, Ronfani L, Nibali SC, Tamburlini G; Italian Study Group on Acute Otitis Media. Delayed prescription may reduce the use of antibiotics for acute otitis media: a prospective observational study in primary care. Arch Pediatr Adolesc Med 2005;159(7):679–684

23. Hoberman A, Paradise JL, Reynolds EA, Urkin J. Efficacy of Auralgan for treating ear pain in children with acute otitis media. Arch Pediatr Adolesc Med 1997;151(7):675–678

24. Chonmaitree T, Saeed K, Uchida T, et al. A randomized, placebo-controlled trial of the effect of antihistamine or corticosteroid treatment in acute otitis media. J Pediatr 2003;143(3):377–385

25. American Academy of Family Physicians; American Academy of Otolaryngology-Head and Neck Surgery; American Academy of Pediatrics Subcommittee on Otitis Media With Effusion. Otitis media with effusion. Pediatrics 2004;113(5):1412–1429

26. Perera R, Haynes J, Glasziou P, Heneghan CJ. Autoinflation for hearing loss associated with otitis media with effusion. Cochrane Database Syst Rev 2006;18(4):CD006285

27. Gonzalez C, Arnold JE, Woody EA, et al. Prevention of recurrent acute otitis media: chemoprophylaxis versus tympanostomy tubes. Laryngoscope 1986;96(12):1330–1334

28. Casselbrant ML, Kaleida PH, Rockette HE, et al. Efficacy of antimicrobial prophylaxis and of tympanostomy tube insertion for prevention of recurrent acute otitis media: results of a randomized clinical trial. Pediatr Infect Dis J 1992;11(4):278–286

29. Paradise JL, Bluestone CD, Rogers KD, et al. Efficacy of adenoidectomy for recurrent otitis media in children previously treated with tympanostomy-tube placement. Results of parallel randomized and nonrandomized trials. JAMA 1990;263(15):2066–2073

30. Burston BJ, Pretorius PM, Ramsden JD. Gradenigo's syndrome: successful conservative treatment in adult and paediatric patients. J Laryngol Otol 2005;119(4):325–329

31. Agarwal A, Lowry P, Isaacson G. Natural history of sigmoid sinus thrombosis. Ann Otol Rhinol Laryngol 2003;112(2):191–194

32. Bradley PJ, Manning KP, Shaw MD. Brain abscess secondary to otitis media. J Laryngol Otol 1984;98(12):1185–1191

2 The Work-Up of Childhood Sensorineural Hearing Loss

Jonathan M. Sherman, Eliot Shearer, Richard J.H. Smith, and Dana Suskind

The Problem

Hearing loss in children is common in the United States with an estimated incidence of 1 to 2 per 1000 live births.[1,2] During childhood, the prevalence increases. A 2010 report suggests that by adolescence, nearly 20% of children have a significant degree of at least unilateral hearing loss.[3] This striking estimate, which has increased by a third in just a decade, places childhood hearing loss among the major public health concerns in the United States.[4]

Historically, delays in hearing loss diagnosis resulted in lost opportunity to intervene at a critical time in listening and spoken language development. Compelling evidence has linked timely identification and treatment to improved communication and school performance.[5-7] Citing this data, the Joint Committee on Infant Hearing endorsed the concept of a Universal Newborn Hearing Screening (UNHS) in 2000.[8] Soon after, the U.S. Department of Health and Human Services' initiative, Healthy People 2010, reinforced this goal, advocating nationwide UNHS by 1 month, diagnostic confirmation by 3 months, and early intervention enrollment by 6 months of age.[9] UNHS expanded rapidly, and by 2005, every state had implemented a UNHS program. By 2006, approximately 95% of newborns in the United States were screened before hospital discharge.[10]

One of the challenges created by UNHS is that as more children are identified with hearing loss, no clear approach exists for determining the cause and identifying important associated medical conditions. In 2002, approximately 40,000 children were diagnosed each year in the United States alone, so that the classification of and medical work-up for a child identified with hearing loss is a dilemma that will be increasingly faced by not only tertiary care centers but by community otolaryngologists.[11] At the same time, the number of diagnostic tests available are constantly increasing, resulting from ongoing strides in our understanding of disease pathogenesis and our ability to detect genetic determinants of disease. Experts feel that within the next decade, specific genetic testing which is being developed now will become the most important tool after history and physical examination in the work-up of a child with hearing loss, completely changing the diagnostic approach.

In this chapter we will attempt to provide a modern framework for approaching the medical work-up of a child identified with sensorineural hearing loss (SNHL).

Classifying Hearing Loss

Hearing loss is classically defined as conductive (involving the transmission of sound from the outside world to the oval window), sensorineural (involving the function of the cochlea, eighth cranial nerve, and central nervous system [CNS]), or mixed. The differential diagnosis of a child with conductive hearing loss is beyond the scope of this chapter, but it is important to recognize that conductive losses account for a substantial fraction of children identified with hearing loss. More than half of children aged 1 to 24 months, nearly a quarter of all UNHS failures, and up to 15% neonatal intensive care unit (NICU) babies with hearing loss have purely conductive loss.[12]

Hearing loss can also be classified as either bilateral or unilateral. While some controversy existed earlier regarding clinical significance, more than 2 decades of convincing evidence now shows that children with unilateral SNHL, such as those with bilateral disease, have significant deficits in psycholinguistic stills and school performance, as well as problems with sound localization and discerning speech-in-noise.[13,14] Unilateral SNHL is caused by many of the same disease processes that lead to bilateral loss, and in fact, 20% of children identified with unilateral disease have progressive disease and 10% go on to develop hearing loss in the contralateral ear.[15]

Hearing loss is also characterized by the degree of severity. Like children with unilateral loss, those with mild and moderate hearing loss in one or both ears were once thought to be immune to the struggles of children with severe bilateral disease, but now several authors have shown that even mild hearing loss affects school performance, and that mild and moderate loss may be associated with learning disabilities.[16,17] Severity of loss can be stable or progressive.

Etiology of Hearing Loss

In developed countries, it is estimated that two-thirds of childhood SNHL has a genetic etiology, 70% of which is not associated with any other phenotype and is therefore termed nonsyndromic hearing loss (NSHL) (**Fig. 2.1**).[18] To date more than 59 genes have been implicated in nonsyndromic SNHL and more than 100 deafness loci have been determined where the gene has not yet been determined (http://hereditaryhearingloss.org/). SNHL that is not related to a genetic cause can be the result of prenatal and perinatal infection, exposure to ototoxic medicines in utero or in the postnatal period, NICU-related exposures and other perinatal conditions, autoimmune disease, or noise exposure (**Fig. 2.1**).

Genetic Nonsyndromic Hearing Loss

Eighty percent of genetic nonsyndromic hearing loss is autosomal recessive (autosomal recessive nonsyndromic hearing loss [ARNSHL], termed DFNB hearing loss), with the rest being mostly autosomal dominant (autosomal dominant nonsyndromic hearing loss [ADNSHL], termed DFNA), while X-linked and mitochondrial causes contribute less than 1%.[19] Therefore, most children with genetic hearing loss otherwise appear normal and have parents with normal hearing. ARNSHL is generally prelingual and profound across all frequencies.[20] To date, 38 genes and more than 60 loci have been causally implicated in ARNSHL.[21] The single most common causative gene—*GJB2* (DFNB1), encoding gap junction protein connexin 26—accounts for approximately half of ARNSHL in many populations, and has been shown to account for approximately 25% of ARNSHL in the United States.[22] Many mutations in *GJB2* have been identified, including mutations that cause dominant deafness. Due to the diversity of mutations and the possibility of either other genetic or environmental modifiers, generalizations about hearing loss caused by *GJB2* are difficult to make. However, it is clear that genotype–phenotype correlations exist based on the specific mutation.[22–24] These data have shown that DFNB1 hearing loss is generally prelingual and ranges from mild to severe in degree.

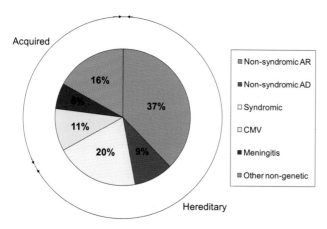

Figure 2.1 Classification of sensorineural hearing loss (SNHL) by cause. Whereas the numbers vary from study to study, it is clear that at least two-thirds of childhood SNHL can be attributed to specific genetic causes. Clearly genetic factors also contribute to hearing loss in children with "acquired SNHL," including susceptibility to ototoxicity of certain drugs. Regardless of the system used to classify etiologies, experts agree that the largest group among children with SNHL is inherited in an autosomal recessive pattern with no associated syndrome—children with no obvious cause by history or examination and normal hearing parents. AD, autosomal dominant; AR, autosomal recessive; CMV, cytomegalovirus.

Autosomal dominant mutations are diagnosed in a significantly smaller fraction of children with nonsyndromic SNHL. To date, 25 genes and more than 50 loci have been identified as causative for ADNSHL.[21] Hearing loss in patients affected by ADNSHL is often progressive and postlingual although there are clear exceptions.

> ### Genetic Nonsyndromic SNHL
>
> Consider these diagnostic tests: *GJB2* (connexin 26) testing, large throughput multiple gene assays in all children with SNHL with a clear family history or for whom an obvious cause is not readily apparent after physical examination, history, and audiologic evaluation (**Table 2.1**).

Genetic Syndromic Hearing Loss

Over 200 syndromes include hearing loss.[25] Most are very rare, but several are important contributors to the overall incidence of SNHL.

Autosomal Dominant Syndromes

Some of the important autosomal dominant syndromes include branchio-oto-renal (BOR) syndrome, Waardenburg syndrome (WS), Stickler syndrome (STL), neurofibromatosis type 2 (NF2), and CHARGE (*C*oloboma, *H*eart defects, *A*tresia, *R*etardation of growth and development, *G*enitourinary disorders, and *E*ar abnormalities) syndrome.

Children with BOR syndrome have branchial cleft, otologic, and renal anomalies. Otologic findings include preauricular pits and tags and auricular abnormalities; middle ear anomalies including ossicular malformation, facial nerve dehiscence, and absence of the oval window; and inner ear anomalies including cochlear hypoplasia, lateral canal hypoplasia, or enlargement of the cochlear or vestibular aqueducts.[26,27] Hearing impairment may be purely sensorineural or conductive, but most often is mixed. BOR is most frequently caused by mutations in the *EYA1* gene.

> ### BOR Syndrome
>
> Consider these diagnostic tests: genetic consultation/testing for *EYA1* mutations, renal ultrasound, urinalysis, computed tomography (CT) head in children with suggestive family history, external ear abnormalities, and branchial cleft anomalies.

Children with WS are classically described as having SNHL, a white forelock, heterochromia of the irises, and dystopia canthorum (lateral displacement of the medial canthi).[28] There are four subtypes with a combined prevalence of 1:10,000. WS type 1 is classical WS, type 2 lacks the dystopia canthorum, type 3 (also called Klein-Waardenburg syndrome) has upper limb hypoplasia or contracture, and type 4 (also called Waardenburg-Shah syndrome) is associated with Hirschsprung disease. Hearing loss is usually congenital, can be bilateral, and is stable over time.[29] Nearly 90% of WS type 1 is caused by mutations in *PAX3*; genetic contribution to the other types, however, is more uncertain.

WS

Consider these diagnostic tests: genetic consultation/testing for *PAX3* mutations in children with suggestive physical examination or family history.

STL has variable presence of SNHL, midline clefting, childhood myopia (except STL3, which is caused by mutations in *COL11A2*), joint hypermobility, and retinal detachment. The cluster of symptoms is related to abnormal collagen synthesis. Hearing loss is present in 40 to 60%, is often delayed in its presentation, preferentially affects high frequencies, and is most often mild. Despite this, a priority in STL (and any syndrome causing concomitant deafness and vision loss) is early identification for maximum efficacy of cochlear implantation if this becomes necessary.[30]

STL

Consider these diagnostic tests: genetic consultation/testing for *COL2A1* (STL1), *COL11A1* (STL2), *COL11A2* (STL3) mutations, ophthalmology evaluation in children with personal/family history of visual problems, craniofacial anomalies, and joint abnormalities.

NF2 is a cause of progressive SNHL characterized by the development of bilateral vestibular schwannomas. These patients often have other benign CNS tumors and posterior subcapsular lenticular opacities. Hearing loss is usually high-frequency, progressive, delayed until the second decade, and may be associated with vertigo, tinnitus, and facial nerve palsy.[31]

NF2

Consider these diagnostic tests: genetic consultation/testing for NF2 mutations, magnetic resonance imaging (MRI) brain, ophthalmology evaluation in children with family history, other cranial nerve abnormalities, headache, and visual complaints.

CHARGE syndrome, affecting 1 in 10,000 children, may be inherited in an autosomal dominant pattern, but the majority of cases result from de novo mutations in the chromodomain helicase DNA-binding protein-7 gene (*CHD7*). Typically, infants with CHARGE syndrome have bilateral mixed type hearing loss with a wedge-shaped audiogram having a flat air conduction curve intersecting at low frequencies with a descending bone conduction and have specific ear anomalies seen on imaging studies (**Fig. 2.2**).[32]

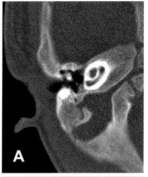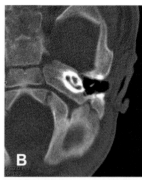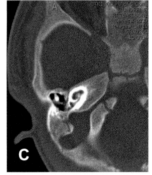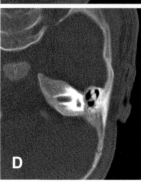

Figure 2.2 Temporal bone computed tomography scan of a child with CHARGE (*C*oloboma, *H*eart defects, *A*tresia, *R*etardation of growth and development, *G*enitourinary disorders, and *E*ar abnormalities) syndrome. Common inner ear anomalies typically seen in CHARGE syndrome include (A, B) underdevelopment or agenesis of the cochlea beyond the basal turn and (C, D) hypoplastic vestibule and semicircular canals.

CHARGE Syndrome

Consider these diagnostic tests: genetic consultation/testing for *CHD7* mutations, then pediatric cardiology, urology consultations, and CT head in children with suggestive physical examination result, growth delay, history of feeding difficulties due to choanal atresia, cryptorchidism, undescended testes, hypospadias, or external ear anomalies.

Autosomal Recessive Syndromes

Syndromes causing SNHL inherited in an autosomal recessive pattern include Pendred syndrome (PS), Usher syndrome (USH), and Jervell and Lange-Nielsen syndrome (JLNS).

PS accounts for roughly 10% of all hereditary deafness with an estimated prevalence of 1 in 10,000 individuals.[33] PS is caused by a mutation in the *PDS* (SLC26A4) gene that encodes an anion transporter present in the inner ear and thyroid. *PDS* mutations are also found in 86% of patients with enlarged vestibular aqueducts (EVA), leading authors to suggest that EVA is the most consistent finding in PS. Because of this, CT scan abnormalities are often the first clue toward PS diagnosis after SNHL diagnosis (**Fig. 2.3**).[34] In the past, a perchlorate discharge test was done to confirm PS, but low sensitivity has made genetic testing the preferred examination in suspected patients.[35] Most children with PS respond to cochlear implantation favorably.[36]

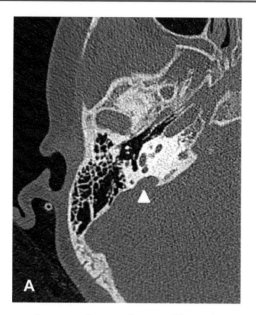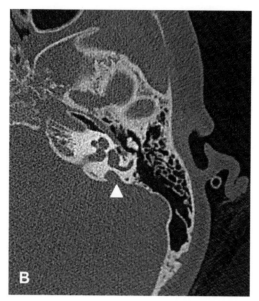

Figure 2.3 Computed tomography scan of temporal bone of a patient with Pendred syndrome (A) shows typical enlarged vestibular aqueducts (B) bilaterally (arrowheads).

PS

Consider these diagnostic tests: genetic consultation/testing for *SLC26A4* mutations, thyroid function tests, CT head in children with EVA, cochlear anomalies on CT scan, goiter, and suggestive family history.

USH is characterized by SNHL, retinitis pigmentosa, and vestibular dysfunction, and taken together are the most common cause of deafness-blindness in the United States.[37] There are three types of USH. USH1 is characterized by severe congenital hearing loss, vestibular dysfunction, and retinitis pigmentosa developing in early childhood; USH2 has hearing loss that is moderate, no vestibular dysfunction, and later onset of retinal degeneration; and USH3 is characterized by progressive hearing loss and vestibular dysfunction with variable retinal disease. Because USH is relatively common and cannot otherwise be differentiated from ARNSHL early on, and because early bilateral implantation is critical for children with USH in light of the vision deficits, all children with bilateral SNHL and without obvious cause after history and examination should have an ophthalmological examination which may include electroretinography (ERG).

USH

Consider these diagnostic tests: genetic consultations/testing for *CDH23, CLRN1, GPR98, MYO7A, PCDH15, USH1C, USH1G,* and *USH2A* mutations, ophthalmology consultation, and ERG in any child with presumed bilateral, symmetric ARNSHL, or history or examination suggestive of USH.

JLNS is a form of congenital deafness that is associated with a prolonged QT interval seen on electrocardiogram.

Hearing loss in children with JLNS is most commonly profound, bilateral, and present at birth. Like other long QT syndromes, syncope is sometimes present in affected children, but the presenting symptom may be ventricular arrhythmia and sudden death, thus making this condition an important one to rule out in congenitally deaf children.[38]

JLNS

Consider these diagnostic tests: genetic testing/consultation, electrocardiography (EKG), pediatric cardiology consultation in any child with personal/family history of syncope, long QT syndrome, or family history of sudden death.

X-linked Syndromes

Syndromes causing SNHL inherited in an X-linked pattern include Alport syndrome (AS) and X-linked deafness syndrome.

AS is a common disease affecting renal function. Its prevalence is estimated to be 1 in 5000. This disease can be inherited in an autosomal recessive or dominant pattern, but sex-linked inheritance accounts for 80% of patients. In addition to hematuric nephritis, patients with AS suffer from congenital cataracts and progressive SNHL. The hearing loss is present in 55% of affected patients, is high-frequency, and typically presents in the second decade of life.[39]

AS

Consider these diagnostic tests: genetic testing/consultation, urinalysis, renal electrolytes, complete blood count (CBC), ophthalmology consultation in children (mostly male) with hematuria, suggestive eye abnormalities, personal/family history of other renal disease, and thrombocytopenia.

DFN3, an X-linked form of deafness, is characterized by malformation of the labyrinth, creating an abnormal communication between the cerebrospinal fluid (CSF) and perilymph. The cochlea is shortened and lacks bony separation from the internal auditory canal and the facial nerve course is altered. Although patients usually have mixed hearing loss, stapes surgery is not recommended due to the risk for a perilymphatic gusher.[40]

X-linked Deafness Syndrome

Consider these diagnostic tests: genetic consultation, MRI in males with a suggestive family history and progressive mixed-type hearing loss.

Syndromes Related to Mitochondrial Disorders

Maintenance of ionic potentials is fundamentally important to cochlear function and the demand for energy in this tissue is high. Therefore, mitochondrial diseases can be associated with SNHL. Examples include mitochondrial encephalopathy, lactic acidosis, stroke syndrome, Kearns-Sayre syndrome (heart block and progressive ophthalmoplegia), and MERRF (myoclonic epilepsy and red ragged fibers) syndrome. Patients with these disorders are prone to late-onset, progressive, and bilateral high-frequency hearing loss.[3]

Mitochondrial Disorders

Consider these diagnostic tests: genetic, ophthalmology, neurology, and cardiology consultations in children with suggestive histories, retinitis pigmentosa, and suggestive family histories.

Nongenetic Hearing Loss

There are a large number of insults that occur during fetal life, in the peri- and postnatal periods, and later that cause SNHL. The largest nongenetic cause of SNHL is infection—both in children identified by failed UNHS and among children who develop hearing loss later. Cytomegalovirus (CMV) is the most common intrauterine infection and a major cause of sensorineural deafness worldwide.[41,42] The prevalence of CMV infection is so high (1% of all live births in the United States) that even with only 14% of infected children developing SNHL, CMV accounts for 15 to 20% of all bilateral moderate to profound loss.[43] Ten percent of CMV-infected neonates are symptomatic at birth, and most will fail UNHS. Of the remaining 90% who are normal at birth, between 7.5 and 10% will eventually develop hearing impairment. Many also eventually develop cognitive delay and other neurological disease, vision loss, growth retardation, hepatosplenomegaly, hematological abnormalities, and various cutaneous manifestations. The median age of detection is 27 months among children who originally passed newborn hearing screens.[44]

CMV Infection

Consider these diagnostic tests: CMV titers in mother and child, CMV quantitative polymerase chain reaction, then CT head, infectious disease and developmental pediatric consults in any child diagnosed with SNHL presenting in the first 3 weeks of life.

Other important intrauterine infections include toxoplasmosis, rubella, and syphilis. Treatment is available and effective if administered early for many infectious causes of neonatal SNHL, making selective screening important.

Congenital TORCH Infection

Consider these diagnostic tests: toxoplasmosis, Rubella, CMV, herpes simplex virus, syphilis, vericella-zoster virus titers in neonates with suggestive physical examination results and pregnancy history.

Another important risk factor for SNHL is NICU admission. Before universal screening, directed hearing screens were administered to neonates in the intensive care unit because of their high risk status, with prevalence of 3.2%.[45] Several environmental risk factors and associated conditions are hypothesized as causative, including increased ambient noise, perinatal complications such as hypoxia and acidosis, inherited syndromes, hyperbilirubinemia, meningitis, extended positive pressure ventilation, extracorporeal membrane oxygenation (ECMO) requirement, and ototoxic drug administration. In a recent, large retrospective study, neonates from the NICU who failed UNHS were found to be significantly more likely to have dysmorphic features, low appearance, pulse, grimace, activity, respiration (Apgar) score at 1 minute, sepsis, meningitis, cerebral bleeding, and cerebral infarction compared with controls.[46]

Severe hyperbilirubinemia and the resultant kernicterus have been long established as an important cause of SNHL in neonates. The proposed mechanism of injury in this case is auditory nerve myelinopathy.[47] The hearing loss that results falls into a subclass of SNHL called auditory neuropathy (AN)—an SNHL that is defined by normal outer hair cell function with an abnormal auditory brainstem response (ABR). AN is an abnormality in the neural processing of auditory stimuli. AN was first described in 1996, and since then its identification has increased dramatically. Classically, AN is diagnosed when children have speech recognition scores which are disproportionately low representing an inability to decode speech and language in the setting of normal or slightly elevated audiogram pure-tone thresholds. In fact, AN as it is defined is a group of hearing losses that are diverse in pathophysiology and treatment. Abnormalities in synchronizing inner hair cell firing and nerve conduction—now more appropriately termed "auditory dyssynchrony"—make up a form of AN for which implantation is clearly beneficial.[48]

The fact that children in the NICU are at higher risk for developing AN has implications for UNHS protocols. The Joint Committee on Infant Hearing in 2007 recommended screening these high-risk neonates with ABR, as AN is missed with screens that only test outer hair cell function. NICU graduates are also at increased risk for delayed, progressive hearing loss, and so they must be carefully screened for changes in hearing during childhood.

Auditory Dyssynchrony/Neuropathy

Consider these diagnostic tests: CT internal auditory canals (IACs) or MRI IACs in children with suggestive ABR or audiogram, history of NICU admission or hyperbilirubinemia and who are cochlear implant candidates.

Bacterial meningitis is the most common cause of acquired SNHL in the postnatal period. Roughly a third of affected children develop at least a mild hearing loss.[46] This fact and the risk of postinfectious cochlear ossification make close audiological follow-up and early cochlear implant evaluation critical.

Ototoxic drugs can affect hearing in utero and at any point during childhood. Drugs that pose a risk include aminoglycosides, for which there is a genetic predisposition[47,49]; other antibiotics such as erythromycin, vancomycin, and tetracycline, which have a more pronounced ototoxic affect in children with renal impairment; certain chemotherapeutic agents, including cisplatin, 5-fluorouracil, bleomycin, and nitrogen mustard; salicylates, which cause SNHL that is completely reversible with discontinuation of the drug; and high-dose intravenous loop diuretics, in which the effect is largely temporary and potentiated by other ototoxins.[50] Maternal use of alcohol and illicit drugs during pregnancy may also affect a child's ability to hear. Of all these drugs, cisplatin is generally accepted as the most ototoxic, causing hearing impairment in up to 25% of patients.[51]

Another important nonhereditary cause of SNHL is noise. While increased noise exposure in the NICU is one theoretical risk factor, of greater concern is noise trauma in older children. The prevalence of noise-induced hearing loss among children has increased dramatically in the last several decades, with most recent estimates approaching 20%.[3,4] An increase in use of personal listening devices has been blamed. With supra-aural headphones, recommendations limit noise exposure to 1 hour daily at 60% maximal volume. These types of headphones are clearly safer than insert headphones (earbuds).[52] Noise-induced hearing loss is typically sensorineural and often shows frequency dip at 4 kHz, the resonant frequency of the external canal.

Cogan's syndrome is an autoimmune rheumatic condition causing SNHL in older children and young adults. Following recovery from an influenza-like infection, affected individuals develop interstitial keratitis, vasculitis, and vestibuloauditory symptoms including progressive bilateral SNHL. No definitive test exists, but when symptoms and an elevated erythrocyte sedimentation rate (ESR), leukocytosis, and thrombocytosis are suggestive, prompt treatment should be initiated with steroids and other immunosuppressants to halt progress of hearing and vision loss.[53] Other autoimmune conditions associated with SNHL—also found in older children—include systemic lupus erythematosus, juvenile rheumatoid arthritis, and juvenile diabetes.

Autoimmune-Related Childhood SNHL

Consider these diagnostic tests: ESR, antinuclear antibody, rheumatoid factor, CBC, ophthalmology consultation, glucose testing in older children with suggestive history, particularly with personal/family history of autoimmune disorders.

It is important to note that anatomic anomalies of the inner ear—often unrelated to any known underlying genetic cause—are a major cause of SNHL in children. In fact, roughly a quarter of all children with congenital SNHL have some inner ear malformation detectable by modern imaging.[54,55] The most common is Scheibe dysplasia, or cochleosaccular dysplasia. The most severe bony anomaly is Michel aplasia, or complete labyrinthian aplasia. Incomplete partition, or Mondini dysplasia, is characterized by only 1.5 turns in the cochlea, is the most common congenital cochlear malformation, and is associated with PS and EVA.

Anatomical Anomalies of the Inner Ear

Consider these diagnostic tests: genetic testing/consultation, CT temporal bones in all children with SNHL for whom an obvious cause is not readily apparent after physical examination history, and audiologic evaluation and connexin 26 testing is negative.

Medical Evaluation of a Child with SNHL

Increasing numbers of children with SNHL are being identified through screening, and the tests available to classify the underlying cause of that hearing loss are growing in number and becoming more complex. In the current environment of increasingly limited resources, this has created a dilemma for which there is still no clear answer.

Each provider or institution approaches the work-up of SNHL differently. In general, a great deal of information is gained through a thorough history and physical examination including complete audiographic analysis, and some experts suggest that this is the only universally required step. Others weigh the yield of each test and the danger of a missed diagnosis against its cost, and choose from a variety of blood tests, genetic tests, imaging, other ancillary examinations and specialist consults.

In the next several years, as we have an exponentially improved understanding of the genetic determinants of hearing loss and methods for determining them, the most efficient work-up of children with SNHL will change so that genetic testing will become the most important part of a diagnostic work-up of a child with SNHL after history, physical examination, and audiometry.

History

A complete history is imperative and should address multiple issues including: (1) exposure to intrauterine infections (toxoplasma, rubella, CMV, herpes simplex virus, human immunodeficiency virus, and syphilis); (2) maternal and child vaccination history; (3) maternal metabolic disorders including diabetes or hyperthyroidism; and (4) the use of toxic agents during pregnancy (ethanol, tobacco, illicit drugs, ototoxic medications). The birth history should include Apgar scores, episodes of hypoxia, hyperbilirubinemia, pulmonary hypertension, low birth weight, and ECMO requirement. Any history of head trauma or noise exposure, meningitis history, fainting spells, or visual problems should also be noted.

Family history is essential and may help identify a genetic basis for the hearing loss. A history of consanguinity increases the possibility of an autosomal recessive disorder.

Physical Examination

A thorough physical examination first must rule out conductive components to the hearing loss. Possible syndromes should be ruled out with attention to the presence of endocrine abnormalities (thyroid nodules, diabetes), visual anomalies (retinitis pigmentosa, retinal detachment), craniofacial anomalies (dystopia canthorum, aural atresia, branchial anomalies, cleft palate), cardiac anomalies, other cranial nerve palsies, and pigmentary anomalies (heterochromic irides, white forelock).

Audiologic Analysis

Aside from the history and physical examination a complete audiologic evaluation is the only testing that some experts feel is uniformly required in the work-up of childhood SNHL. If there is a family history of dominant hearing loss, the audiogram often displays characteristic gene-specific patterns (**Fig. 2.4**). For example, a "cookie-bite" pattern can be caused by mutations in *COL11A2* (DFNA13), while mutations in *WFS1* usually cause low-frequency hearing loss that rises to normal in the high frequencies (DFNA6/14/38). These differences are exploited by an online resource called AudioGene. AudioGene is a support vector machine trained to predict the genetic cause of hearing loss in dominant families by using pattern recognition or audioprofiling[56] (**Table 2.2**).

Blood Tests

The SNHL-specific diagnostic yield of laboratory testing has been shown to be as low as 0 to 2%[57] and is generally not recommended. One notable exception is in the evaluation for

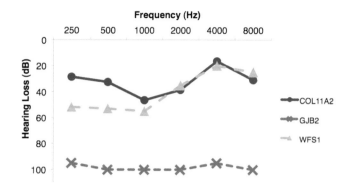

Figure 2.4 Typical audiogram appearances of selected causative mutations.

intrauterine CMV infection. In several European countries, CMV screening is part of a routine prenatal work-up for all pregnant women, but at present, this policy has not been adapted in the United States. Because CMV is causative in 15% of bilateral hearing loss in childhood, efforts are being made to develop an acceptable neonatal CMV screen, a CMV vaccine, and CMV treatment for infected neonates.[58,59] At present, CMV culture of saliva, urine, or serum can confirm CMV infection in 6% of neonates failing UNHS.[60] All children presenting before 3 weeks of age should be tested for CMV titers (with maternal testing as well).

EKG

The role of EKG as a screening examination for all children after confirmed SNHL is an area of contention and most experts recommend an EKG only with a family history of syncope, arrhythmia, or sudden death.[61]

Genetic Testing

The role of genetic testing is growing as comprehensive testing becomes accessible and cheaper. These changes reflect the concurrent development of high-throughput genetic screening by multiple centers.[62–70] At the same time, the fraction of SNHL attributed to known, testable genetic defects is growing.

Several investigators have suggested that because 20% of children with severe-to-profound bilateral SNHL have causative mutations in *GJB2*, a cost-effective paradigm in the face of this type of hearing loss begins with mutation screening of *GJB2*. The identification of mutations in this gene would obviate other ancillary tests, saving health care dollars while at the same time practicing evidence-based medicine.[66] In 2007, a nationwide survey to pediatric otolaryngologists showed that nearly 70% follow this paradigm and order *GJB2* testing routinely on the first visit.

In the future, the most cost-effective evaluation of childhood SNHL will likely involve a permutation of this paradigm, with more extensive genetic testing as the first test ordered. Recent advances in genetic screening methods now allow sequencing of millions of bases simultaneously

Table 2.1   High-Throughput Genetic Tests Currently Reported

Test Name	Location of Development	DNA Sequencing Technology	Screened	Advantages	Disadvantages	Reference
HHLAPEM	Stanford University	Single base-pair primer extension	198 deafness mutations	Inexpensive	Only screens 198 mutations, not direct sequencing	Rodriguez-Paris et al, PLoS One 2010
OtoChip™	Harvard University	Resequencing microarray	13 deafness genes	Inexpensive	Only examines 13 of >60 known deafness genes	Kothiyal et al, BMC Biotechnology 2010
OtoSCOPE®	University of Iowa	Sequence capture followed by massively parallel sequencing	66 deafness genes	Examines all known deafness genes	More expensive	Shearer et al, PNAS 2010

HHLAPEM: hereditary hearing loss arrayed primer extension microarray.

thus making comprehensive genetic testing possible for deafness. The emerging screening methods are summarized in **Table 2.1**.[63–65]

Radiologic Imaging

The need for imaging in all patients with SNHL and the ideal imaging modality for these children remain controversial topics. Imaging is essential when a child is a candidate for cochlear implantation, and the complementary information provided by CT and MRI makes both tests helpful for treatment planning.[61]

High-resolution CT scanning is thought by many to be the preferred modality in evaluating nonacute SNHL as it allows for evaluation of bony abnormalities of the cochlea, vestibular apparatus, internal auditory canal, or temporal bone otherwise. A review of 351 children with SNHL in 2009 showed that 31% had abnormalities on CT, the most common being EVA (15%).[54] A recent CT and MRI comparison in a series of children with unilateral and asymmetric SNHL advocated CT, as 41% of CTs showed abnormalities while only 30% of MRIs were read as abnormal.

MRI, however, offers benefits of increased soft tissue resolution, which is important in evaluating the cochlear nerve and membranous labyrinth. A 2008 retrospective evaluation of 170 children with SNHL showed that MRI demonstrated inner ear abnormalities in 38% of children with bilateral moderate to profound hearing loss and in 62% of children with unilateral disease. Absence of the cochlea nerve was seen in 21 children in this study, one-third of whom would be missed by CT. By CT size criteria, one-third of these would have been missed.[67]

MRI is particularly useful in patients with AN/auditory dysynchrony.[68] A review of 118 children with this diagnosis demonstrated at least one MRI abnormality in two-thirds of patients. Common abnormalities that became apparent with MRI (and not with CT) in these patients were cochlear nerve deficiencies (28%), brain abnormalities (40%), and prominent temporal horns (16%).

Specialist Consults

Half of pediatric otolaryngologists order ophthalmologic consultation as part of a routine SNHL evaluation, and half order a genetic consultation.[61]

The role for ophthalmologic evaluation is supported by a 2002 study which reported ocular abnormalities in 31% of children referred after SNHL diagnosis. As a result of an evaluation of 49 patients, 4 children underwent nonoperative intervention, 2 had surgery, 2 received prescription lenses, and 2 received diagnosis of a hearing loss related syndrome.[69] In the algorithm suggested below, only some children are referred for formal ophthalmologic consultation as a part of the diagnostic process, but all children with SNHL should undergo vision screening as part of treatment to optimize sensory input.

Otolaryngologists refer families for genetic consultation not only because such an evaluation can be helpful in identifying syndromic causes of SNHL, but also because explaining the genetics of SNHL and its implications for future children is complex. The overall recurrence chance for a normal hearing couple to have an additional child with hearing loss after the birth of one child with presumed ARNSHL is 17.5%,[70] but that estimate changes in various situations, and most otolaryngologists are unable to provide accurate data to families.[61,71]

Table 2.2   Audiogram Profiles of Common Types of Hereditary, Nonsyndromic Sensorineural Hearing Loss

Class	Gene	Locus	Audio Phenotype
Autosomal recessive	*GJB2*	DFNB1	Hearing loss varies from mild to profound. Several large studies that have demonstrated good phenotype–genotype correlations for *GJB2*-related deafness.
	SLC26A4	DFNB4	DFNB4 is allelic; hearing loss is associated with dilatation of the vestibular aqueduct, and it can be unilateral or bilateral. In high frequencies, it is generally at least severe, while it is highly variable at low frequencies. Onset can be either congenital or progressive and postlingual.
Autosomal dominant	*DIAPH1*	DFNA1	Low-frequency loss beginning in the first decade and progressing to profound loss at all frequencies.
	KCNQ4	DFNA2	Symmetrical high-frequency loss beginning in the first decade and progressing over all frequencies.
	WFS1	DFNA6/14/38	Early-onset low-frequency hearing loss.
	EYA4	DFNA10	Hearing loss beginning in the second decade with a gently sloping audio profile that becomes steeply sloping with age.
	COL11A2	DFNA13	Congenital mid-frequency sensorineural loss that shows progression across the auditory range.
	POU4F3	DFNA15	Progressive sensorineural loss beginning in the second decade which is generally symmetrical.
	ACTG1	DFNA20/26	Bilateral, progressive hearing loss beginning in the second decade and eventually yielding hearing loss across all frequencies, although a sloping configuration is maintained in most cases.
X-linked	*POU3F4*	DFN3	Conductive hearing loss that mimics otosclerosis with superimposed progressive sensorineural loss.
Mitochondrial	*12S rRNA*	mtDNA1555A>G	Symmetric hearing loss with variable severity; loss in hearing can occur after aminoglycoside therapy.

Adapted from: Smith RJ, Bale JF Jr, White KR. Sensorineural hearing loss in children. *Lancet* 2005;365(9462):879–890.

Suggested Algorithm for Medical Work-Up of a Child with Newly Diagnosed SNHL

All children with newly diagnosed SNHL should have a complete history (including family history), physical examination, and complete audiology evaluation (**Fig. 2.5**). Siblings and parents of all children without an obvious nonhereditary cause of SNHL should get audiograms, both for their own care and to aid the diagnostic process. All children identified before 3 weeks of age should be evaluated for CMV infection. If a syndrome is suggested by the basic evaluation, additional syndrome-specific testing should be considered.

If the SNHL is mild and unilateral, the child should be followed carefully for progression of the hearing loss, obtaining a CT if necessary. CT scan should be considered for fluctuating hearing loss as well. If the child has unilateral SNHL that is at least moderate in severity, MRI should be completed.

If the child has bilateral SNHL of any degree, genetic testing should be obtained. In the near future, this will include all genes known to cause nonsyndromic hearing loss. An ophthalmological examination should be completed if history, physical examination, and family history are not helpful. CT should also be considered in these children.

If the child is a candidate for cochlear implantation, both MRI and CT should be completed.

Conclusion

The evaluation of childhood SNHL is evolving. This change is seen most clearly in the increasing role played by genetic

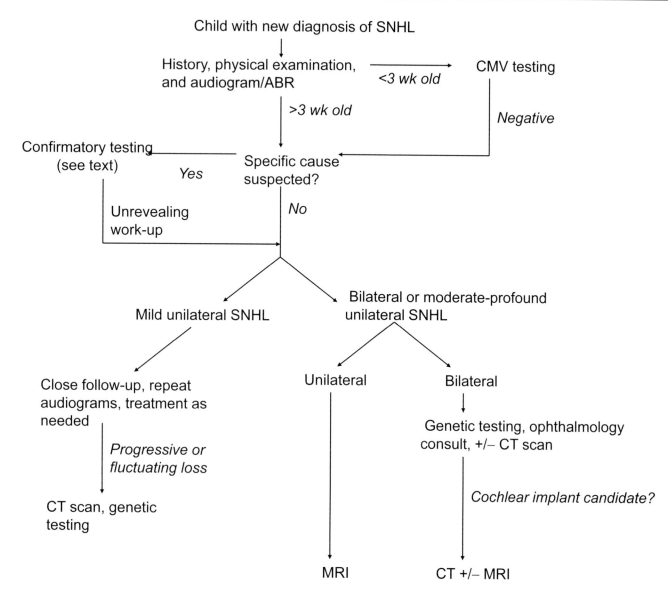

Figure 2.5   Suggested algorithm for the work-up of children with sensorineural hearing loss. ABR, auditory brainstem response; CMV, cytomegalovirus; CT, computed tomography; MRI, magnetic resonance imaging; SNHL, sensorineural hearing loss; wk, week(s).

testing. As this type of testing becomes cheaper, it can be used as a platform from which other informed and evidence-based decisions can be made in the appropriate evaluation of the child with hearing loss.

References

1. Mehl AL, Thomson V. Newborn hearing screening: the great omission. Pediatrics 1998;101(1):E4
2. Brookhouser PE. Sensorineural hearing loss in children. Pediatr Clin North Am 1996;43(6):1195–1216
3. Shargorodsky J, Curhan SG, Curhan GC, Eavey R. Change in prevalence of hearing loss in US adolescents. JAMA 2010;304(7):772–778
4. Niskar A, Kieszak S, Holmes A, Esteban E, Rubin C, Brody D. Estimated prevalence of noise-induced hearing threshold shifts among children 6 to 19 years of age: the Third National Health and Nutrition Examination Survey, 1988–94, US. Pediatrics 2001;108(1):40–43

5. Vohr B, Jodoin-Krauzyk J, Tucker R, Johnson MJ, Topol D, Ahlgren M. Early language outcomes of early-identified infants with permanent hearing loss at 12 to 16 months of age. Pediatrics 2008;122(3):535–544
6. Watkin P, McCann D, Law C, et al. Language ability in children with permanent hearing impairment: the influence of early management and family participation. Pediatrics 2007;120(3):e694–e701
7. Yoshinaga-Itano C, Sedey AL, Coulter DK, Mehl AL. Language of early- and later-identified children with hearing loss. Pediatrics 1998;102(5):1161–1171
8. Joint Committee on Infant Hearing; American Academy of

Audiology; American Academy of Pediatrics; American Speech-Language-Hearing Association; Directors of Speech and Hearing Programs in State Health and Welfare Agencies. Year 2000 position statement: principles and guidelines for early hearing detection and intervention programs. Joint Committee on Infant Hearing, American Academy of Audiology, American Academy of Pediatrics, American Speech-Language-Hearing Association, and Directors of Speech and Hearing Programs in State Health and Welfare Agencies. Pediatrics 2000;106(4):798–817

9. US Department of Health and Human Services. Office of Disease Prevention and Health Promotion. Healthy People 2010. Washington DC. Available at: http://www.cdc.gov/nchs/healthy-people/hp2010/hp2010-final-review.htm. Accessed 2/11

10. Morton CC, Nance WE. Newborn hearing screening—a silent revolution. N Engl J Med 2006;354(20):2151–2164

11. Greinwald JH Jr, Hartnick CJ. The evaluation of children with sensorineural hearing loss. Arch Otolaryngol Head Neck Surg 2002;128(1):84–87

12. Holster IL, Hoeve LJ, Wieringa MH, Willis-Lorrier RM, de Gier HH. Evaluation of hearing loss after failed neonatal hearing screening. J Pediatr 2009;155(5):646–650

13. Bess FH, Tharpe AM. Case history data on unilaterally hearing-impaired children. Ear Hear 1986;7(1):14–19

14. Lieu JE. Speech-language and educational consequences of unilateral hearing loss in children. Arch Otolaryngol Head Neck Surg 2004;130(5):524–530

15. Uwiera TC, DeAlarcon A, Meinzen-Derr J, et al. Hearing loss progression and contralateral involvement in children with unilateral sensorineural hearing loss. Ann Otol Rhinol Laryngol 2009;118(11):781–785

16. Teasdale TW, Sorensen MH. Hearing loss in relation to educational attainment and cognitive abilities: a population study. Int J Audiol 2007;46(4):172–175

17. Gilbertson M, Kamhi AG. Novel word learning in children with hearing impairment. J Speech Hear Res 1995;38(3):630–642

18. Morton NE. Genetic epidemiology of hearing impairment. Ann N Y Acad Sci 1991;630:16–31

19. Smith RJ, Bale JF Jr, White KR. Sensorineural hearing loss in children. Lancet 2005;365(9462):879–890

20. Sundstrom RA, Van Laer L, Van Camp G, Smith RJ. Autosomal recessive nonsyndromic hearing loss. Am J Med Genet 1999;89(3):123–129

21. Vancampg G, Smith R. Hereditary Hearing Loss Homepage. Available at: http://hereditary hearingloss.org. 2011. Accessed 2/11

22. Apps SA, Rankin WA, Kurmis AP. Connexin 26 mutations in autosomal recessive deafness disorders: a review. Int J Audiol 2007;46(2):75–81

23. Cryns K, Orzan E, Murgia A, et al. A genotype-phenotype correlation for GJB2 (connexin 26) deafness. J Med Genet 2004;41(3):147–154

24. Bartsch O, Vatter A, Zechner U, et al. GJB2 mutations and genotype-phenotype correlation in 335 patients from germany with nonsyndromic sensorineural hearing loss: evidence for additional recessive mutations not detected by current methods. Audiol Neurootol 2010;15(6):375–382

25. Mhatre AN, Lalwani AK. Molecular genetics of deafness. Otolaryngol Clin North Am 1996;29(3):421–435

26. Kalatzis V, Petit C. Branchio-oto-oenal syndrome. Adv Otorhinolaryngol 2000;56:39–44

27. Chen A, Francis M, Ni L, et al. Phenotypic manifestations of branchio-oto-renal syndrome. Am J Med Genet 1995;58(4):365–370

28. Newton VE. Clinical features of the Waardenburg syndromes. Adv Otorhinolaryngol 2002;61:201–208

29. Read AP, Newton VE. Waardenburg syndrome. J Med Genet 1997;34(8):656–665

30. Webb AC, Markus AF. The diagnosis and consequences of Stickler syndrome. Br J Oral Maxillofac Surg 2002;40(1):49–51

31. Bance M, Ramsden RT. Management of neurofibromatosis type 2. Ear Nose Throat J 1999;78(2):91–94, 96

32. Arndt S, Laszig R, Beck R, et al. Spectrum of hearing disorders and their management in children with CHARGE syndrome. Otol Neurotol 2010;31(1):67–73

33. Everett LA, Glaser B, Beck JC, et al. Pendred syndrome is caused by mutations in a putative sulphate transporter gene (*PDS*). Nat Genet 1997;17(4):411–422

34. Reardon W, OMahoney CF, Trembath R, Jan H, Phelps PD. Enlarged vestibular aqueduct: a radiological marker of pendred syndrome, and mutation of the PDS gene. QJM 2000;93(2):99–104

35. Stinckens C, Huygen PL, Van Camp G, Cremers CW. Pendred syndrome redefined. Report of a new family with fluctuating and progressive hearing loss. Adv Otorhinolaryngol 2002;61:131–141

36. Harker LA, Vanderheiden S, Veazey D, Gentile N, McCleary E. Multichannel cochlear implantation in children with large vestibular aqueduct syndrome. Ann Otol Rhinol Laryngol Suppl 1999;177:39–43

37. Petit C. Usher syndrome: from genetics to pathogenesis. Annu Rev Genomics Hum Genet 2001;2:271–297

38. Komsuoğlu B, Göldeli O, Kulan K, et al. The Jervell and Lange-Nielsen syndrome. Int J Cardiol 1994;47(2):189–192

39. Meyers KE. Evaluation of hematuria in children. Urol Clin North Am 2004;31(3):559–573

40. Aschendorff A, Maier W, Jaekel K, et al. Radiologically assisted navigation in cochlear implantation for X-linked deafness malformation. Cochlear Implants Int 2009;10 (S 1):14–18

41. Li XC, Friedman RA. Nonsyndromic hereditary hearing loss. Otolaryngol Clin North Am 2002;35(2):275–285

42. Weller TH. The cytomegaloviruses: ubiquitous agents with protean clinical manifestations. I. N Engl J Med 1971;285(4):203–214

43. Ogawa H, Suzutani T, Baba Y, et al. Etiology of severe sensorineural hearing loss in children: independent impact of congenital cytomegalovirus infection and GJB2 mutations. J Infect Dis 2007;195(6):782–788

44. Grosse SD, Ross DS, Dollard SC. Congenital cytomegalovirus (CMV) infection as a cause of permanent bilateral hearing loss: a quantitative assessment. J Clin Virol 2008;41(2):57–62

45. Hille ET, van Straaten HI, Verkerk PH; Dutch NICU Neonatal Hearing Screening Working Group. Prevalence and independent risk factors for hearing loss in NICU infants. Acta Paediatr 2007;96(8):1155–1158

46. Coenraad S, Goedegebure A, van Goudoever JB, Hoeve LJ. Risk factors for sensorineural hearing loss in NICU infants compared to normal hearing NICU controls. Int J Pediatr Otorhinolaryngol 2010;74(9):999–1002 epub ahead of print

47. Vlastarakos PV, Nikolopoulos TP, Tavoulari E, Papacharalambous G, Korres S. Auditory neuropathy: endochlear lesion or temporal processing impairment? Implications for diagnosis and management. Int J Pediatr Otorhinolaryngol 2008;72(8):1135–1150

48. Berlin C, Hood L, Rose K. On renaming auditory neuropathy as auditory dyssynchrony: implications for a clear understanding of underlying mechanisms and management options. Audiology Today 2001;13:15–17

49. Casano RA, Johnson DF, Bykhovskaya Y, Torricelli F, Bigozzi M, Fischel-Ghodsian N. Inherited susceptibility to aminoglycoside ototoxicity: genetic heterogeneity and clinical implications. Am J Otolaryngol 1999;20(3):151–156

50. Gallagher KL, Jones JK. Furosemide-induced ototoxicity. Ann Intern Med 1979;91(5):744–745

51. Berg AL, Spitzer JB, Garvin JH Jr. Ototoxic impact of cisplatin in pediatric oncology patients. Laryngoscope 1999;109(11):1806–1814

52. Fligor BJ, Cox LC. Output levels of commercially available portable compact disc players and the potential risk to hearing. Ear Hear 2004;25(6):513–527

53. Grasland A, Pouchot J, Hachulla E, Blétry O, Papo T, Vinceneux P; Study Group for Cogan's Syndrome. Typical and atypical Cogan's syndrome: 32 cases and review of the literature. Rheumatology (Oxford) 2004;43(8):1007–1015

54. Antonelli PJ, Varela AE, Mancuso AA. Diagnostic yield of high-resolution computed tomography for pediatric sensorineural hearing loss. Laryngoscope 1999;109(10):1642–1647

55. McClay JE, Tandy R, Grundfast K, et al. Major and minor temporal bone abnormalities in children with and without congenital sensorineural hearing loss. Arch Otolaryngol Head Neck Surg 2002;128(6):664–671

56. Hildebrand MS, DeLuca AP, Taylor KR, et al. A contemporary review of AudioGene audioprofiling: a machine-based candidate gene prediction tool for autosomal dominant nonsyndromic hearing loss. Laryngoscope 2009;119(11):2211–2215

57. Mafong DD, Shin EJ, Lalwani AK. Use of laboratory evaluation and radiologic imaging in the diagnostic evaluation of children with sensorineural hearing loss. Laryngoscope 2002;112(1):1–7

58. Boppana SB, Ross SA, Novak Z, et al; National Institute on Deafness and Other Communication Disorders CMV and Hearing Multicenter Screening (CHIMES) Study. Dried blood spot real-time polymerase chain reaction assays to screen newborns for congenital cytomegalovirus infection. JAMA 2010;303(14):1375–1382

59. Kimberlin DW, Lin CY, Sánchez PJ, et al; National Institute of Allergy and Infectious Diseases Collaborative Antiviral Study Group. Effect of ganciclovir therapy on hearing in symptomatic congenital cytomegalovirus disease involving the central nervous system: a randomized, controlled trial. J Pediatr 2003;143(1):16–25

60. Stehel EK, Shoup AG, Owen KE, et al. Newborn hearing screening and detection of congenital cytomegalovirus infection. Pediatrics 2008;121(5):970–975

61. Duncan RD, Prucka S, Wiatrak BJ, Smith RJ, Robin NH. Pediatric otolaryngologists' use of genetic testing. Arch Otolaryngol Head Neck Surg 2007;133(3):231–236

62. Gardner P, Oitmaa E, Messner A, Hoefsloot L, Metspalu A, Schrijver I. Simultaneous multigene mutation detection in patients with sensorineural hearing loss through a novel diagnostic microarray: a new approach for newborn screening follow-up. Pediatrics 2006;118(3):985–994

63. Rodriguez-Paris J, Pique L, Colen T, Roberson J, Gardner P, Schrijver I. Genotyping with a 198 mutation arrayed primer extension array for hereditary hearing loss: assessment of its diagnostic value for medical practice. PLoS One 2010;5(7):e11804

64. Kothiyal P, Cox S, Ebert J, et al. High-throughput detection of mutations responsible for childhood hearing loss using resequencing microarrays. BMC Biotechnol 2010;10:10

65. Shearer AE, DeLuca AP, Hildebrand MS, et al. Comprehensive genetic testing for hereditary hearing loss using massively parallel sequencing. Proc Natl Acad Sci U S A 2010;107(49):21104–21109

66. Preciado DA, Lawson L, Madden C, et al. Improved diagnostic effectiveness with a sequential diagnostic paradigm in idiopathic pediatric sensorineural hearing loss. Otol Neurotol 2005;26(4):610–615

67. McClay JE, Booth TN, Parry DA, Johnson R, Roland P. Evaluation of pediatric sensorineural hearing loss with magnetic resonance imaging. Arch Otolaryngol Head Neck Surg 2008;134(9):945–952

68. Roche JP, Huang BY, Castillo M, Bassim MK, Adunka OF, Buchman CA. Imaging characteristics of children with auditory neuropathy spectrum disorder. Otol Neurotol 2010;31(5):780–788

69. Mafong DD, Pletcher SD, Hoyt C, Lalwani AK. Ocular findings in children with congenital sensorineural hearing loss. Arch Otolaryngol Head Neck Surg 2002;128(11):1303–1306

70. Green GE, Scott DA, McDonald JM, Woodworth GG, Sheffield VC, Smith RJ. Carrier rates in the midwestern United States for GJB2 mutations causing inherited deafness. JAMA 1999;281(23):2211–2216

71. Robin NH, Dietz C, Arnold JE, Smith RJ. Pediatric otolaryngologists' knowledge and understanding of genetic testing for deafness. Arch Otolaryngol Head Neck Surg 2001;127(8):937–940

3 Pediatric Vestibular Dysfunction

Manali Shailesh Amin

Vestibular dysfunction in children is a commonly underdiagnosed problem. It is characterized by an inability to maintain visual acuity during movement. This impairment results in motor incoordination and places children at risk of injuries during normal play. Furthermore, vestibular dysfunction may impair a child's ability to integrate sensory stimuli.[1]

For a problem with such great health implications, vestibular dysfunction in the pediatric population is poorly understood. This is in large part the result of multiple barriers to diagnosis. To obtain a better understanding of pediatric vestibular dysfunction, one must first understand normal maturation and development of the vestibular system.

The vestibular system is the first of the sensory systems to develop. Embryologically, the membranous vestibular apparatus and the membranous cochlea both develop from ototcysts. The bony labyrinth develops from the surrounding mesoderm. Morphologically, the vestibular system is fully developed by the 49th day of gestation.[2] Connections between the peripheral vestibular system and the central system and myelination continues until birth. The vestibular system is fully developed at birth but continues to mature with age. This maturation process is greatest during the toddler years and continues well into childhood. For instance, although the optokinetic response is present by 3 to 6 months of age, eye drift in a direction opposite to the rotating drum is seen up to 5 months of age when myelination of the visual pursuit system is completed. The saccadic system continues to develop until the age of 2. Furthermore, the ability to isolate these systems during routine activities and use them to complete more complex tasks such as reaching for an object while maintaining postural control continues to evolve into school age.[3] An understanding of this maturation process is important when determining whether an abnormality exists.

In obtaining a history and performing a physical examination, one will often want to know if there are discrete vertiginous spells or an underlying balance disorder and whether the symptoms are associated with a hearing loss. This chapter is designed to provide an overview of some of the conditions that can present with a complaint of dizziness or balance dysfunction. It has been organized into two sections: (1) conditions associated with a hearing loss and (2) those conditions without a hearing loss. Knowing whether the vertigo spells are of an acute or chronic nature and whether or not they are episodic is also important. Time is often the best determinant of a diagnosis as some conditions may not become apparent until several spells have occurred.

Vestibular Disorders Associated with a Hearing Loss

It has been long known that children with hearing loss are more likely to have a vestibular problem. Unilateral or bilateral vestibular hypofunction may be seen with a congenital sensorineural hearing loss (SNHL) as well as some progressive mixed hearing losses. Vestibular hypofunction is seen in more than 30% of children with an autosomal dominant congenital hearing loss.[1] Certain syndromes are associated with both vestibular dysfunction and hearing loss, such as Waardenburg syndrome, branchiootorenal syndrome, Pendred syndrome, Klippel–Feil syndrome, and Usher syndrome.

Acoustic Neuroma

Acoustic neuromas are the most common posterior fossa tumor in children. They may present rather insidiously. High frequency hearing loss and tinnitus often precede the vestibular complaints. Additional cranial nerve findings may also be apparent. In children, acoustic neuromas are most often associated with neurofibromatosis type 2. Audiologic testing may show worse speech discrimination than would be expected based upon pure-tone thresholds or auditory brainstem response (ABR) abnormalities. On ABR testing, an abnormal waveform or wave V latency of ≥ 0.2 ms may be noted. ABR abnormalities may not be apparent until the tumor is fairly large. By contrast, a magnetic resonance imaging (MRI) with gadolinium can detect tumors as small as 2 mm in size. The preferred treatment option in children is surgical excision. Gamma knife, which has been used in older adults, is not a good option in children given the effects of radiation over time.

Autoimmune Inner Ear Disease

Autoimmune inner ear disease (AIED) is characterized by a fluctuating, often progressive hearing loss, vertigo, lightheadedness, ataxia, and motion intolerance. Although it usually affects both ears, unilateral presentation may be seen. Patients will occasionally complain of tinnitus and/or aural fullness, making it difficult to distinguish from Ménière disease. AIED is associated with a systemic autoimmune disease in 15 to 30%. Symptoms generally progress over weeks to months and may improve on steroid treatment. There are isolated reports of vestibular dysfunction in the absence of hearing loss. Electronystagmogram (ENG) findings vary depending on whether one or both ears are affected. Partial recovery of vestibular function after steroid administration as measured in caloric testing and regression upon discontinuation has been reported. There are no definitive tests to diagnose AIED. Treatment of this relatively rare disease may be with steroids or chemotherapeutic agents.

Enlarged Vestibular Aqueduct

An enlarged vestibular aqueduct (EVA) is associated with a mixed or SNHL that may be mild to profound, fluctuating to progressive, or even sudden in presentation. Vestibular dysfunction ranges from mild clumsiness or imbalance to true vertigo and may be associated with oscillopsia or a tullio phenomenon. An EVA can be unilateral or bilateral and may be isolated or associated with a Mondini dysplasia of the cochlea. The mechanism for vestibular dysfunction is not well understood but is felt to result from a third window effect similar to the effect seen in superior canal dehiscence syndrome (SCDS). In fact, on vestibular-evoked myogenic potential (VEMP) testing, the thresholds may be lowered and amplitudes higher just as one would see in SCDS.

Eustachian Tube Dysfunction and Middle Ear Effusion

Eustachian tube dysfunction and middle ear effusion (MEE) are among the most common diagnoses resulting in a complaint of imbalance in younger children. A child may present with symptoms of clumsiness, unsteadiness, and falls. MEE generally presents with limited tympanic membrane mobility on pneumatic otoscopy, conductive hearing loss (CHL), and middle ear dysfunction on tympanometry. Vestibular dysfunction is equally likely with a unilateral effusion as it is with bilateral effusions. An ENG is not necessary for diagnosis. Treatment consists of watchful waiting for spontaneous resolution of the effusions or myringotomy and extraction of effusion with or without tube placement.

Labyrinthine Concussion

A labyrinthine concussion can follow some forms of head injury, especially one to the temporoparietal and occipitoparietal areas. Symptoms can include headaches, nausea/vomiting, visual disturbances, irritability, personality changes, and sleep disturbances. Vestibular symptoms include vertigo, a tilting sensation, dizziness, and unsteadiness. Vertigo will sometimes present as recurrent attacks which last 5 to 10 seconds and are associated with nausea. Unsteadiness usually manifests as sway to the affected side. Symptoms are usually present for a few days and then subside over a 4- to 6-week period but balance problems may be seen for years, especially with tandem gait and on Romberg testing

with eyes closed. Dix–Hallpike testing may be positive for a nystagmus, consistent with an associated benign paroxysmal positional vertigo (BPPV). Rotational chair testing is usually normal.

Ménière Disease/Endolymphatic Hydrops

Ménière disease is extremely rare in children. Symptoms include recurrent paroxysmal vertigo, SNHL, aural fullness, and tinnitus. Hearing loss may be fluctuating to progressive and unilateral or bilateral. In adults, the hearing loss is often reported to be a low frequency loss. By contrast, in children, the hearing loss may initially be high frequency. There is often a positive family history for Ménière and a personal history of allergic rhinitis and/or AIED.

Hydrops can also manifest in individuals with congenital cytomegalovirus (CMV) or otosyphilis. Children with congenital CMV have variable vestibular function. Some may have normal function while others have unilateral or bilateral peripheral hypofunction and delayed ambulation. Alternatively, vestibular symptoms may not present for many years. Vestibular testing including cochlear hydrops analysis masking procedure and electrocochleography can assist in making the diagnosis.[4] In addition, a unilateral weakness on caloric testing and asymmetry on rotational chair testing may be seen if only one ear is affected.

Ototoxicity

Many medications are alleged to produce vestibular ototoxicity including aminoglycosides, various other antibiotics (such as minocycline, erythromycin, polymyxin, and chloramphenicol), loop diuretics, salicylates, quinidine, barbiturates, and certain chemotherapeutic agents including cisplatin. In addition to vestibulotoxicity, most of these medications typically destroy the outer hair cells in the basal turn of the cochlea leading to a high frequency SNHL. Patients may present with disequilibrium, an ataxic gait, and oscillopsia. Both the vestibulo-ocular reflex (VOR) and vestibulospinal reflexes are affected. Therefore, rotational chair testing may show reduced gains and time constant. Posturography will usually result in falls on sensory organization test 6.[5] When oscillopsia occurs, it is generally with severe damage secondary to a loss of the VOR. These patients may have significant difficulty walking in the dark or on uneven surfaces and may have to navigate by holding onto walls and furniture.

Perilymph Fistula

Perilymph fistula (PLF) may result from a direct injury to the labyrinth or as a result of barotrauma or otologic surgery. Patients present with imbalance, vertigo, progressive SNHL, tinnitus, and nystagmus. The injury can be either unilateral or bilateral. On examination, positive pressure may result in nystagmus and is present in approximately 25% of patients. A computed tomography (CT) scan may show an anatomic abnormality which may predispose a child to a PLF such as a Mondini deformity. The definitive diagnosis is made by seeing perilymph on middle ear exploration.

Superior Semicircular Canal Dehiscence

In the late 1990s, Dr. Lloyd Minor first described the condition now commonly known as SSCD. This disorder was considered to be primarily one that affects adults. Children, like adults, present with symptoms of vertigo and oscillopsia with or without an associated nystagmus that may be induced by loud sounds (Tullio sign) or changes in pressure (Hennebert sign). Others may complain of autophony or hearing their own pulse or eye movements. On examination with Valsalva or holding their breath against a closed glottis, one may see vertical torsional eye movements. On audiogram, one may see a pseudo CHL in which bone conduction thresholds are better than 0 dB with normal pure tone averages or a CHL with air bone gaps at the lower frequencies. The stapedius reflex is usually normal. The dehiscence can be seen on high-resolution computed tomography (HRCT) scanning. VEMPs will almost always show a low threshold and high amplitude.

Temporal Bone Fractures

Temporal bone fractures are traditionally described as either transverse or longitudinal. Fractures which are parallel to the petrous bone are considered longitudinal while those which are perpendicular are transverse, although in reality most fractures are oblique. Transverse fractures may violate the internal auditory canal, semicircular canals, vestibule, cochlea, or facial nerve. Symptoms include hearing loss, vertigo, nausea, and vomiting. A spontaneous nystagmus may be seen. Hearing loss is usually immediate and severe but can be progressive if there is a PLF or if a patient develops endolymphatic hydrops. There are several theories on how hydrops may develop after a fracture including possible fracture and secondary occlusion of the vestibular aqueduct. Other mechanisms of injury that may result in vertigo include disruption of the membranous labyrinth, vascular vasospasm, thrombosis or hemorrhage, and disruption of the endosteum of the round window or oval window with resulting PLF. HRCT can establish the diagnosis. On vestibular function testing, one may see a spontaneous nystagmus toward the good ear. Sway on posturography is usually toward the injured ear and if rotary chair or caloric testing is done, abnormalities of the VOR may be seen.

Vestibular Labyrinthitis/Neuronitis

Vestibular neuronitis and labyrinthitis are characterized by sudden onset of vertigo that lasts for a few days with unsteadiness persisting for weeks to months. If it is associated with an acute hearing loss, it is considered vestibular labyrinthitis. In the absence of hearing loss, it is vestibular neuronitis. A horizontal nystagmus beating toward the healthy ear may be seen. It often follows an upper respira-

tory tract infection and is considered to have a viral etiology, possibly herpes simplex virus, measles, or mumps. The viral infection is felt to cause damage to the superior branch of the superior vestibular nerve. Utricular dysfunction can be seen in both while saccular dysfunction is seen primarily with labyrinthitis. Caloric testing will often show a decreased response in the affected ear. Rotational chair testing may show asymmetry and VEMPs may be absent in about one-third of patients. Subjective visual horizontal testing may show a deviation of the line from the horizontal with the affected side down.

Whiplash Injury

Whiplash can result in symptoms of dizziness, tinnitus, and occasionally hearing loss and visual disturbance. It typically follows a motor vehicle accident. The mechanism of action is not understood but theorized to result from cervical muscle spasm or decreased blood flow through the vertebrobasilar circulation as a result of sudden acceleration and deceleration. Before proceeding with any testing, it is important to ensure that the C-spine has been cleared. This injury is felt to primarily affect the cervico-ocular reflex (COR). COR gains are likely to be reduced generally as a result of reduced neck movements. A positional nystagmus may be seen with the head hyperextended. A spontaneous nystagmus or gaze-evoked nystagmus may also be seen as well as VOR abnormalities. Otolithic dysfunction has only been sporadically reported.

Dizziness with Normal Hearing

A majority of the children who present to an otolaryngology practice with complaints of dizziness or vertigo do not have an associated hearing loss. In fact, most will not have a vestibular problem. However, it is important to understand some of the other common disorders that may result in a consultation to appropriately manage the patient. Often, a neurology, ophthalmology, or cardiac evaluation may provide additional information.

BPPV

BPPV, the most common vestibular etiology for dizziness in the adult, is an uncommon finding in children. When it is seen, it most often follows a traumatic event in older children. Some theorize that the otoconia in children are more tightly adherent to the macula and, therefore, less likely to become dislodged. The classic description is of posterior canal BPPV and is characterized by sudden attacks of vertigo, nausea, and vomiting triggered by certain head movements and positions. A Dix–Hallpike maneuver will result in a rotary nystagmus which begins after a latency of a few seconds and is of limited duration. It fatigues with repeated provocation. The proposed mechanisms are canalithiasis, in which otoconial debris floats freely within the semicircular canal and cupulolithiasis, in which the debris adheres to the cupula of the canals. In both situations, the resulting disruptions of endolymphatic flow within the semicircular canal leads to a nystagmus and sensation of vertigo with head movement. Treatment consists of an Epley maneuver or one of its many modifications. In rare cases, surgical intervention with canal plugging, singular neurectomy, vestibular nerve section, or labyrinthectomy may be considered for intractable vertigo.

Chiari Type I Malformation

Chiari type I malformation is characterized by a herniation of the cerebellar tonsils through the foramen magnum. Before the availability of MRI, this was an uncommon diagnosis. The age of onset of symptoms is variable. Children with a Chiari malformation often present with torticollis, headaches, vocal cord paralysis, swallowing difficulties, ataxia, and opisthotonus. Vestibular symptoms are variable and can include oscillopsia, diplopia, blurred vision, and vertigo. On examination, horizontal or downbeat nystagmus is most commonly seen. Other findings include a jerky motion on pursuit and abducens palsy. Chiari malformation results in oculomotor and central vestibular dysfunction. Central abnormalities may be seen on electronystagmography. An MRI showing herniation of the cerebellar tonsils is diagnostic and posterior fossa decompression may result in improvement and/or resolution of symptoms.

Migraine/Migraine Variant

Migraine and migraine variants are the most common etiology of pediatric dizziness. A possible etiology for this condition may arise from paroxysmal ischemia of the vestibular nuclei. Paroxysmal torticollis and benign paroxysmal vertigo (BPV) of childhood are childhood periodic syndromes that are felt to be migraine precursors. In fact, some children who initially present with paroxysmal torticollis will later go on to develop BPV and possibly migraines or migraine variants as an older child. These children should generally be referred to a neurologist.

Paroxysmal torticollis is characterized by episodic torticollis which lasts between 4 hours and 4 days and can be associated with pallor, vomiting, and behavioral changes. It typically presents between the age of 2 to 8 months and has a female predilection. The frequency and duration of the episodes decline as a child grows older. Treatment includes watchful waiting, avoidance of triggers if they can be identified, and in rare cases, pharmacologic intervention.

BPV of childhood begins before the age of 5 and resolves within 2 years of onset. Unlike migraines, males and females are affected equally. It is characterized by rotary vertigo lasting from seconds up to 5 minutes. It may be associated with pallor, nausea, vomiting, and diaphoresis. There are usually no complaints of headaches or tinnitus. Younger children may cry inconsolably and appear frightened.

Episodes eventually resolve spontaneously. Treatment consists of watchful waiting and avoidance of identifiable triggers. In severe cases, prophylactic cyproheptadine may be considered.

Migraine variant vertigo typically begins around the age of 8 and is characterized by vertigo of several minutes' duration. Children may have associated pallor, nausea, vomiting, and noise or light sensitivity. There is usually a family history of migraines. Triggers are similar to migraine triggers and include fatigue, stress, missing a meal, travel, climate changes, and bright lights. Symptoms usually resolve with sleep but can be severe enough to warrant medication.

Finally, no discussion on migraines and dizziness is complete without a mention of basilar migraines. Basilar migraines present in older children and adolescents. Symptoms include vertigo, tinnitus, decreased hearing, headaches, ataxia, dysarthria, visual symptoms, diplopia, paresthesias, and decreased level of consciousness. It is felt to be secondary to decreased blood flow through the basilar artery and resulting ischemia of the occipital lobe and brainstem.

Ocular Abnormality

Vision problems should not be overlooked in children who complain of dizziness. In one study, 5% of children referred for vestibular testing had an ocular disorder.[6]

Posttraumatic Epilepsy/Epileptic Vertigo

Posttraumatic epilepsy presents in 5 to 7% of children after a closed-head injury. The central vestibular system is affected including the frontal, parietal, and temporal lobes. In particular, damage is most often seen in the superior temporal lobe, middle temporal gyrus, and supramarginal and angular gyrus. The resulting epileptic discharges often present as vertigo. Hearing is usually normal. In some instances, the seizure may stem from pursuit eye movements rather than presenting as vestibular dysfunction. An electroencephalography will be abnormal but may need to be completed in the sleep-deprived state. Finally, an ENG may show directional or labyrinthine preponderance.

Vertebrobasilar Insufficiency

Vertebrobasilar insufficiency (VBI) is the result of occlusion of a vertebral artery or of one of the posterior inferior cerebellar arteries or its branches. Lateral medullary infarction (also known as Wallenberg syndrome) or cerebellar infarction can result. Although less likely, VBI may also occur secondary to an arterial dissection. Patients complain of vertigo and headache on examination, they may be ataxic, dysarthric, and exhibit a nystagmus. Several types of nystagmus have been described including horizontal, horizonto-rotary, torsional, see-saw, and others. A lateral medullary infarct, in particular, is characterized by a horizontal nystagmus that beats away from the side of the lesion. Vestibular testing may show multiple abnormalities. On VEMP testing, one may see normal latencies but contralateral large amplitude. Dysmetria may be seen on saccade testing. Usually the patient overshoots to the side of the infarct and undershoots to the contralateral side. On smooth pursuit testing, mildly saccadic eye movements are noted and the child may fall on sensory organization tests 5 and 6 on posturography. The results of caloric testing when done are usually normal.

References

1. Phillips JO, Backous DD. Evaluation of vestibular function in young children. Otolaryngol Clin North Am 2002;35(4): 765–790

2. Nandi R, Luxon LM. Development and assessment of the vestibular system. Int J Audiol 2008;47(9):566–577

3. Saavedra S, Woollacott M, van Donkelaar P. Effects of postural support on eye hand interactions across development. Exp Brain Res 2007;180(3):557–567

4. Lee JB, Choi SJ, Park K, et al. Diagnostic efficiency of the cochlear hydrops analysis masking procedure in Ménière's disease. Otol Neurotol 2011;32(9):1486–1491

5. Black FO, Pesznecker SC. Vestibular ototoxity. Clinical considerations. Otolaryngol Clin North Am 1993;26(5):713–736

6. Anoh -Tanon MJ, Bremond-Gignac D, Wiener-Vacher SR. Vertigo is an underestimated symptom of ocular disorders: dizzy children do not always need MRI. Pediatr Neurol 2000;23(1):49–53

Bibliography

Bachor E, Wright CG, Karmody CS. The incidence and distribution of cupular deposits in the pediatric vestibular labyrinth. Laryngoscope 2002;112(1):147–151

Bovo R, Ciorba A, Martini A. The diagnosis of autoimmune inner ear disease: evidence and critical pitfalls. Eur Arch Otorhinolaryngol 2009; 266(1):37–40

Choung YH, Park K, Kim CH, Kim HJ, Kim K. Rare cases of Ménière's disease in children. J Laryngol Otol 2006;120(4):343–352

Cuvellier JC, Lépine A. Childhood periodic syndromes. Pediatr Neurol 2010;42(1):1–11

Eviatar L, Bergtraum M, Randel RM. Posttraumatic vertigo in children: a diagnostic approach. Pediatr Neurol 1986;2(2):61–66

Golz A, Netzer A, Angel-Yeger B, Westerman ST, Gilbert LM, Joachims HZ. Effects of middle ear effusion on the vestibular system in children. Otolaryngol Head Neck Surg 1998;119(6):695–699

Huygen PLM, Admiraal RJC. Audiovestibular sequelae of congenital cytomegalovirus infection in 3 children presumably representing 3 symptomatically different types of delayed endolymphatic hydrops. Int J Pediatr Otorhinolaryngol 1996;35(2):143–154

Kluge M, Beyenburg S, Fernández G, Elger CE. Epileptic vertigo: evidence for vestibular representation in human frontal cortex. Neurology 2000; 55(12):1906–1908

Korres S, Balatsouras DG, Zournas C, Economou C, Gatsonis SD, Adamopoulos G. Periodic alternating nystagmus associated with Arnold-Chiari malformation. J Laryngol Otol 2001;115(12):1001–1004

Liebenberg WA, Georges H, Demetriades AK, Hardwidge C. Does posterior fossa decompression improve oculomotor and vestibulo-ocular manifestations in Chiari 1 malformation? Acta Neurochir (Wien) 2005;147(12):1239–1240, discussion 1240

Lundy L, Zapala D, Olsholt K. Dorsolateral medullary infarction: a neurogenic cause of a contralateral, large-amplitude vestibular evoked myogenic potential. J Am Acad Audiol 2008;19(3):246– 256, quiz 275

Lyos AT, Marsh MA, Jenkins HA, Coker NJ. Progressive hearing loss after transverse temporal bone fracture. Arch Otolaryngol Head Neck Surg 1995;121(7):795–799

Maire R, Van Melle G. Horizontal vestibulo-ocular reflex dynamics in acute vestibular neuritis and viral labyrinthitis: evidence of otolith-canal interaction. Acta Otolaryngol 2004;124(1):36–40

Montfoort I, Van Der Geest JN, Slijper HP, De Zeeuw CI, Frens MA. Adaptation of the cervico- and vestibulo-ocular reflex in whiplash injury patients. J Neurotrauma 2008;25(6):687–693

Murofushi T, Halmagyi GM, Yavor RA, Colebatch JG. Absent vestibular evoked myogenic potentials in vestibular neurolabyrinthitis. An indicator of inferior vestibular nerve involvement? Arch Otolaryngol Head Neck Surg 1996;122(8):845–848

Murofushi T, Ushio M, Takai Y, Iwasaki S, Sugasawa K. Does acute dysfunction of the saccular afferents affect the subjective visual horizontal in patients with vestibular neurolabyrinthitis? Acta Otolaryngol Suppl 2007;127(559):61–64

Parnes LS, McCabe BF. Perilymph fistula: an important cause of deafness and dizziness in children. Pediatrics 1987;80(4):524–528

Sheykholeslami K, Schmerber S, Habiby Kermany M, Kaga K. Vestibular-evoked myogenic potentials in three patients with large vestibular aqueduct. Hear Res 2004;190(1-2):161–168

Silverboard G, Tart R. Cerebrovascular arterial dissection in children and young adults. Semin Pediatr Neurol 2000;7(4):289–300

Soliman AM. Immune-mediated inner ear disease. Am J Otol 1992;13(6): 575–579

Spiegel JH, Lalwani AK. Large vestibular aqueduct syndrome and endolymphatic hydrops: two presentations of a common primary inner-ear dysfunction? J Laryngol Otol 2009;123(8):919–921

Versino M, Sances G, Anghileri E, et al. Dizziness and migraine: a causal relationship? Funct Neurol 2003;18(2):97–101

Vibert D, Häusler R. Acute peripheral vestibular deficits after whiplash injuries. Ann Otol Rhinol Laryngol 2003;112(3):246–251

Zhou G, Gopen Q. Characteristics of vestibular evoked myogenic potentials in children with enlarged vestibular aqueduct. Laryngoscope 2011; 121(1):220–225

4 Cochlear Implants

Greg R. Licameli and Frank W. Virgin

Permanent sensorineural hearing loss (SNHL) in the moderate-to-severe range is reported to occur in approximately 1 to 3 of every 1000 children born in the United States and other developed countries.[1] Hearing loss that is presumed to be late in onset and at least moderate in severity is diagnosed in 1.2 to 3.3 per 10,000 school-aged children.[2] Approximately 50% of congenital hearing loss is associated with environmental factors such as infection, prematurity, or other perinatal insults. Genetic factors account for the other 50%, of which 15% are associated with syndromes and 35% are nonsyndromic with autosomal inheritance being the most common form.

The cost to society of severe-to-profound hearing loss is significant. These costs include the negative effects in productivity as well as direct costs such as education and spending to provide equal access to services. It is estimated that approximately 42% of individuals with severe-to-profound hearing loss between the ages of 18 and 44 years are unemployed compared with 18% of the general population.[3] Despite substantial expenditures in the education of severe-to-profoundly deaf children, 44% fail to graduate from high school as compared with 19% of normal-hearing population. Only 5% of severe-to-profoundly deaf children graduate from college as compared with 13% of the normal-hearing population. Much work has been done to evaluate the cost-effectiveness of cochlear implantation. Overall, including indirect costs such as reduced educational spending, cochlear implants provide a savings exceeding US$ 50,000 per child.[4,5]

Cochlear implants were first approved for use in adults in the United States by the Food and Drug Administration in 1984 and for children 2 years of age or older in 1990. Subsequently, the age was lowered to 1 year in 2002. With the benefits of cochlear implantation becoming established and experience gained in patient selection, device development, and programming, cochlear implantation is become an increasingly common method of treating children with profound SNHL.

Technology of Cochlear Implants

These devices function primarily by stimulating surviving neural elements within the inner ear and provide auditory stimulation that aids in the development and/or maintenance of the spoken language. There are several manufacturers of cochlear implants and each device has subtle differences, the details of which are beyond the scope of this chapter. The most commonly implanted systems include the cochlear implants systems manufactured by Cochlear Corporation, Advanced Bionics, and Medical Electronic (Med-El). Each of the devices currently available has several essential components. An external microphone picks up pressure differences in a sound field and converts it to electrical signals. An externally worn processor then processes the signal according to a predefined strategy and then transmits stimuli to the electrode array which is surgically implanted in the scala tympani of the cochlea.

Signal Processing

The speech-coding strategy of an implant defines the method by which pitch, loudness, and timing of sound are translated into a series of electrical pulses. Each implant in the market today is capable of using a variety of algorithms but in general there are two major coding strategies. The first is called "simultaneous strategy" in which a device is capable of simultaneous stimulation. The second coding strategy is "continuous interleaved sampling," which stimulates each electrode serially, with no stimulation out of order. Signal processing strategies such as feature extraction, spectral peak, and above combination encoder are included in this category. Programming of cochlear implants is an area of ongoing research and is largely responsible for the gains made in obtaining successful outcomes in implant patients.

Candidate Assessment

Identification of appropriate cochlear implant candidates is critical to the overall success of implantation. In countries with universal newborn screening, the early identification of hearing loss has produced a significant increase in the number of implant candidates, making selection criteria increasingly more important. Papsin and Gordon reported that a child's duration of deafness; age at receipt of cochlear implantation; educational setting; form of communication; cognitive, motor, and social development; speech language development; family structure and support; intelligence; and socioeconomic status all play a critical role in the outcome for each implant recipient.[1] Use of a preimplant questionnaire can be useful in the evaluation of a patient's candidacy and in predicting communication outcomes.[6]

Children undergoing evaluation for cochlear implantation fall into several broad categories of patients. The most common are children with prelingual deafness, usually congenitally acquired. A second group is of children with hearing loss, who have developed spoken language with the use of hearing aids, but have undergone deterioration of hearing over time to a point where hearing aids are no longer beneficial. Children with auditory neuropathy spectrum disorders make up the third category. The fourth category includes children with significant medical or developmental disorders in whom a lack of hearing may not be their greatest challenge. The final group of children is of those who are deaf and primarily use other nonverbal methods to communicate. Each of these groups presents its own set of challenges and highlights the need for a comprehensive team approach for implant selection.

Audiologic Evaluation

Audiologic evaluation will consist of auditory brainstem response (ABR), otoacoustic emissions, and verification of hearing aid fitting. It is of benefit for the audiologist who will perform preoperative behavioral audiologic examination after surgery to become familiar with a child's response style. In addition to standard audiologic testing, there are other testing criteria for children based on their individual language achievement. Children who have not developed word-recognition ability can meet the audiologic criteria by showing a lack of progress or developmental lag on a scale such as the Infant-Toddler Meaningful Auditory Integration Scale or the Meaningful Auditory Integration Scale.[7] Young children may meet the criteria with best-aided, word-recognition ability no greater than 20% for the Advanced Bionics and Med-El devices and no greater than 30% for the Cochlear Corporation device using the Multisyllabic Lexical Neighborhood Test or the Lexical Neighborhood Test.[8] Older children who are able to repeat sentences completely, but have had progressive hearing loss can meet the criteria by using the adult criteria, which is no more than 60% best-aided word score on a sentence recognition test such as the Hearing in Noise Test.[9] In the future there will be continued evolution of the audiologic evaluation and criteria for cochlear implantation.

Age of Implantation

There is clear evidence that implanting children early in life is advantageous.[10] Language development begins at birth and develops rapidly during the early childhood years. Speech, vocabulary, and language skills are enhanced by early auditory stimulation. In 2001, Kileny et al published data which demonstrated that children who were implanted between the ages of 12 and 36 months outperformed children implanted between the ages of 37 and 60 months.[11] With the exception of patients with postmeningitic hearing loss where there is concern for cochlear ossification if surgery is delayed, implantation in the less than 12-month population is not universally performed.

Special Populations

Auditory neuropathy is a form of hearing impairment that is characterized by moderate-to-profound SNHL in which the function of the outer hair cells is preserved, but afferent neural activity in the cochlear nerve and central auditory pathways is disordered.[12] These patients warrant a thorough evaluation including electrocochleography, ABR, and magnetic resonance imaging (MRI) in an attempt to identify the underlying pathological condition.[13]

Developmental disability coexists with hearing loss in 30 to 40% of cases.[14] Cochlear implant centers see these children for evaluation in increasing numbers. This population of patients epitomizes the need for a comprehensive evaluation with a multidisciplinary team approach. Additionally, it is important to give realistic expectations of success to family and caregivers.

Medical Evaluation

The medical evaluation should include a determination of the patient's ability to undergo a surgical procedure as well as radiologic evaluation to determine anatomical abnormalities that may preclude implantation or result in variation of normal surgical technique. Traditionally, high resolution computed tomography (HRCT) has been used for radiologic examination of patients being evaluated for cochlear implantation. However, recent investigations have assessed the usefulness of MRI in conjunction with HRCT or alone. HRCT provides a superior evaluation of the boney anatomy whereas MRI can provide improved evaluation of soft tissues including evaluation of the cochlear nerve and membranous portion of the cochlea. Currently, HRCT is the imaging modality of choice in all age groups, including children, to identify cochlear dysplasia, labyrinthine ossification, and other temporal bone anomalies associated with congenital hearing loss, which might contribute to intraoperative complications (**Fig. 4.1**).[15–17] Although MRI has the advantage of providing improved resolution of soft tissue structures, it has the disadvantage of higher cost and longer image acquisition times requiring general anesthesia in the pediatric population. However, it has been clearly shown that HRCT is not capable of demonstrating early cochlear obliteration nor is it capable of detecting cochlear nerve aplasia (**Fig. 4.2**).[16] In 2007, Trimble et al assessed the usefulness of HRCT and MRI in the evaluation of cochlear implant candidates. The results of their work proposed a model that would use either imaging modality based on a patient's history. These authors concluded that selective use of each imaging modality would not miss any findings relevant to implantation and would result in cost improvements.[18] Currently, the majority of centers use HRCT on all patients and MRI in the setting of postmeningitic hearing loss and in cases where there is concern for cochlear nerve aplasia.[19]

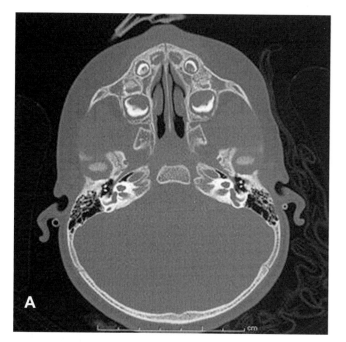
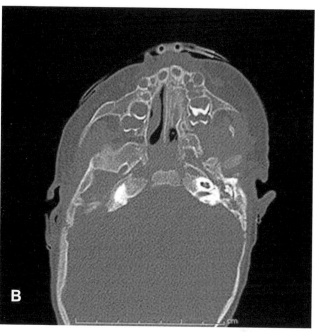

Figure 4.1 Examples of abnormalities that can be identified on a computed tomography scan. (A) Bilateral dysmorphic cochlea with absent modiolus, small and narrow basal turn and complete absence of separation of the middle and apical turns as well as stenosis of the cochlear aperture. (B) Severe stenosis of the cochlear aperture raising the question of cochlear nerve aplasia.

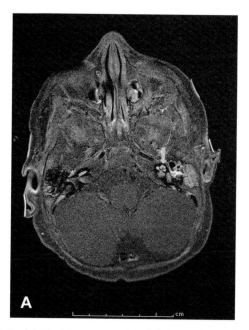
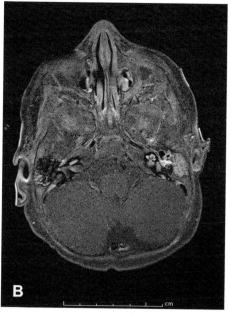

Figure 4.2 (A) T1-, fat-suppressed, gadolinium-enhanced magnetic resonance image demonstrating cochlear enhancement (arrow) in an infant with bacterial meningitis. (B) Computed tomography scan was normal in appearance.

Surgical Technique

The patient is placed under general anesthesia and is positioned with the operative ear up. Preoperative antibiotics are given based on institutional guidelines. Skin incisions for cochlear implants have evolved and vary widely. In our institution, a lazy-S incision is used and infiltrated with 0.5% lidocaine with 1:200,000 epinephrine to aid in hemostasis.

The incision is planned so that it is no less than 1 cm from the edge of the implant at any given site. An anteriorly based periosteal flap is elevated to expose the mastoid and skull. A subperiosteal pocket is made to house both the device and ground electrode depending on the device to be implanted. Mastoidectomy is performed and the facial recess is identified and opened. It is essential to obtain a view of the stapes to provide perspective used in accurately identifying the round window niche. The superior portion of the round window niche is frequently drilled away to provide a clear view of the round window membrane.

Once the round window is identified, a well is developed to house the device and provide a channel for the electrode to travel to the mastoid. The well is carefully developed and in young children it is often necessary to expose dura to facilitate a good implant fit. It is important to ensure that there are no sharp edges and that the electrode can pass freely from the stimulator/receiver into the mastoid. Cochleostomy is generally performed in the anterior inferior portion of the round window to provide direct exposure of the scala tympani for electrode insertion. The size of the cochleostomy ranges from 1 to greater than 2 mm depending on the type of implant being inserted. Care is taken to keep the cochlea clear of blood and to avoid trauma to the basilar membrane from aggressive suctioning.

The implant is then brought into the field and placed in the well. The device may or may not be secured with sutures or mesh to the skull, depending on the surgeon's preference. The electrode is inserted into the scala tympani to the full extent atraumatically and in accordance with the manufacturer's specifications. Once the electrode is inserted, the extra length is coiled into the attic and attempts are made to keep the electrode out of the mastoid tip to avoid the theoretical risk of electrode migration as the patient grows and the mastoid tip enlarges. The periosteum is then closed over the electrode and implant, and the skin is closed ideally with offset suture lines. In our institution the integrity of the implant is tested intraoperatively by a member of the audiological team. Additionally, an anterior–posterior film of the skull may be taken to confirm placement before awaking the patient from anesthesia.

Outcomes

Cochlear implantation has become an established intervention in children with severe-to-profound SNHL. Clear benefit has been established and great strides have been made in predicting which candidates will succeed with cochlear implantation. The primary goal in cochlear implantation is the development of spoken language, however, children vary greatly in their performance. In general, the most successful patients are those with congenital hearing loss that are cognitively normal, who are implanted early, and are in an environment with motivated families, educators, and an environment rich in oral communication.

Multiple factors seem to influence the outcomes in cochlear implant recipients. Shorter duration of deafness before cochlear implantation has been demonstrated to be a positive predictor of better outcome.[20] Additionally, an implant recipient's method of communication and educational environment also influence outcome. When compared with patients who use total communication (oral and sign language), those who use oral communication only achieved higher in speech perception, speech intelligibility, verbal rehearsal skills, and literacy.[21] Children with cognitive

delay have been shown to demonstrate some forms of measurable postimplant gains in speech perception and word or sentence recognition, but these gains are slower than in typically developing children.[22] Although auditory gains in the medically complex patient may be slower, spoken language as a primary mode of communication may be attainable in some patients and even if spoken language does not develop, speech production is not the only indication of benefit from cochlear implantation.[6]

Many children with cochlear implants achieve open-set speech recognition within the first year of implantation.[23] In one long-term study, 67% of patients developed intelligible speech, 78% attended mainstream school, and 79% were able to use the telephone. On average, recipients had 72% open-set word recognition in quiet and 45% in noise. Implanted children have also demonstrated increased difficulty with receptive language when compared with their normal hearing peers with 75% scoring below the mean. These differences have been shown to persist into adolescence.[24,25]

There is growing group of patients who have received bilateral cochlear implants, either simultaneously or sequentially placed. Bilateral implant users have the advantage of spatial separation between target and competing speech.[26–28] Additionally, it has been shown that bilaterally implanted children also demonstrate a significant increase in speech discrimination when compared with the best-performing unilateral implant.[29,30]

There have been significant advancements in cochlear implantation since the first devices were designed. In a recent study that evaluated the Advanced Bionics cochlear implant systems, one group of patients used the Clarion 1.2 system and the other group used the newer CII/HiRes 90K system. When the two groups were compared it was clearly demonstrated that the children who used the newer system developed better speech perception skills.[31] Over the past two decades there have been advances in cochlear implant devices as well as processing and rehabilitation strategies. Currently, the first groups of children implanted are entering adulthood. Although clear benefits of cochlear implantation have been established, it is still to be determined how these effects translate into adulthood. It is anticipated that as device processing strategies and rehabilitation improves, outcomes for children receiving cochlear implants will continue to improve.

Future Directions

Cochlear implant programs have significantly evolved over the past 20 years and great strides have been made in the identification and rehabilitation of this unique group of patients. Significant socioeconomic gains have been demonstrated in the implanted patient, which has led to greater utilization of this technology over time. As the implant field moves forward, advances in candidate selection, rehabilitation, device production, programming strategies, and surgical technique will continue to provide robust areas of research and innovation.

References

1. Papsin BC, Gordon KA. Cochlear implants for children with severe-to-profound hearing loss. N Engl J Med 2007;357(23):2380–2387

2. Smith RJ, Bale JF Jr, White KR. Sensorineural hearing loss in children. Lancet 2005;365(9462):879–890

3. Mohr PE, Feldman JJ, Dunbar JL. The societal costs of severe to profound hearing loss in the United States. Policy Anal Brief H Ser 2000;2(1):1–4

4. Cheng AK, Rubin HR, Powe NR, Mellon NK, Francis HW, Niparko JK. Cost-utility analysis of the cochlear implant in children. JAMA 2000;284(7):850–856

5. Palmer CS, Niparko JK, Wyatt JR, Rothman M, de Lissovoy G. A prospective study of the cost-utility of the multichannel cochlear implant. Arch Otolaryngol Head Neck Surg 1999;125(11):1221–1228

6. O'Brien LC, Kenna M, Neault M, et al. Not a "sound" decision: is cochlear implantation always the best choice? Int J Pediatr Otorhinolaryngol 2010;74(10):1144–1148

7. Robbins AM, Renshaw JJ, Berry SW. Evaluating meaningful auditory integration in profoundly hearing-impaired children. Am J Otol 1991;12(Suppl):144–150

8. Kirk KI, Pisoni DB, Sommers MS, Young M, Evanson C. New directions for assessing speech perception in persons with sensory aids. Ann Otol Rhinol Laryngol Suppl 1995;166:300–303

9. Dowell RC, Hollow R, Winton E. Outcomes for cochlear implant users with significant residual hearing: implications for selection criteria in children. Arch Otolaryngol Head Neck Surg 2004;130(5):575–581

10. Arts HA, Garber A, Zwolan TA. Cochlear implants in young children. Otolaryngol Clin North Am 2002;35(4):925–943

11. Kileny PR, Zwolan TA, Ashbaugh C. The influence of age at implantation on performance with a cochlear implant in children. Otol Neurotol 2001;22(1):42–46

12. Starr A, Picton TW, Sininger Y, Hood LJ, Berlin CI. Auditory neuropathy. Brain 1996;119(Pt 3):741–753

13. Gibson WP, Graham JM. Editorial: 'auditory neuropathy' and cochlear implantation - myths and facts. Cochlear Implants Int 2008;9(1):1–7

14. Meinzen-Derr J, Wiley S, Grether S, Choo DI. Language performance in children with cochlear implants and additional disabilities. Laryngoscope 2010;120(2):405–413

15. Arriaga MA, Carrier D. MRI and clinical decisions in cochlear implantation. Am J Otol 1996;17(4):547–553

16. Nikolopoulos TP, O'Donoghue GM, Robinson KL, Holland IM, Ludman C, Gibbin KP. Preoperative radiologic evaluation in cochlear implantation. Am J Otol 1997;18(6, Suppl)S73–S74

17. Woolley AL, Oser AB, Lusk RP, Bahadori RS. Preoperative temporal bone computed tomography scan and its use in evaluating the pediatric cochlear implant candidate. Laryngoscope 1997;107(8):1100–1106

18. Trimble K, Blaser S, James AL, Papsin BC. Computed tomography and/or magnetic resonance imaging before pediatric cochlear implantation? Developing an investigative strategy. Otol Neurotol 2007;28(3):317–324

19. Licameli G, Kenna MA. Is computed tomography (CT) or magnetic resonance imaging (MRI) more useful in the evaluation of pediatric sensorineural hearing loss? Laryngoscope 2010;120(12):2358–2359

20. Geers AE, Sedey AL. Language and verbal reasoning skills in adolescents with 10 or more years of cochlear implant experience. Ear Hear 2011;32(1, Suppl)39S–48S

21. Geers AE, Strube MJ, Tobey EA, Pisoni DB, Moog JS. Epilogue: factors contributing to long-term outcomes of cochlear implantation in early childhood. Ear Hear 2011;32(1, Suppl)84S–92S

22. Edwards LC. Children with cochlear implants and complex needs: a review of outcome research and psychological practice. J Deaf Stud Deaf Educ 2007;12(3):258–268

23. Yoon PJ. Pediatric cochlear implantation. Curr Opin Pediatr 2011;23(3):346–350

24. Beadle EA, McKinley DJ, Nikolopoulos TP, Brough J, O'Donoghue GM, Archbold SM. Long-term functional outcomes and academic-occupational status in implanted children after 10 to 14 years of cochlear implant use. Otol Neurotol 2005;26(6):1152–1160

25. Uziel AS, Sillon M, Vieu A, et al. Ten-year follow-up of a consecutive series of children with multichannel cochlear implants. Otol Neurotol 2007;28(5):615–628

26. Gantz BJ, Tyler RS, Rubinstein JT, et al. Binaural cochlear implants placed during the same operation. Otol Neurotol 2002;23(2):169–180

27. Litovsky R, Parkinson A, Arcaroli J, Sammeth C. Simultaneous bilateral cochlear implantation in adults: a multicenter clinical study. Ear Hear 2006;27(6):714–731

28. Müller J, Schön F, Helms J. Speech understanding in quiet and noise in bilateral users of the MED-EL COMBI 40/40+ cochlear implant system. Ear Hear 2002;23(3):198–206

29. Kühn-Inacker H, Shehata-Dieler W, Müller J, Helms J. Bilateral cochlear implants: a way to optimize auditory perception abilities in deaf children? Int J Pediatr Otorhinolaryngol 2004;68(10):1257–1266

30. Peters BR, Litovsky R, Parkinson A, Lake J. Importance of age and postimplantation experience on speech perception measures in children with sequential bilateral cochlear implants. Otol Neurotol 2007;28(5):649–657

31. Bosco E, D'Agosta L, Mancini P, Traisci G, D'Elia C, Filipo R. Speech perception results in children implanted with Clarion devices: Hi-Resolution and Standard Resolution modes. Acta Otolaryngol 2005;125(2):148–158

5 Facial Nerve Paralysis in Children

Myriam Loyo, Margaret L. Skinner, and David E. Tunkel

Paralysis of the facial nerve, cranial nerve VII (CN VII), can cause dramatic changes in the appearance with obvious concern to the affected child and parents. In addition to the significant functional, social, and psychological impact, severe or persistent facial palsy can lead to deformity, loss of oral competency, and visual impairment due to impaired corneal protection.

Facial nerve paralysis is uncommon in children. The estimated annual incidence in the entire population is 15 to 40 per 100,000.[1] Children are two to four times less likely than adults to be affected by facial paralysis. While the most common cause of adult-onset facial nerve paralysis is idiopathic facial paralysis (Bell palsy), facial paralysis in children is more likely a result of infections, inflammation, or trauma.[2,3] Early recognition and treatment are particularly important in the pediatric population. We provide a review of the relevant anatomy, clinical presentations, etiologies, diagnostic studies, and treatments for facial nerve paralysis in children.

Anatomy and Function

In addition to providing motor innervation to the facial muscles of expression, the facial nerve also serves other important functions such as salivation, lacrimation, and taste. A discussion of the anatomical course of the facial nerve and functions of the components of this nerve, from brainstem through the temporal bone and into the face allows understanding of the localization of different injuries and prediction of expected deficits.[4]

The facial nerve carries three distinct types of fibers: (1) efferent motor fibers from the motor nuclei that provide facial expression; (2) efferent secretory fibers from the superior salivary nucleus that provide preganglionic parasympathetic innervation to the lacrimal, sublingual, and submandibular glands; and (3) afferent fibers that provide both specialized taste sensation from the anterior two-thirds of the tongue and sensation of the external auditory canal. It is important to mention that the motor fibers that innervate the forehead receive bilateral cortical input while the lower facial expression muscles receive only contralateral innervation. This feature helps differentiate central from peripheral lesions.

The facial nerve emerges from the caudal border of the pons at the cerebellopontine angle (CPA) and enters the internal auditory canal (IAC). The facial nerve and the vestibulocochlear nerve, CN VIII, travel in proximity to each other within the temporal bone. The sensory fibers of CN VII travel between the motor component of CN VII and CN VIII; these fibers are known as nervus intermedius. Leaving the IAC, the facial nerve has labyrinthine, tympanic, and mastoid segments. This intratemporal course is encased in a bony canal that makes the nerve susceptible to compression. The labyrinthine segment is the narrowest segment and the most susceptible to compression by edema. It is at the level of the labyrinthine segment that the greater superficial petrosal nerve, carrying the preganglionic parasympathetic innervation to the lacrimal gland, arises. Congenital dehiscence of the facial canal is common in the tympanic segment—an area susceptible to injury from middle-ear infection, cholesteatoma, or even surgical trauma.

The mastoid portion of the facial nerve contains the origins of the nerve to the stapedius muscle as well as the chorda tympani. The chorda tympani supplies afferent taste to the anterior two-thirds of the tongue as well as parasympathetic innervation of the submandibular and sublingual glands. The facial nerve exits the temporal bone via the stylomastoid foramen and courses through the parotid gland to supply the muscles of facial expression. Within the parotid gland, the nerve lies between the deep and superficial lobes. The nerve usually branches at the pes anserinus into the superior temporal facial branch and inferior cervicofacial branch, which subsequently branch into the temporal or frontal, zygomatic, buccal, marginal mandibular, and cervical branches (**Fig. 5.1**).

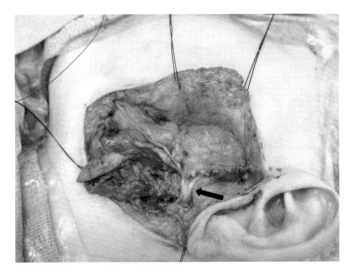

Figure 5.1 Dissection of the left intraparotid facial nerve in a child who has a first branchial cleft sinus running from the cartilaginous ear canal to the upper neck, directly beneath the main trunk and pes anserinus. Arrow points to the main trunk.

Table 5.1   The House-Brackmann Facial Nerve Scale

Grade	Description	Characteristics
I	Normal	Normal facial function in all areas
II	Mild dysfunction	Gross: slight weakness noticeable on close inspection; may have very slight synkinesis At rest: normal symmetry and tone Motion: forehead—moderate to good function; eye—complete closure with minimum effort; and mouth—slight asymmetry
III	Moderate dysfunction	Gross: obvious but not disfiguring difference between two sides; noticeable but not severe synkinesis, contracture, or hemifacial spasm At rest: normal symmetry and tone Motion: forehead—slight to moderate movement; eye—complete closure with effort; and mouth—slightly weak with maximum effort
IV	Moderately severe dysfunction	Gross: obvious weakness and/or disfiguring asymmetry At rest: normal symmetry and tone Motion: forehead—none; eye—incomplete closure; and mouth: asymmetric with maximum effort
V	Severe dysfunction	Gross: only barely perceptible motion At rest: asymmetry Motion: forehead: none; eye: incomplete closure; and mouth: slight movement
VI	Total paralysis	No movement

Assessment of Facial Nerve Dysfunction

The assessment of facial nerve function in children may require careful observation during rest as well as during crying, if the child is too young to follow commands to move portions of the face. The House-Brackmann scale is the most widely used system to grade facial nerve function. The scale ranges from normal function (Grade I) to complete paralysis (Grade VI).[5] Examining for full-eye closure is critical as incomplete eye closure can lead to eye dryness, corneal abrasion, and vision loss. Failure to achieve full-eye closure differentiates Grades III and IV of facial nerve dysfunction on the House-Brackmann scale (**Table 5.1**). Facial photography has been recommended to objectively document the degree of facial nerve dysfunction.

Assessments of lacrimal function, the stapedius reflex, taste deficits, and salivary flow have been used to predict the site of facial nerve lesions, but these tests are of limited value in children. Imaging studies and electrodiagnostic tests are more commonly used to investigate facial nerve dysfunction when the etiology is not clear.

Etiology of Facial Nerve Paralysis

Idiopathic paralysis (Bell palsy) has long been regarded as the most common cause of facial paralysis in adults and children, with up to half of the cases diagnosed as Bell palsy.[6,7] Recent investigations have been more fruitful in identifying specific causes of facial paralysis in children. A retrospective study over an 8-year period at Children's National Medical Center in Washington, DC, found a specific etiology for 84% of children with facial paralysis, with the leading causes being infections (28%) and trauma (24%).[3] A review from the Boston Children's Hospital published in 2005 found an identifiable cause of facial paralysis in 86% of children, with infections (36%) and trauma (19%) again being most common etiologies.[2]

Infectious Causes of Facial Paralysis in Children

The infections that cause facial paralysis in children are most commonly acute otitis media (AOM), followed by Lyme disease and varicella zoster infection.[6,8] These infectious causes are often identified by a thorough clinical and otologic evaluation. More unusual infectious causes of facial paralysis in children include tuberculosis, Mycobacterium avium-intracellulare, and viral infections that include mumps, rubella, cytomegalovirus, coxsackievirus, and herpes simplex virus (HSV). Some of these infections may present with isolated facial paralysis, while others may present as disseminated disease with multiple neurologic deficits. Additionally, immunologic responses associated with known or presumed infectious agents can cause facial paralysis as cranial-specific or generalized neuropathies. Some examples include Guillain-Barré syndrome, Kawasaki disease, human immunodeficiency virus infection, and sarcoidosis.

Otitis Media

AOM is common in children, but the likelihood of facial paralysis arising from AOM is low. The Early Childhood

Longitudinal Study, Birth Cohort, which constituted a national prospective study in the United States and followed 8000 children born in 2001 for 2 years, determined that 62% of the children were diagnosed with AOM by 2 years of age.[9] Facial paralysis occurred as a complication of otitis media in only 0.2% of the cases.[10] The mechanism for facial nerve paralysis involves inflammatory spread from middle ear into the facial nerve canal through vascular pathways and bony dehiscences, with edema and compression of the nerve. The pathogens causing AOM complicated by facial paralysis are similar to those in noncomplicated cases: *Haemophilus influenzae, Streptococcus pneumoniae, Moraxella catarrhalis,* and *Staphylococcus* species.[11] The treatment of AOM with facial paralysis includes oral or parenteral antibiotics. Myringotomy, with or without ventilation tube insertion, may be indicated as well, for drainage of the middle ear space and culture of the infected material. Facial paralysis from AOM is not usually treated with mastoidectomy with or without facial nerve decompression. Such surgery is reserved for patients who do not improve with antibiotics and middle-ear drainage. The prognosis for recovery of facial nerve paralysis associated with AOM appears to be favorable. In one retrospective study of 40 patients with facial nerve paralysis and AOM, 85% of the patients had facial nerve recovery to House-Brackmann Grade I and the remaining 15% to Grade II functions.[11]

Facial paralysis can also be caused by chronic otitis media. In chronic otitis media, with or without associated cholesteatoma, direct inflammatory involvement or compression/invasion of the facial nerve is more likely than in cases of AOM (**Fig. 5.2**). More aggressive and earlier surgical intervention with mastoidectomy with possible facial nerve decompression may be needed. Chronic otitis media and/or cholesteatoma should be suspected and ruled out for any child with facial paralysis, particularly those who have a history of ear infections, hearing loss, or otorrhea. Medical therapy should include coverage for gram-negative organisms, including *Pseudomonas aeruginosa, Proteus* species, *Klebsiella* species, and *Escherichia coli,* and anaerobes such as *Bacteroides, Peptococcus,* and *Peptostreptococcus* that are more common in chronic ear disease.[12]

Lyme Disease

Lyme disease, an infection with the spirochete *Borrelia burgdorferi,* is the most common cause of facial paralysis in children in areas endemic for this infection.[8,13] Northern Hemisphere regions with temperate weather are endemic for Lyme disease. While Lyme disease has been reported in every state of the United States, it is most prevalent in the New England and Mid-Atlantic regions. In Europe, the disease is common in central countries such as Austria and Slovenia. The disease vector in the United States is the *Ixodes scapularis,* commonly known as deer tick. In the United States, most cases occur from late spring through early fall, the period of peak exposure to ticks. Facial paralysis is the most common

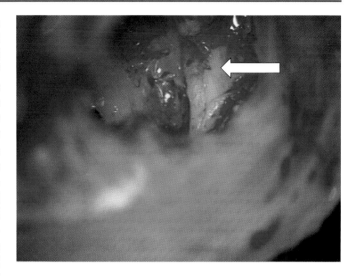

Figure 5.2   Facial nerve dehiscence in the left middle ear, with erosion of the bony fallopian canal just superior to the oval window. This 6-year-old child had cholesteatoma that eroded the stapes suprastructure as well as the fallopian canal, but did not have clinical evidence of facial nerve weakness. Arrow points to the tympanic facial nerve.

cranial neuropathy associated with Lyme disease, and it can occur on one or both sides. In some patients, facial paralysis may be the only sign of Lyme disease, and progression to more diffuse or chronic central nervous system (CNS) disease can occur without treatment.[13] Facial paralysis usually arises in the ipsilateral side of the bite, suggesting direct involvement by the spirochete. Approximately 50% of the patients will fail to demonstrate the dermatological lesions, requiring a high index of suspicion in endemic regions.[14] The neurologic stage can present as early as within the first days of the disease. Other neurologic symptoms range from painful radiculitis to diffuse meningitis and/or encephalitis. Cardiac conduction defect may occur during this stage. Marked arthritic and chronic CNS involvement characterize the final, more advanced stage.

The Centers for Disease Control and Prevention recommends a two-step approach to Lyme diagnosis with initial enzyme-linked immunosorbent assay followed by Western blot. Patients with Lyme disease and facial paralysis often undergo lumbar puncture with examination of cerebrospinal fluid (CSF). CSF pleocytosis and elevated protein levels can be seen, and testing of CSF should be performed for specific antibodies and polymerase chain reaction (PCR) analysis for DNA from *B. burgdorferi.* Treatment for Lyme-associated facial paralysis includes antibiotic treatment against *B. burgdoferi,* usually for 10 to 20 days. The recommended regimen for children older than 8 years of age is doxycycline 100 mg twice a day, while children under 8 years of age are usually treated with amoxicillin 50 to 60 mg/kg/d. Parenteral ceftriaxone is used for disseminated infection.[8] Some authors advocate the use of parenteral antibiotics for all cases of Lyme-associated facial paralysis. In general, the prognosis for facial nerve recovery is good, with recovery rates higher than 90% and mean duration of paralysis of 5 weeks.[14]

Ramsay Hunt Syndrome

Reactivation of dormant varicella zoster virus (VZV) can cause Ramsay Hunt syndrome (RHS) with facial paralysis. After primary infection, the VZV lies dormant in sensory ganglia such as the geniculate ganglia. Reactivation leads to facial paralysis and vestibulocochlear dysfunction as well as to a painful herpetic vesicular eruption within the external auditory canal known as herpes zoster oticus. In a retrospective study of children with facial paralysis, Hato et al found RHS in 16% of children.[15] These authors found less severe symptoms of RHS as well as better prognosis in children when compared with adults—25% of children had hearing loss and 17% had vestibular hypofunction, whereas 52% of adults had hearing loss and 31% had vestibular hypofunction. Complete recovery of hearing was seen in 66% of affected children.

RHS tends to affect children older than 6 years of age who have had chickenpox in the past. Maximal facial weakness usually occurs within 1 week of onset of symptoms. Facial paralysis may precede development of any skin lesion in up to 50% of children.[15] History and physical examination remain the key for diagnosis of RHS. Laboratory testing for VZV from swabs of the skin lesions is available, using direct fluorescent antigen assays and PCR.[16] Current recommendations for treatment of RHS include use of both steroids and antiviral agents. A large review of RHS evaluated 80 patients, all older than 15 years of age, and showed statistically significant improved outcomes in those patients treated with prednisone and acyclovir within 3 days of onset of facial paralysis.[17] The recovery from RHS is usually favorable, although perhaps not as encouraging as following idiopathic facial paralysis. Approximately 80% of patients will have complete recovery.[18] In March 1995, the U.S. Food and Drug Administration approved the Oka varicella vaccine for routine administration in the pediatric age group of 19 to 35 months. Although the incidence and epidemiology of RHS might change following the widespread use of the varicella vaccine, RHS has been reported in immunized children.

Trauma and Facial Paralysis

Trauma is the second most common cause of facial paralysis in children. Fortunately, birth trauma-related facial paralysis usually resolves if the birth trauma is not severe. Blunt head trauma can result in facial paralysis from swelling or disruption of CN VII within the temporal bone. Penetrating trauma to the head and face can damage the facial nerve and its branches near the ear and in the face. Iatrogenic injuries to the facial nerve can occur in tympanomastoidectomy, parotid gland surgery, and intracranial surgery. While all intratemporal portions of the facial nerve are at risk during ear surgery, the tympanic segment is particularly at risk

when dissecting inflamed tissues or cholesteatoma in the middle ear. While facial paralysis of varying extents is not uncommon after parotidectomy, recovery is expected unless CN VII or one of the branches was transected.

Birth Trauma

The incidence of facial paralysis as a result of birth trauma has decreased due to a decline in the use of delivery forceps. The reported incidence in the 1980s was as high as 1.8%, whereas the incidence has been as low as 0.003% in the 1990s.[18] Although the use of obstetric forceps continues to be a risk factor for facial paralysis, most cases occur in vaginal deliveries without instrumentation. Intrauterine trauma may occur as a result of pressure of the infant's face on the sacral promontory of the ischial spine resulting in nerve injury. Neonatal facial paralysis from intracranial hemorrhage has also been described.

The distinction between acquired and developmental causes of congenital facial paralysis is important because acquired facial paralysis carries an excellent prognosis and developmental paralysis is usually permanent. Obstetric-related risk factors are prolonged labor, primiparity, newborn's weight greater than 3500 g, and use of obstetric instrumentation.[18,19] The face should be carefully inspected for signs of trauma including the presence of facial bruises. Nearly 90% of the infants exhibit complete recovery of facial nerve function, usually before 4 months of age.[18]

Temporal Bone Trauma

Temporal bone fractures are the most common traumatic base of skull fracture and occur in 4 to 16% of cases of blunt trauma to the head in children.[20] Temporal bone fractures present with hemotympanum or blood in the external auditory canal. More than half of the children will have other intracranial injuries. Temporal bone fractures may cause facial paralysis, hearing loss (conductive, sensorineural, or mixed), dysequilibrium, and/or CSF otorrhea or rhinorrhea. Facial nerve paralysis appears to be more common in adults with temporal bone fractures than in children. Facial weakness has been described in 38% of these fractures in adults compared with only 7% in children with these fractures.[20]

Facial nerve paralysis can occur immediately at the time of trauma, or may develop later. Incomplete and delayed paralyses usually recover, with observation and/or steroid treatment. Complete and immediate facial paralyses may benefit from surgical exploration for reanastomosis of a transected nerve or decompression of the nerve. Darrouzet et al conducted a retrospective study on 115 cases of facial paralysis from temporal bone trauma in children and adults identifying complete transection and a nerve gap in 14% of cases.[21] Identification of those patients who may benefit from surgery remains problematic. In addition to facial paralysis, temporal bone fracture can cause hearing loss and CSF leaks. Hearing loss has been reported in 16 to 81% of temporal bone fractures; this wide variation probably reflecting the difficulties of hearing evaluation in the acute setting. Most series report complete resolution of hearing loss in 60 to 80% of patients with temporal bone fractures.[20] Persistent conductive hearing loss may be an indication for middle-ear exploration to identify and repair abnormalities such as incudostapedial dislocation or stapes fracture. Persistent sensorineural hearing loss has also been described in a minority of patients.[2] CSF otorrhea is rare and seen in approximately 7% of patients; it usually resolves without operative interventions.

Congenital/Developmental and Syndromic Facial Palsies

Congenital/developmental facial nerve paralysis may occur from agenesis of the nerve or motor nuclei, or agenesis of the muscles of expression. Rehabilitation of the congenitally paralyzed face usually relies on a combination of muscle and nerve-transfer procedures. The mildest form of congenital facial paralysis is agenesis of depressor labii inferioris or depressor anguli oris, causing asymmetry of lips in the crying newborn. Möbius syndrome is a rare disorder characterized by paralysis of facial and abducens nerves.[22] Bilateral facial paralysis can be seen in the syndrome as well as involvement of other cranial nerves such as trigeminal, glossopharyngeal, and vagus nerve. Möbius syndrome results as a developmental disorder of the rhombencephalon, where magnetic resonance imaging (MRI) suggests absence of CN VII within the IAC.

Children with CHARGE syndrome (*c*olobomata, *h*eart disease, *a*tresia or choanae, *r*etarded growth, *g*enital hypoplasia, and *e*ar abnormalities) can have varying degrees of facial weakness. In this syndrome, involvement of the vestibulocochlear nerve (CN VIII) is seen in 60%, facial nerve involvement in 43%, and glossopharyngeal or vagus involvement in 30%.[23] Hemifacial microsomia, often evidenced by microtia and facial asymmetries as well as eye and vertebral abnormalities, is the second most common congenital facial anomaly after cleft lip and palate. Over 25% of these patients have facial paralysis.

Melkersson-Rosenthal syndrome is a disorder that typically affects teenagers characterized by the triad of recurrent episodes of orofacial swelling, recurrent facial paralysis, and lingua plicata or fissured tongue. The complete triad is present in only 25% of the patients, and more commonly patients present with recurrent facial edema involving the cheek, lips, and tongue. The site of facial paralysis corresponds with the area of facial swelling, and management is often symptomatic. Residual facial paralysis may persist after recurrent episodes.[24]

Facial Paralysis from Neoplasms

Primary tumors of the facial nerve, such as schwannomas and hemangiomas, are rare in children. Vestibular schwannomas classically present with bilateral involvement in children with neurofibromatosis type 2. Such schwannomas can lead to facial paralysis by direct involvement of the facial nerve or compression within the IAC. Children can suffer facial nerve paralysis secondary to other tumors that involve the facial nerve, such as rhabdomyosarcoma, parotid tumors, lymphoma or leukemia, and CNS tumors (**Fig. 5.3 A–C**). Parotid gland masses are rare in children, with the majority representing benign lesions. Malignancy should be suspected in parotid masses when facial paralysis is seen.

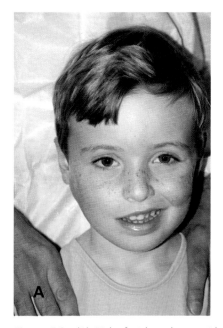 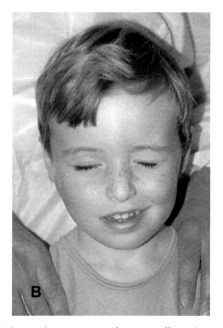 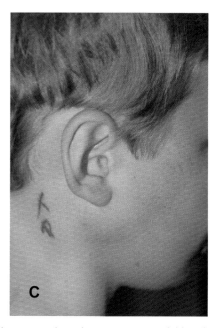

Figure 5.3 (A) Right facial weakness with (B) lower division motor function affected more than upper branches, in a young child with (C) a parotid and parapharyngeal mass. Pathology was consistent with a pseudosarcoma lesion.
Printed with permission.

Bell Palsy (Idiopathic Facial Paralysis)

Bell palsy refers to idiopathic peripheral facial nerve paralysis of acute onset in the absence of other neurologic signs. The diagnosis of Bell palsy in a child should be a diagnosis of exclusion, as the frequency of infectious, traumatic, and other defined causes of facial palsy merits a full diagnostic work-up for any child with facial weakness. The incidence of Bell palsy is of 2.7 per 100,000 under the age of 10 and 10.1 per 100,000 between the age of 10 and 20 years.[25] The proposed etiologies of Bell palsy include microvascular abnormalities, viral infection, and autoimmune reactions. Reactivation of HSV infection is a widely accepted hypothesis. Serologic studies showing seroconversion to HSV after episodes of Bell palsy have been inconsistent. Some patients complain of otalgia before the onset of facial paralysis. Viral prodromes may precede the paralysis.

The onset tends to be rapid with the majority of the patients progressing to maximal facial paralysis within 24 hours of onset; however, progression may occur over several hours or up to 1 week. Approximately two-thirds of the patients will progress to complete facial paralysis.[26] Bilateral Bell palsy is rare (0.3%) as is recurrence of more than one episode of facial paralysis (9%). Familiar history of Bell paralysis is present in 8% of the patients. The prognosis for facial nerve recovery in Bell palsy is excellent, with 85% of patient exhibiting recovery within 3 weeks of onset.[26] Patient with incomplete paralysis have recovery rates approaching 100%. The Copenhagen Facial Nerve Study is a large retrospective study that evaluated the natural history (without any therapeutic intervention) of 2570 patients with Bell palsy over a 25-year period. The study included 463 children under the age of 15, and 90% exhibited full facial nerve recovery.[26]

Imaging for Facial Paralysis

MRI with intravenous gadolinium contrast is useful in children with facial nerve paralysis, suspected CNS pathology, or tumors of the facial nerve. For slowly progressing or long-standing facial weakness, MRI should be obtained to image the brainstem, temporal bone, and parotid gland. In cases of facial nerve inflammation, such as in Bell palsy or RHS, enhancement of the nerve is seen on MRI—enhancement that may persist for longer than 1 year after presentation.

Computed tomography (CT) is the study of choice to examine the temporal portion of the facial nerve, allowing assessment of the facial nerve in the fallopian canal from the IAC to the stylomastoid foramen. CT should be obtained for facial palsy associated with temporal bone fractures or with middle-ear diseases such as chronic otitis media/mastoiditis or cholesteatoma (**Fig. 5.4**).

Treatment of Facial Paralysis

The etiology, severity, and duration of the paralysis guide the treatment for facial nerve paralysis in children. Specific

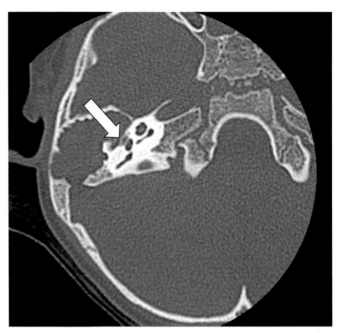

Figure 5.4 Computed tomographic image in the axial plane of a 3-year-old child with a large cholesteatoma that fills the mastoid and middle ear and has eroded the fallopian canal in the tympanic segment of cranial nerve VII. Arrow points to the tympanic segment.

infectious causes should be treated with appropriate antibiotics and even surgical drainage when indicated. Artificial tears, lubricants, and patching/taping of the eye are used with the advice of ophthalmology consultants for patients with impaired eye closure. Bell palsy should be treated with steroids if not otherwise contraindicated, although the benefits of antiviral drugs remain debated. When transection of the facial nerve or a major branch from trauma is likely, exploration and reanastomosis/grafting should be considered. The benefits of facial nerve decompression remain to be determined in the pediatric population. In cases of congenital or permanent paralysis, static and dynamic facial reanimation with muscle transfers and nerve grafts are available options for reconstruction. Reanimation surgery is usually considered after 12 months of facial paralysis when the chance of additional motor recovery is low.

Pharmacological Treatment

Pharmacological treatments for Bell palsy in children have been adopted from studies of these medications in the adult population. Two meta-analyses and two randomized controlled trials have documented improved motor function with the use of corticosteroids for Bell palsy. Therapy is more likely to be effective if started within 72 hours of onset of paralysis, and less effective when started after 7 days.[27,28] Corticosteroid treatment appears to quicken recovery as well as increase the likelihood of recovery. Salinas et al performed a meta-analysis and showed complete motor nerve recovery at 9 months in 77% of the patients treated with corticosteroids and 67% of those who did not receive steroids.[28] Early corticosteroid treatment for children with Bell palsy, using prednisone 1–2 mg/kg daily (up to 80 mg daily) for five to seven days, followed by a taper, has been recommended, despite the paucity of studies of children.[29]

Antiviral medications, administered in conjunction with corticosteroids, may provide additional benefit. While several randomized controlled trials have shown benefit of antivirals in conjunction with steroids, two meta-analyses did not show additional benefit.[27,30] Antiviral therapy alone is less effective than corticosteroids and not more effective than placebo.[30] The addition of acyclovir or valacyclovir for one week may be considered in the treatment of Bell paralysis, particularly in children with severe paralysis.

Surgery for Facial Paralysis in Children

Facial nerve decompression has not been recommended for acute facial paralysis in children, in the absence of an anatomic lesion such as fallopian canal fracture, tumor, or cholesteatoma. Available literature represents case series limited to adults, with inconsistent facial nerve recovery following decompression.[31,32] The role of facial nerve decompression in facial paralysis remains to be determined, particularly in the pediatric population.

Children with penetrating trauma to the face and temporal bone are at increased risk of complete transection of the facial nerve and its branches. In such cases where complete transection is suspected, exploration with direct neural reanastomosis or repair with use of neural grafts is advocated. Surgery within the first 72 hours of injury allows for the use of nerve stimulation to identify distal segments of the transected nerve. Even with anatomic nerve repair, the majority of patients will have unfavorable functional outcomes. About 85% will have recovered function in the House-Brackmann Grades III to IV range, with the remainder having complete paralysis.[32]

Surgical reanimation techniques are divided into (1) dynamic procedures that allow some active facial expression and (2) static procedures that restore facial symmetry at rest. Reanimation should generally be considered only if the paralysis does not improve after 12 months. Facial nerve repair is generally preferred either with end-to-end anastomosis or cable grafts. When use of the ipsilateral proximal nerve is not an option, cross-face grafting and nerve/muscle transfers are considered. These procedures are successful at returning tone and some degree of volitional movement, but cannot provide return to normal function.

References

1. Cha CI, Hong CK, Park MS, Yeo SG. Comparison of facial nerve paralysis in adults and children. Yonsei Med J 2008;49(5):725–734

2. Evans AK, Licameli G, Brietzke S, Whittemore K, Kenna M. Pediatric facial nerve paralysis: patients, management and outcomes. Int J Pediatr Otorhinolaryngol 2005;69(11):1521–1528

3. Grundfast KM, Guarisco JL, Thomsen JR, Koch B. Diverse etiologies of facial paralysis in children. Int J Pediatr Otorhinolaryngol 1990;19(3):223–239

4. Flint PW, Cummings CW. Cummings Otolaryngology–Head & Neck Surgery, 5th ed. Philadelphia, PA: Mosby/Elsevier; 2010

5. House JW, Brackmann DE. Facial nerve grading system. Otolaryngol Head Neck Surg 1985;93(2):146–147

6. Manning JJ, Adour KK. Facial paralysis in children. Pediatrics 1972;49(1):102–109

7. May M, Klein SR. Differential diagnosis of facial nerve palsy. Otolaryngol Clin North Am 1991;24(3):613–645

8. Cook SP, Macartney KK, Rose CD, Hunt PG, Eppes SC, Reilly JS. Lyme disease and seventh nerve paralysis in children. Am J Otolaryngol 1997;18(5):320–323

9. Salinas RA, Alvarez G, Daly F, Ferreira J. Corticosteroids for Bell's palsy (idiopathic facial paralysis). Cochrane Database Syst Rev. 2010;17(3):CD001942

10. Kangsanarak J, Fooanant S, Ruckphaopunt K, Navacharoen N, Teotrakul S. Extracranial and intracranial complications of suppurative otitis media. Report of 102 cases. J Laryngol Otol 1993;107(11):999–1004

11. Yonamine FK, Tuma J, Silva RF, Soares MC, Testa JR. Facial paralysis associated with acute otitis media. Braz J Otorhinolaryngol 2009;75(2):228–230

12. Lee SK, Lee MS, Jung SY, Byun JY, Park MS, Yeo SG. Antimicrobial resistance of *Pseudomonas aeruginosa* from otorrhea of chronic suppurative otitis media patients. Otolaryngol Head Neck Surg 2010;143(4):500–505

13. Tveitnes D, Øymar K, Natås O. Acute facial nerve palsy in children: how often is it Lyme borreliosis? Scand J Infect Dis 2007;39(5):425–431

14. Moscatello AL, Worden DL, Nadelman RB, Wormser G, Lucente F. Otolaryngologic aspects of Lyme disease. Laryngoscope 1991;101(6 Pt 1):592–595

15. Hato N, Kisaki H, Honda N, Gyo K, Murakami S, Yanagihara N. Ramsay Hunt syndrome in children. Ann Neurol 2000;48(2):254–256

16. Vázquez M, LaRussa PS, Gershon AA, Steinberg SP, Freudigman K, Shapiro ED. The effectiveness of the varicella vaccine in clinical practice. N Engl J Med 2001;344(13):955–960

17. Murakami S, Hato N, Horiuchi J, Honda N, Gyo K, Yanagihara N. Treatment of Ramsay Hunt syndrome with acyclovir-prednisone: significance of early diagnosis and treatment. Ann Neurol 1997;41(3):353–357

18. Falco NA, Eriksson E. Facial nerve palsy in the newborn: incidence and outcome. Plast Reconstr Surg 1990;85(1):1–4

19. McHugh HE. Facial paralysis in birth injury and skull fractures. Arch Otolaryngol 1963;78:443–455

20. McGuirt WF Jr, Stool SE. Temporal bone fractures in children: a review with emphasis on long-term sequelae. Clin Pediatr (Phila) 1992;31(1):12–18

21. Darrouzet V, Duclos JY, Liguoro D, Truilhe Y, De Bonfils C, Bebear JP. Management of facial paralysis resulting from temporal bone fractures: our experience in 115 cases. Otolaryngol Head Neck Surg 2001;125(1):77–84

22. Kremer H, Kuyt LP, van den Helm B, et al. Localization of a gene for Möbius syndrome to chromosome 3q by linkage analysis in a Dutch family. Hum Mol Genet 1996;5(9):1367–1371

23. Blake KD, Hartshorne TS, Lawand C, Dailor AN, Thelin JW. Cranial nerve manifestations in CHARGE syndrome. Am J Med Genet A 2008;146A(5):585–592

24. Zimmer WM, Rogers RS III, Reeve CM, Sheridan PJ. Orofacial manifestations of Melkersson-Rosenthal syndrome. A study of 42 patients and review of 220 cases from the literature. Oral Surg Oral Med Oral Pathol 1992;74(5):610–619

25. Katusic SK, Beard CM, Wiederholt WC, Bergstralh EJ, Kurland LT. Incidence, clinical features, and prognosis in Bell's palsy, Rochester, Minnesota, 1968-1982. Ann Neurol 1986;20(5):622–627

26. Peitersen E. Natural history of Bell's palsy. Acta Otolaryngol Suppl 1992;492:122–124

27. de Almeida JR, Al Khabori M, Guyatt GH, et al. Combined corticosteroid and antiviral treatment for Bell palsy: a systematic review and meta-analysis. JAMA 2009;302(9):985–993

28. Engström M, Berg T, Stjernquist-Desatnik A, et al. Prednisolone and valaciclovir in Bell's palsy: a randomised, double-blind, placebo-controlled, multicentre trial. Lancet Neurol 2008; 7(11):993–1000

29. De Diego JI, Prim MP, De Sarriá MJ, Madero R, Gavilán J. Idiopathic facial paralysis: a randomized, prospective, and controlled study using single-dose prednisone versus acyclovir three times daily. Laryngoscope 1998;108(4 Pt 1):573–575

30. Lockhart P, Daly F, Pitkethly M, Comerford N, Sullivan F. Antiviral treatment for Bell's palsy (idiopathic facial paralysis). Cochrane Database Syst Rev 2009; (4):CD001869

31. Gantz BJ, Rubinstein JT, Gidley P, Woodworth GG. Surgical management of Bell's palsy. Laryngoscope 1999;109(8):1177–1188

32. Coker NJ, Kendall KA, Jenkins HA, Alford BR. Traumatic intratemporal facial nerve injury: management rationale for preservation of function. Otolaryngol Head Neck Surg 1987;97(3):262–269

SECTION II: Pharynx, Nose, and Sinuses

6 Infectious and Inflammatory Disorders of the Tonsils and Adenoid

David H. Darrow

The tonsils and adenoid are anatomic structures that are highly predisposed to infectious and inflammatory processes. These areas are exposed to external influences during speech, mastication, deglutition, and respiration. Additionally, children use the oral and nasal cavities as areas of exploration. The immaturity of the immune system in children also places them at even greater risk for local infection and inflammation. This chapter reviews the diagnosis and management of the infectious and inflammatory disorders in children that are of the greatest importance to the otolaryngologist.

Functions of the Tonsils and Adenoid

The palatine tonsils and adenoid are tissues of "Waldeyer ring," a group of lymphoepithelial tissues that also includes the tubal tonsils in the nasopharynx and the lingual tonsil. Collectively, these tissues participate in the mucosal immune system of the pharynx. Positioned strategically at the entrance of both the gastrointestinal and the respiratory tracts, the tonsils and adenoid serve as secondary lymphoid organs, initiating immune responses against antigens entering the body through the mouth or nose. The size of the tonsils appears to correlate with their level of immunological activity, peaking between the ages of 3 and 10 years, and demonstrating age-dependent involution. There is also some evidence that their size increases with the bacterial load.

The tonsils are covered by a nonkeratinizing stratified squamous epithelium featuring some 10 to 30 deep crypts that effectively increase the surface area exposed to incoming antigens. The crypts occasionally harbor degenerated cells and debris that give rise to so-called "tonsilloliths," in which the presence of biofilms has also been implicated. Although the tonsils lack afferent lymphatics, the epithelium contains a system of specialized channels lined by "M" cells that take up antigens into vesicles and transport them to the intraepithelial and subepithelial spaces where they are presented to lymphoid cells. The transport function of M cells also serves as a portal for mucosal infections and immunizations, and M cells also can initiate immunologic responses within the epithelium, introducing foreign antigens to lymphocytes and antigen-presenting cells (APCs).

After passing through the crypt epithelium, inhaled or ingested antigens reach the extrafollicular region or the lymphoid follicles. In the extrafollicular region, APCs process the antigens and present them to helper T lymphocytes that stimulate proliferation of follicular B lymphocytes. The B lymphocytes ultimately develop into one of two types of cell: antibody-expressing B memory cells capable of migration to the nasopharynx and other sites, or plasma cells that produce antibodies and release them into the crypt lumen. Tonsillar plasma cells can produce all five immunoglobulin (Ig) classes that help combat and prevent infection. In addition, the contact of memory B-cells in the lymphoid follicles with antigen is an essential part of the generation of a secondary immune response.[1,2]

Among the Ig isotypes, IgA may be considered the most important product of the adenotonsillar immune system. In its dimeric form, IgA can attach to the transmembrane secretory component (SC) to form secretory IgA, a critical component of the mucosal immune system of the upper airway. This component is necessary for binding of IgA monomers to each other and to the SC, and is an important product of B-cell activity in the tonsil follicles. While the tonsils produce immunocytes bearing the joining (J) chain carbohydrate, SC is produced only in the adenoid and extratonsillar epithelium, and therefore only the adenoid possesses a local secretory immune system.[3]

Overview of Infectious and Inflammatory Diseases of the Tonsils and Adenoid

Pharyngotonsillitis is a general term used to describe diffuse inflammation of the structures of the oropharynx, including the tonsils. The disorder presents with symptoms of sore throat; however, objective signs of inflammation must be present to make the diagnosis. Pharyngotonsillitis may be classified based on duration of symptoms as acute, subacute, or chronic, with most patients presenting acutely. Alternatively, inflammatory disease of the nasopharynx may be considered *nasopharyngitis*, in which common symptoms include rhinorrhea, nasal congestion, sneezing, and cough. Inflammation limited to the adenoid pad (adenoiditis) is difficult to diagnose in the primary care setting due to the inaccessibility of this tissue to direct visualization.

Common Viral Infection of the Tonsils and Adenoid

Nasopharyngitis typically occurs during the cold weather months among young children during their early exposures to respiratory viruses. Adenoviruses, influenza viruses, parainfluenza viruses, and enteroviruses are the most common etiologic agents. Rhinovirus and respiratory syncytial virus occur almost exclusively in preschool children and are rarely associated with overt signs of pharyngeal inflammation. Adenoviruses are more common among older children and adolescents. Nasopharyngitis of viral etiology may also cause a concomitant pharyngotonsillitis. The infection is most commonly acute and self-limited, with symptoms resolving within 10 days. Nonviral agents are less frequently associated with nasopharyngitis, but may include *Corynebacterium diphtheriae, Neisseria meningitidis, Haemophilus influenzae,* and *Coxiella burnetii.*

The viruses responsible for pharyngotonsillitis are more diverse than those in nasopharyngitis; adenoviruses, influenza viruses, parainfluenza viruses, enteroviruses, Epstein-Barr virus (EBV), and *Mycoplasma* account for some 70% of these infections. As in nasopharyngitis, most viral pharyngotonsillitis requires no specific therapy.

Group A β-Hemolytic and Other Streptococci

The group A β-hemolytic *Streptococcus* (GABHS) is the most common bacterium associated with pharyngotonsillitis in children. In the 70 years since the advent of antibiotics, most pharyngeal infections by GABHS have been benign, self-limited, and uncomplicated processes. In fact, most patients improve symptomatically without any medical intervention whatsoever. However, a small number of affected children continue to develop renal and cardiac complications following GABHS infection, and some authors have implicated GABHS in the development of common childhood neuropsychiatric disorders. In addition, there is evidence that early antibiotic therapy may be useful in treating the symptoms of GABHS. As a result, appropriate diagnosis and treatment is imperative.

The incidence of GABHS pharyngitis has not been estimated on the basis of population-based data. Nevertheless, "strep throat" is well recognized as a common disease among children and adolescents. The incidence peaks during the winter and spring seasons, and is more common in cooler, temperate climates. Close interpersonal contact in schools, military quarters, dormitories, and families with several children appears to be a risk factor for the disease.

Transmission of GABHS is believed to occur through droplet spread. Individuals are most infectious early in the course of the disease, and the risk of contagion depends on the inoculum size and the virulence of the infecting strain. The incubation period is usually between 1 and 4 days. After starting antimicrobial therapy, most physicians will allow affected children to return to school within 36 to 48 hours. The role of individuals colonized with GABHS in the spread of the disease is uncertain, although data suggest that carriers rarely spread the disease to close contacts.[4]

The streptococci are gram-positive, catalase-negative cocci, characterized by their growth in long chains or pairs in culture. These organisms are traditionally classified into 18 groups with letter designations (Lancefield groups) on the basis of the antigenic carbohydrate component of their cell walls. While the GABHS is isolated from most patients with streptococcal pharyngitis, groups C, G, and B streptococci may also occasionally cause this disorder. Further subclassification of streptococci is made based on their ability to lyse sheep red blood cells in culture; the β-hemolytic strains cause hemolysis associated with a clear zone surrounding their colonies, while α-hemolytic strains cause partial hemolysis and gamma-hemolytic strains cause no hemolysis. The α-hemolytic strains are normal flora of the oral cavity and pharynx and should not be confused with the more pathogenic β-hemolytic strains.

The primary determinant of streptococcal pathogenicity is an antigenically distinct protein known as the M protein. This molecule is found within the fimbriae, which are finger-like projections from the cell wall of the organism that facilitate adherence to pharyngeal and tonsillar epithelium. Over 120 M serotypes are known. The M protein allows *Streptococcus* to resist phagocytosis in the absence of type-specific antibody. In the immunocompetent host, the synthesis of type-specific anti-M and other antibodies confers long-term serotype specific immunity to the particular strain in question. In laboratory-produced penicillin-resistant strains of GABHS, the M protein is absent, thereby rendering these strains more vulnerable to phagocytosis. This finding may help explain why no naturally occurring penicillin-resistant GABHS have yet been isolated.

GABHS are capable of elaborating at least 20 extracellular substances that affect host tissue; the interested reader may find a complete discussion of these substances elsewhere. Among the most important are streptolysin O, an oxygen-labile hemolysin, and streptolysin S, an oxygen-stable hemolysin, which lyse erythrocytes and damage other cells such as myocardial cells. Streptolysin O is antigenic, while streptolysin S is not. GABHS also produce three erythrogenic or pyrogenic toxins (A, B, and C) whose activity is similar to that of bacterial endotoxin. Other agents of significance include exotoxin A, which may be associated with toxic shock syndrome, and bacteriocins, which destroy other gram-positive organisms. Spread of infection may be facilitated by a variety of enzymes elaborated by GABHS, which attack fibrin and hyaluronic acid.

Signs and symptoms of GABHS pharyngotonsillitis are acute in onset, usually characterized by high fever, odynophagia, headache, and abdominal pain. However, the presentation may vary from mild sore throat and malaise (30 to 50% of cases) to high fever, nausea and vomiting, and dehydration (10%).[4] The pharyngeal and tonsillar mucosa are typically erythematous and occasionally edematous, with exudate present in 50 to 90% of cases. Cervical adenopathy is seen in 30 to 60% of cases. Most patients improve spontaneously in 3 to 5 days, unless otitis media, sinusitis, or peritonsillar abscess (PTA) occur secondarily.

The risk of rheumatic fever following GABHS infection of the pharynx is approximately 0.3% in endemic situations, and 3% under epidemic circumstances.[4] A single episode of rheumatic fever places an individual at high risk for recurrence following additional episodes of GABHS pharyngitis. Acute glomerulonephritis occurs as a sequelae in 10 to 15% of those infected with nephritogenic strains.[4] In patients who develop these sequelae, there is usually a latent period of 1 to 3 weeks.

Pediatric autoimmune neuropsychiatric disorder associated with group A streptococcal infection (PANDAS) has been described as a selective immunopathy similar to Sydenham chorea in which the response to streptococcal infection leads to dysfunction in the basal ganglia, resulting in tic, obsessive–compulsive, and affective disorders.[5] Classically, the behaviors are abrupt in onset and must have some temporal relationship to infection by GABHS. Clinical improvement has been reported among some patients treated with antibiotics, particularly as prophylaxis against recurrence. However, a cause-and-effect association of PANDAS with GABHS infection has yet to be established. Many experts believe that, as has been observed with other stressors, infection of any kind may provoke the neuropsychiatric phenomena.[6]

Early diagnosis of streptococcal pharyngitis has been a priority in management of the disease, primarily due to the risk of renal and cardiac sequelae. Several studies of the predictive value of various combinations of signs and symptoms to distinguish streptococcal from nonstreptococcal pharyngitis have found no clinically reliable predictors. Taken together, these studies demonstrate a false-negative rate of approximately 50% and a false-positive rate of 75%.[7] Adenopathy, fever, and pharyngeal exudate have the highest predictive value for a positive culture and rise in antistreptolysin O (ASO) titer, and absence of these findings in the presence of cough, rhinorrhea, hoarseness, or conjunctivitis most reliably predicts a negative culture, or positive culture without rise in ASO.[7]

Most clinicians advocate throat culture as the gold standard for diagnosis and treatment of GABHS. However, the tonsils, tonsillar crypts, or posterior pharyngeal wall must be swabbed for greatest accuracy. Tests for rapid detection of the group-specific carbohydrate simplify the decision to treat at the time of the office visit, and often eliminate the need for additional postvisit communication. However, while these tests have demonstrated a specificity of greater than 95%, their sensitivity is generally in the 70 to 90% range. As a result, many clinicians advocate throat culture for children with suspected streptococcal disease and negative rapid strep tests. Rapid antigen detection is usually more expensive than throat culture, and this technique must still be interpreted with care given the high incidence of posttreatment carriers. Studies also suggest possible clinician bias in interpretation of this test.

Carriage of GABHS may be defined as a positive culture for the organism in the absence of a rise in ASO convalescent titer, or in the absence of symptoms. The prevalence of GABHS carriers has been estimated at anywhere from 5 to 50% depending on the time of year and location, but this may be an overestimate as some antibiotics may occasionally interfere with the rise in ASO titer. Carriers are at low risk to transmit GABHS or to develop symptoms or sequelae of the disease. The importance of this condition is in the distinction of true acute streptococcal pharyngitis from nonstreptococcal sore throat in a carrier. When this distinction is important, a baseline convalescent ASO titer should be drawn. A subsequent positive test may be defined as a twofold dilution increase in titer between acute and convalescent serum, or any single value above 333 Todd units in children.[7] However, a low titer does not rule out acute infection, and a high titer may represent infection in the distant past. As a result, the American Academy of Pediatrics and the Infectious Disease Society of America recommend that testing for GABHS should not be performed in children with conjunctivitis, cough, hoarseness, coryza, diarrhea, oral ulcerations, or other clinical manifestations highly suggestive of viral infection. Furthermore, it is critical that patients referred to for potential tonsillectomy for "recurrent strep" be ruled out as carriers before they are considered candidates for surgery.

Although most upper respiratory infections by GABHS resolve without treatment, antimicrobial therapy likely prevents suppurative and nonsuppurative sequelae, including rheumatic fever, and may also hasten clinical improvement.[8,9] Treatment is therefore indicated for most patients with positive rapid tests for the group A antigen. When the test is negative or not available, one may be treated for a few days while formal throat cultures are incubating.

GABHS is sensitive to several antibiotics, including penicillins, cephalosporins, macrolides, and clindamycin. Expert panels have designated penicillin the drug of choice in managing GABHS owing to its track record of safety, efficacy, and narrow spectrum.[10,11] To date, no strains of GABHS acquired in vivo have demonstrated penicillin resistance or increased minimum inhibitory concentrations in vitro.[12] Beginning in the 1980s, several studies reporting a decrease in bacteriologic control rates, attributed primarily to inoculum effects and to increased tolerance to penicillin.[13,14] Whether cephalosporins may achieve greater eradication of GABHS than penicillin remains controversial.[15,16]

Depot benzathine penicillin G is still advocated by the American Heart Association for primary treatment of GABHS pharyngitis; however, a 10-day course of penicillin given orally is the most widely prescribed regimen. Twice-daily dosage by the enteral route yields results similar to those obtained with four-times-a-day dosage. Courses of shorter duration are associated with bacteriologic relapse and are less efficacious in the prevention of rheumatic fever. Amoxicillin appears to have efficacy equal to that of penicillin.[14] In poorly compliant or penicillin-allergic patients, azithromycin given once daily for 5 days may be a reasonable alternative. Erythromycin is now used less commonly than in the past due to its gastrointestinal side effects.

Most patients with positive cultures following treatment

are GABHS carriers; these individuals need not be re-treated if their symptoms have resolved. For patients in whom complete bacteriologic clearance is desirable, such as those with a family member with a history of rheumatic fever, a course of clindamycin or a second course of penicillin combined with rifampin may yield increased success. In patients with recurrent symptoms, serotyping may aid in distinguishing bacterial persistence from recurrence. There are no data available regarding the use of antibiotic prophylaxis in these patients, and in such cases tonsillectomy may sometimes be advantageous. During antimicrobial therapy, patients must be monitored carefully for fluid intake, pain control, and impending suppurative complications such as PTA.

Infectious Mononucleosis

Pharyngitis is one of the hallmarks of infectious mononucleosis (IM), a disorder associated with primary infection by the EBV. Worldwide, some 80 to 95% of adults exhibit serologic reactivity to EBV antigens. However, while primary infection by EBV occurs during the second and third decade in developed nations and regions of high socioeconomic status, young children may still be exposed, especially in developing countries and regions of low socioeconomic status. When the virus is acquired at a younger age, symptoms are generally less severe.

The incidence of IM in the United States is approximately 1 per 50 to 100,000 per year, but increases to approximately 100 per 100,000 among adolescents and young adults. Infected individuals transmit EBV by way of saliva exchanged during kissing or other close contact.

EBV is a member of the herpes virus family that preferentially infects and transforms human B lymphocytes. The virus enters the cell by attaching to a receptor designed for proteins of the complement chain, and its genetic material is transported by vesicles to the nucleus, where it dwells as a plasmid and maintains a "latent" state of replication. An incubation period of 2 to 7 weeks follows initial exposure, during which EBV induces a proliferation of infected B cells. This process is subsequently countered by a potent cellular immune response, characterized by the appearance of atypical lymphocytes (most likely T lymphocytes responding to the B-cell infection) in the blood. The number of infected circulating B cells is reduced during this 4- to 6-week period.

IM is characterized by a prodrome of malaise and fatigue, followed by the acute onset of fever and sore throat. Physical examination typically reveals enlarged, erythematous palatine tonsils, in most cases with yellow–white exudate on the surface and within the crypts. Cervical adenopathy is present in nearly all patients, and involvement of the posterior cervical nodes often helps distinguish EBV infection from that by streptococcus or other organisms. Between the second and fourth weeks of illness, about 50% of patients develop splenomegaly, and 30 to 50% develop hepatomegaly. Rash, palatal petechiae, and abdominal pain may also be present in some cases. The fever and pharyngitis generally subside within 2 weeks, while adenopathy, organomegaly, and malaise may last as long as 6 weeks.

Diagnosis of IM can usually be made on the basis of clinical presentation, absolute lymphocytosis, the presence of atypical lymphocytes in the peripheral smear, and detection of Paul-Bunnell heterophile antibodies. The latter is the basis of the Mono-Spot, Mono-Diff, and Mono-Test assays, which test for agglutination of horse erythrocytes. Children under 5 years of age may not develop a detectable heterophile antibody titer; in these patients, it is possible to determine titers of IgG antibodies to the viral capsid antigen, as well as antibodies to the "early antigen" complex. Antibodies to EBV nuclear antigen appear late in the course of the disease (**Table 6.1**).

In most cases of IM, treatment is supportive. In severe cases, particularly those with respiratory compromise due to severe tonsillar enlargement and those with hematologic or neurologic complications, a course of systemic steroids may hasten resolution of the acute symptoms. Placement of a nasopharyngeal trumpet or endotracheal intubation may be necessary on rare occasions when severe airway compromise occurs. Antibiotics may be useful in cases of concomitant group A β-hemolytic pharyngotonsillitis; however, ampicillin can cause a rash in this setting.

The use of antiviral agents in IM has yielded disappointing results. In clinical trials, acyclovir reduced viral shedding in the pharynx but demonstrated little efficacy in the treatment of symptoms. Other agents have exhibited greater in vitro effect than acyclovir but have yet to be tested clinically.

Exposure to EBV has been implicated in the development of posttransplantation lymphoproliferative disorder (PTLD). Children who have received bone marrow and solid organ transplants may develop abnormal proliferation of lymphoid cells in the setting of immunosuppression; approximately 80% of affected individuals have a history of EBV infection.[17] EBV seronegative transplant recipients may develop acute

Table 6.1 Expected Results of Serologic Testing for EBV

	Never Been EBV Infected	EBV Infected Now	EBV Infected in the Past
Anti-VCA	Negative	Positive	Positive
Anti-EBNA	Negative	Negative	Positive

EBV: Epstein-Barr virus; VCA: viral capsid antigen; EBNA: Epstein-Barr nuclear antigen.

EBV infection from environmental exposure or from the EBV seropositive donor once they become immunosuppressed.[17] The clinical presentation is variable and can mimic graft-versus-host disease, graft rejection, or more conventional infections. Signs and symptoms may resemble an IM-like illness or an extranodal tumor, commonly involving the gut, brain, or the transplanted organ. Mononucleosis-like presentations typically occur in children within the first year after transplant, and are often associated with primary EBV infection after transfer of donor virus from the grafted organ. Extranodal tumors are more common among EBV-seropositive recipients several years after the transplant.[18] Studies have shown that young age at the time of transplant and EBV seronegativity conferred increased risk of adenotonsillar hyperplasia, which may be a precursor to PTLD.[17] A higher incidence of PTLD has also been demonstrated with use of more potent immunosuppressive agents.

Initial management involves reduction of immunosuppression with care to preserve the transplanted organ. Patients who do not tolerate or respond to reduction of immunosuppression require more aggressive therapy and often have a poorer prognosis. Additional treatments include antivirals, such as acyclovir and ganciclovir, antibody therapy, interferon, chemotherapy, and radiation therapy with varying results. Prognosis is poor with mortality rates as high as 50 to 90%.[18] Novel forms of immunotherapy have been tested in PTLD, including both antibody and cell-mediated approaches.

Peritonsillar Infection

Peritonsillar infection may present as either cellulitis or abscess. Most cases are thought to represent a suppurative complication of tonsil infection. Peritonsillar infection occurs more commonly in adolescents and young adults than in young children. Affected patients present with symptoms of sore throat, odynophagia, fever, voice change, and otalgia. Common physical findings include fever, drooling, trismus, muffled "hot potato" voice, and pharyngeal asymmetry with inferior and medial displacement of the tonsil. Radiographic evaluation is usually not necessary, but may be useful in young or uncooperative children or in equivocal cases. Although some authors have found intraoral ultrasound to be useful in adults, computed tomography with contrast remains the imaging modality of choice in children.

While patients with peritonsillar cellulitis may be treated with antibiotics alone, most abscesses require removal of the pus as definitive therapy. Evacuation of PTA can be managed by needle aspiration, incision and drainage, or immediate ("quinsy") tonsillectomy with nearly equivalent efficacy.[19] In very young or poorly cooperative patients, or in those in whom an abscess has been inadequately drained, tonsillectomy is curative and essentially eliminates any chance of recurrence.

Abscess cultures usually reveal a polymicrobial infection, often containing gram-positive organisms and anaerobes.

Appropriate antimicrobial therapy in the emergency room or office setting would include initial parenteral administration of penicillin with or without metronidazole, clindamycin, or ampicillin–sulbactam. Options for oral therapy include amoxicillin–clavulanate, penicillin, and clindamycin, although children may resist taking the latter due to its taste. Intravenous hydration should also be considered for those individuals who have not been able to take liquids orally.

The efficacy of tonsillectomy in the prevention of recurrent PTA has now been compared with that of watchful waiting in a prospective, controlled trial. Studies demonstrate an increased rate of recurrent PTA among those who also had recurrent tonsillitis. A case series suggests that recurrence may be predicted based on a history of two to three episodes of acute tonsillitis in the year before the initial episode[20]; such a history has been elicited in 15 to 30% of patients with PTA.[19–21] Based on the available evidence, it has been suggested that routine elective tonsillectomy or quinsy tonsillectomy is not indicated for patients who present with their first PTA. However, if a patient is a candidate for elective tonsillectomy for other reasons (i.e., two to three tonsillitis events in the previous 12 months), then it seems rational to perform a quinsy tonsillectomy for treatment, or to proceed with planned elective tonsillectomy after successful abscess drainage.[19–21]

"Chronic" Tonsillitis

Chronic tonsillitis is poorly defined in the literature but may be the appropriate terminology for sore throat for at least 3 months accompanied by tonsillar inflammation. Affected individuals may report symptoms of chronic sore throat, halitosis, or debris or concretions in the tonsil crypts known as "tonsilloliths." Affected patients may also have persisting cervical adenopathy. Throat culture in such cases is usually negative. Although no clinical trials exist to help guide medical management of such patients, tonsillectomy seems reasonable for those patients who do not respond to improved oropharyngeal hygiene and aggressive antibiotic therapy.

Recurrent Tonsillitis and Tonsillectomy

When tonsils have been recurrently or chronically infected, the controlled process of antigen transport and presentation is altered due to shedding of the transporting M cells from the tonsil epithelium.[1] As a result, tonsillar lymphocytes can theoretically become overwhelmed with persistent antigenic stimulation, rendering them unable to respond to antigens or to function adequately in local protection or reinforcement of the upper respiratory secretory immune system. Furthermore, the direct influx of antigens disproportionately expands the population of mature B-cell clones and, as a result, fewer early memory B cells go on to become J-chain-positive IgA immunocytes.[1] There would therefore appear to be a therapeutic advantage to removing recurrently or chronically diseased tonsils. The surgeon should bear in mind, however, that tonsillectomy and adenoidectomy procedures remove a source of immunocompetent cells, and some studies demonstrate minor alterations of Ig concentrations in the adjacent tissues following tonsillectomy.[2,22]

Cultures from the deeper tissues of recurrently infected tonsils frequently reveal unusual pathogens including *Staphylococcus aureus*, *H. influenzae*, *Actinomycetes*, *Chlamydia*, *Mycoplasma*, and anaerobes; however, it remains unclear whether such cultures truly represent the offending organisms. Several studies suggest that bacteria in biofilms may be more important in recurrent tonsillitis than their planktonic counterparts.

Recurrent sore throat of a noninfectious nature is a hallmark of Marshall syndrome. This disorder is characterized by periodic fever, aphthous stomatitis, pharyngitis, and adenitis (PFAPA), occurring primarily in children less than 5 years of age. The illness usually lasts more than 5 days and recurs at regular intervals of 3 to 6 weeks.[23] Systemic steroids and cimetidine have demonstrated efficacy in controlling the events.[23] Two small randomized controlled trials demonstrated that tonsillectomy was effective in treating PFAPA syndrome, but children in the control groups also showed improvement.[24] Tonsillectomy may be considered based on the frequency of illness, severity of infection, and the child's response to medical management.

Appropriate medical and surgical management of children with recurrent infectious pharyngotonsillitis depends on accurate documentation of the cause and severity of the individual episodes as well as the frequency of the events. The clinician should record for each event a subjective assessment of the patient's severity of illness; physical findings including body temperature, pharyngeal and/or tonsillar erythema, tonsil size, tonsillar exudate, cervical adenopathy (presence, size, and tenderness); and the results of microbiologic testing for GABHS. A summary of the documentation should be made available to the consultant to aid in the medical decision-making regarding potential surgical intervention. In children with recurrent sore throat whose tests for GABHS are repeatedly positive, it may be desirable to rule out streptococcal carriage concurrent with viral infection as carriers are unlikely to transmit GABHS or to develop suppurative complications or nonsuppurative sequelae of the disease such as acute rheumatic fever. Supportive documentation in children who meet criteria for tonsillectomy may include absence from school, spread of infection within the family, and a family history of rheumatic heart disease or glomerulonephritis.

In all randomized controlled trials of tonsillectomy for infection, sore throat with each event was a necessary entrance criterion, and in most of these trials sore throat was the primary outcome studied. As a result, no claim can be made that tonsillectomy is indicated for children whose constellation of symptoms does not include sore throat, even when GABHS can be cultured from the throat. These studies also suggest that patients whose events are less severe or well documented do not gain sufficient benefit from tonsillectomy to justify the risk and morbidity of the procedure; in such patients, tonsillectomy should be considered only after a period of observation during which documentation of additional events may be made.

Children with frequent recurrences of throat infection over a period of several months demonstrate high rates of spontaneous resolution.[25] As a result, an observation period of at least 12 months is generally recommended before consideration of tonsillectomy. In rare cases, early surgery may reasonably be considered for severely affected patients, such as those with histories of hospitalization for recurrent severe infections, rheumatic heart disease in the family, or numerous repeat infections in a single household ("ping-pong spread"), or those with complications of infection such as PTA or Lemierre syndrome (thrombophlebitis of the internal jugular vein).

Observation of patients is also a reasonable management strategy in children who have had frequent recurrences of pharyngotonsillitis for more than 1 year. In several studies, children demonstrated spontaneous improvement without surgery during the follow-up period, often with patients no longer meeting the original criteria for study entry. The natural history of recurrent pharyngotonsillitis is also found to be favorable in case series that describes patients on "wait lists" for tonsillectomy; many children who were reevaluated after months on such lists later no longer met the criteria for surgery.

Tonsillectomy has been suggested for centuries as a means of controlling recurrent infection of the throat. However, clinical trials investigating the efficacy of tonsillectomy have had a high risk of bias because of poorly defined entrance criteria, nonrandom selection of operated subjects, exclusion of severely affected patients, or reliance on caregivers for postoperative data collection. In the most frequently cited trial, Paradise and colleagues[25] included patients only if their episodes of throat infection met strict criteria as outlined in **Table 6.2**. The key findings of the study were as follows:

1. A mean rate reduction of 1.9 episodes of sore throat per year among tonsillectomized children during the first year of follow-up compared with controls. However, the sore throat associated with performance of the surgery (which would otherwise count as one episode) was excluded from the data. In the control group, patients also improved compared with their preenrollment frequency of infection, experiencing a mean of only 3.1 annual events. Differences between groups were reduced in the second year and were not significant by the third year of follow-up.

2. For episodes of *moderate or severe* throat infection, the control group experienced 1.2 episodes compared with 0.1 in the surgical group. The rate reductions diminished over the subsequent 2 years of follow-up and were not significant in the third year.

Table 6.2 The "Paradise Criteria" for Tonsillectomy in Recurrent Tonsillitis

Criterion	Definition
Frequency of sore throat events	• Seven or more episodes in the preceding year, or • Five or more episodes in each of the preceding 2 years, or • Three or more episodes in each of the preceding 3 years
Clinical features (one required in addition to sore throat)	• Temperature >38.3°C, or • Cervical lymphadenopathy (tender lymph nodes or >2 cm), or • Tonsillar exudate, or • Positive culture for GABHS
Treatment	Antibiotics are administered at appropriate dose for proven or suspected episodes of GABHS
Documentation	• Each episode and its qualifying characteristics are synchronously documented in the medical record, or • In cases of insufficient documentation, two subsequent episodes of throat infection are observed by the clinician with frequency and clinical features consistent with the initial history

Adapted from: Paradise JL, Bluestone CD, *Bachman* RZ, et al. History of recurrent sore throat as an indication for tonsillectomy. Predictive limitations of histories that are undocumented. *N Engl J Med* 1978;298(8):409–413.

GABHS: group A β-hemolytic *Streptococcus*.

3. Mean days with sore throat in the first 12 months were not statistically different between the two groups, but included a predictable period of sore throat postoperatively.

The Paradise group reported a second study[26] with less rigorous criteria for the number of episodes, clinical features required for diagnosis of pharyngitis, and documentation (i.e., four to six episodes in the last year or three or four episodes per year in the past 2 years). In the two arms of the study (tonsillectomy or adenotonsillectomy vs. control, and adenotonsillectomy vs. control), patients undergoing surgery experienced rate reductions of 0.8 and 1.7 episodes/year, respectively, in the first year. For episodes of moderate or severe sore throat, control subjects in the two arms of the study combined experienced 0.3 episodes/year overall compared with 0.1/year in subjects undergoing surgery. Mean days with sore throat in the first 12 months were not statistically different in either arm of the study. The investigators concluded that the modest benefit conferred by tonsillectomy in children moderately affected with recurrent throat infection did not justify the inherent risks, morbidity, and cost of the surgery.

A randomized controlled trial comparing tonsillectomy with watchful waiting in children aged 2 to 8 years, examined fever >38°C for at least 1 day as the primary outcome measure. During a mean follow-up period of 22 months, children in the tonsillectomy group had 0.2 fewer episodes of fever per person year, and from 6 to 24 months there was no difference between the groups. The surgical group also demonstrated, per person year, mild reductions in throat infections (0.2), sore throats (0.6), days with sore throat (5.9), and upper respiratory tract infections (0.5). Pooled data from these studies were also analyzed in a Cochrane systematic

review.[27] Patients undergoing tonsillectomy experienced 1.4 fewer episodes of sore throat in the first year compared with the control group; however, the "cost" of this reduction was one episode of sore throat in the immediate postoperative period.

Despite the modest advantages conferred by tonsillectomy for sore throat, studies of quality of life universally suggest a significant improvement in patients undergoing the procedure. Only two of these studies enrolled children exclusively and both reported improved scores in nearly all subscales. However, both also had numerous methodological flaws including enrollment of patients with "chronic tonsillitis" without definition based on signs and symptoms, absence of a control group, low response rates with potential selection bias, poor follow-up, and caregiver collection of data.

A 2011 guideline on tonsillectomy suggests that tonsillectomy for severely affected children with recurrent throat infection should be considered an "option."[28] Families of patients who meet the appropriate criteria for tonsillectomy as described above must weigh the modest anticipated benefits of tonsillectomy for this indication against the natural history of resolution and the risk of surgical morbidity and complications.

Recurrent and Chronic Adenoiditis

The disorders characterized in children as adenoiditis, rhinosinusitis, and nasopharyngitis are not easily distinguished from one another on the basis of symptoms. Most individuals in whom the diagnosis is made present with nasal stuffiness, mucopurulent rhinorrhea, chronic cough, halitosis, and "snorting" or "gagging" on mucus throughout the day. However, there are no established criteria for making this diagnosis, or for differentiating it from viral upper respiratory illness or acute sinusitis.

In chronic or recurrent nasopharyngitis, the persistence of disease may be due to colonization by pathogenic bacteria. *H. influenzae, S. pneumoniae, S. pyogenes,* and *S. aureus* are commonly found in adenoid cultures and tissue samples among children so affected. Rates of drug-resistant bacteria may be higher among patients with chronic or recurrent infection. Furthermore, molecular typing of paired bacterial isolates from the adenoid and lateral nasal wall in children undergoing adenoidectomy demonstrates a high degree of correlation, and sinonasal symptom scores appear to correlate with quantitative bacteriology of the adenoid "core" and not with adenoid size. Several studies have demonstrated bacterial biofilm formation in the adenoid; however, it is not clear if this is more common in persistent and recurrent nasopharyngitis than in obstructive adenoid hyperplasia. In some patients, sinonasal infection is more likely due to stasis of secretions secondary to obstructive adenoid tissue rather than bacterial factors, although the two may certainly be related. Gastroesophageal reflux has not been established as a cause of chronic adenoid inflammation.

Data suggest that adenoidectomy may be useful in the management of children with persistent and recurrent sinonasal complaints, although a systematic review indicates the evidence is currently inadequate to firmly establish efficacy.[29] Most clinicians favor adenoidectomy before consideration of endoscopic sinus surgery, especially for those children with recurrent acute symptoms rather than those with more chronic sinonasal disease.

Other Inflammatory Tonsil and Adenoid Disorders

Halitosis

Halitosis may result from food debris and bacteria retained within the crypts of the tonsils and adenoid. However, although bad breath is considered an indication for tonsillectomy by some, the evidence for this practice is lacking. A wide variety of other causes should be investigated including periodontal disease, debris of the tongue or lingual tonsils, sinonasal infection or foreign body, and gastroesophageal reflux.

Gonorrhea

Infection by *Neisseria gonorrhea* is a rare cause of pharyngotonsillitis resulting from orogenital contact. In young children gonococcal infection occurs due to sexual abuse, and adolescent girls may contract this infection from consensual orogenital sex.

Gonococcal infection of the throat most commonly presents as an exudative pharyngitis accompanied by fever and adenopathy, but this infection is symptomatic less than 70% of the time. Urethritis in males, and vulvovaginitis in females, and the presence of concomitant sexually transmitted diseases may be more consistent clinical indicators. The pharyngeal infection usually resolves spontaneously within 10 to 12 weeks but should be treated when diagnosed. In most cases, gonococcal pharyngitis may be adequately treated with a single parenteral administration of ceftriaxone or cefotaxime, although some physicians prefer to continue the injections daily for 7 to 10 days. Treatment should also be offered to the offending individual, and the infections must be reported to the appropriate local and national authorities.

Diphtheria

Diphtheria pharyngitis, caused by the gram-positive bacillus *C. diphtheriae*, is a rare but serious cause of airway obstruction in children acquired via the respiratory passages. With aggressive immunization programs, diphtheria infection has become all but extinct in developed countries; no cases have been reported in the United States since 2003. Nevertheless, scattered cases over earlier decades have been observed among unimmunized or underimmunized individuals in lower socioeconomic groups. In fact, a large proportion of adults in the western world lack protective serum levels of diphtheria immunity.

Following an incubation period of 2 to 4 days, diphtheria exotoxin is released by the organism, initiating local tissue necrosis and exudate. The exudate within the airway turns fibrinous, and develops into an adherent gray membrane containing inflammatory cells, epithelial cells, and red blood cells. Enlargement of the membrane and progressive edema cause airway compromise and stridor, and dislodgement of the membrane may cause frank obstruction. Systemic effects of the toxin include myocarditis, peripheral neuritis, and acute tubular necrosis of the kidneys.

Definitive diagnosis is made on the basis of a culture of the membrane and/or demonstration of toxin production by immunoprecipitation, polymerase chain reaction, or immunochromatography; however, management should not be delayed for culture results. Pharyngeal membranes due to diphtheria are tenacious and difficult to remove; patients with airway compromise may urgently require a more secure airway. Once the airway is established, antitoxin and antibiotic therapy with penicillin or erythromycin are subsequently administered, and nonimmune personal contacts are treated as well. Prognosis depends on the immunization status of the host, the promptness of medical therapy, and the virulence of the infecting organism. Prevention of diphtheria is achieved through immunization during infancy.

Kawasaki Disease (Mucocutaneous Lymph Node Syndrome)

Kawasaki disease (KD) is a multisystem vasculitis characterized by fever, rash, pharyngitis, conjunctival inflammation, edema of the extremities, and cervical adenopathy. Initially reported in the Japanese literature in 1967 as a benign disorder of childhood, KD has been linked over the past three decades to serious cardiac complications, arthritis, and several other manifestations. The etiology of KD remains unknown; epidemiologic and clinical data occurrence of KD support an infectious etiology, but a mode of transmission has not been determined. About 80% of KD cases occur in children below 5 years of age.[30] The disease is slightly more common in males and among individuals of Asian extraction. Between 3000 and 5000 cases occur annually in the United States.[30]

KD occurs in three distinct clinical phases. The acute phase lasts 1 to 2 weeks, and is characterized by prolonged high spiking fever, rash, erythema of the bulbar conjunctiva, swelling and erythema of the extremities, and adenopathy. Oral and oropharyngeal manifestations are also common, including swollen, fissured, and bleeding lips; "strawberry tongue" (resulting from diffuse erythema and prominent papillae); and erythema of the oropharyngeal mucosa. Each of these findings is observed in over 90% of patients, except for adenopathy >1.5 cm, which is seen in 50 to 75%. In the subacute phase, days 10 to 25, most of these signs and symptoms resolve, but irritability and conjunctival changes usually persist. The toes and fingers begin to desquamate

and joint pain is present in approximately 30% of patients. Cardiac dysfunction, including coronary arteritis, vascular dilatation and aneurysm formation, myocarditis, arrhythmia, and coronary insufficiency, occurs in about 20% of children during this period. The third, or convalescent, stage begins when clinical signs of KD have completely resolved and ends when the sedimentation rate returns to normal. KD may also be associated with sterile pyuria, aseptic meningitis, hepatic dysfunction, distension of the gallbladder, diarrhea, uveitis, otitis media, and pneumonitis.

Therapy for KD in the acute phase is directed at prevention of cardiac complications. High-dose aspirin is usually administered (with a watchful eye for signs of Reye syndrome) to decrease myocardial inflammation and prevent thrombosis. Anesthetic and antacid mouthwashes may alleviate odynophagia. Lubrication of the lips may reduce fissuring and bleeding. Intravenous immunoglobulin (IVIG) results in a more rapid anti-inflammatory effect than that seen with aspirin alone. IVIG also appears to lessen the risk of long-term coronary artery abnormalities. Once the convalescent phase is reached, patients are generally monitored at regular intervals for evidence of cardiac complications.

References

1. Brandtzaeg P. Immune functions and immunopathology of palatine and nasopharyngeal tonsils. In: Bernstein JM, Ogra PL, eds. Immunology of the Ear. New York: Raven Press; 1987:63–106

2. Nave H, Gebert A, Pabst R. Morphology and immunology of the human palatine tonsil. Anat Embryol (Berl) 2001;204(5): 367–373

3. Brandtzaeg P. Immunology of tonsils and adenoids: everything the ENT surgeon needs to know. Int J Pediatr Otorhinolaryngol 2003;67(Suppl 1):S69–S76

4. Kaplan EL, Gerber MA. Group A streptococcal infections. In: Feigin RD, Cherry JD, eds. Textbook of Pediatric Infectious Diseases. 4th ed. Philadelphia, PA: W.B. Saunders Co.; 1998:1076–1088

5. Swedo SE, Leonard HL, Garvey M, et al. Pediatric autoimmune neuropsychiatric disorders associated with streptococcal infections: clinical description of the first 50 cases. Am J Psychiatry 1998;155(2):264–271

6. Shulman ST. Pediatric autoimmune neuropsychiatric disorders associated with streptococci (PANDAS): update. Curr Opin Pediatr 2009;21(1):127–130

7. Kline JA, Runge JW. Streptococcal pharyngitis: a review of pathophysiology, diagnosis, and management. J Emerg Med 1994;12(5):665–680

8. Randolph MF, Gerber MA, DeMeo KK, Wright L. Effect of antibiotic therapy on the clinical course of streptococcal pharyngitis. J Pediatr 1985;106(6):870–875

9. Krober MS, Bass JW, Michels GN. Streptococcal pharyngitis. Placebo-controlled double-blind evaluation of clinical response to penicillin therapy. JAMA 1985;253(9):1271–1274

10. Bisno AL, Gerber MA, Gwaltney JM Jr, Kaplan EL, Schwartz RH; Infectious Diseases Society of America. Practice guidelines for the diagnosis and management of group A streptococcal pharyngitis. Clin Infect Dis 2002;35(2):113–125

11. American Academy of Pediatrics Committee on Infectious Diseases. Red Book: Report of the Committee on Infectious Diseases. 27th ed. Elk Grove Village, IL: American Academy of Pediatrics; 2006:610–620

12. Gerber MA. Diagnosis and treatment of pharyngitis in children. Pediatr Clin North Am 2005;52(3):729–747

13. Pichichero ME, Casey JR, Mayes T, et al. Penicillin failure in streptococcal tonsillopharyngitis: causes and remedies. Pediatr Infect Dis J 2000;19(9):917–923

14. Dajani A, Taubert K, Ferrieri P, Peter G, Shulman S. Treatment of acute streptococcal pharyngitis and prevention of rheumatic fever: a statement for health professionals. Committee on Rheumatic Fever, Endocarditis, and Kawasaki Disease of the Council on Cardiovascular Disease in the Young, the American Heart Association. Pediatrics 1995;96(4 Pt 1):758–764

15. Casey JR, Pichichero ME. Meta-analysis of cephalosporin versus penicillin treatment of group A streptococcal tonsillopharyngitis in children. Pediatrics 2004;113(4):866–882

16. Shulman ST, Gerber MA. So what's wrong with penicillin for strep throat? Pediatrics 2004;113(6):1816–1819

17. Shapiro NL, Strocker AM, Bhattacharyya N. Risk factors for adenotonsillar hypertrophy in children following solid organ transplantation. Int J Pediatr Otorhinolaryngol 2003;67(2):151–155

18. Macsween KF, Crawford DH. Epstein-Barr virus-recent advances. Lancet Infect Dis 2003;3(3):131–140

19. Johnson RF, Stewart MG, Wright CC. An evidence-based review of the treatment of peritonsillar abscess. Otolaryngol Head Neck Surg 2003;128(3):332–343

20. Herzon FS. Harris P. Mosher Award thesis. Peritonsillar abscess: incidence, current management practices, and a proposal for treatment guidelines. Laryngoscope 1995;105(8 Pt 3, Suppl 74) 1–17

21. Kronenberg J, Wolf M, Leventon G. Peritonsillar abscess: recurrence rate and the indication for tonsillectomy. Am J Otolaryngol 1987;8(2):82–84

22. Kaygusuz I, Gödekmerdan A, Karlidag T, et al. Early stage impacts of tonsillectomy on immune functions of children. Int J Pediatr Otorhinolaryngol 2003;67(12):1311–1315

23. Feder HM, Salazar JC. A clinical review of 105 patients with PFAPA (a periodic fever syndrome). Acta Paediatr 2010;99(2):178–184

24. Burton MJ, Pollard AJ, Ramsden JD. Tonsillectomy for periodic fever, aphthous stomatitis, pharyngitis and cervical adenitis syndrome (PFAPA). Cochrane Database Syst Rev 2010;8(9):CD008669

25. Paradise JL, Bluestone CD, Bachman RZ, et al. History of recurrent sore throat as an indication for tonsillectomy. Predictive limitations of histories that are undocumented. N Engl J Med 1978;298(8):409–413

26. Paradise JL, Bluestone CD, Colborn DK, Bernard BS, Rockette HE, Kurs-Lasky M. Tonsillectomy and adenotonsillectomy for recurrent throat infection in moderately affected children. Pediatrics 2002;110(1 Pt 1):7–15

27. Burton MJ, Glasziou PP. Tonsillectomy or adeno-tonsillectomy versus non-surgical treatment for chronic/recurrent acute tonsillitis. Cochrane Database Syst Rev 2009;(1, 1, Issue 1)CD001802 10.1002/14651858.CD001802.pub2

28. Baugh RF, Archer SM, Mitchell RB, et al; American Academy of Otolaryngology-Head and Neck Surgery Foundation. Clinical practice guideline: tonsillectomy in children. Otolaryngol Head Neck Surg 2011;144(1, Suppl)S1–S30

29. van den Aardweg MT, Schilder AG, Herkert E, Boonacker CW, Rovers MM. Adenoidectomy for recurrent or chronic nasal symptoms in children. Cochrane Database Syst Rev 2010;201(1):CD008282

30. Newburger JW, Takahashi M, Gerber MA, et al; Committee on Rheumatic Fever, Endocarditis and Kawasaki Disease; Council on Cardiovascular Disease in the Young; American Heart Association; American Academy of Pediatrics. Diagnosis, treatment, and long-term management of Kawasaki disease: a statement for health professionals from the Committee on Rheumatic Fever, Endocarditis and Kawasaki Disease, Council on Cardiovascular Disease in the Young, American Heart Association. Circulation 2004;110(17):2747–2771

7 Pediatric Obstructive Sleep Apnea

Stacey L. Ishman and Christopher R. Roxbury

Sleep disordered breathing (SDB) is now well recognized as a common condition in children, representing a spectrum ranging from simple snoring to upper airway resistance syndrome (UARS) to obstructive sleep apnea syndrome (OSAS). Children with obesity, Down syndrome, and craniofacial abnormalities are at high risk for SDB. While adults with SDB commonly present with excessive daytime sleepiness, daytime signs and symptoms are less apparent in affected children. More commonly, caregivers report signs of SDB such as snoring, gasping for breath at night, and poor school performance.

While milder forms of SDB are not generally associated with airflow restriction or oxygen desaturation, OSAS is characterized by apneas, hypopneas, and respiratory effort-related arousals (RERAs). Severe OSAS in children can lead to cardiovascular and pulmonary complications. SDB, even of milder severity such as primary snoring, has been associated with behavioral and neurocognitive disturbances, decreased school performance, and quality of life impairment. As such, it is important to recognize these entities early and implement proper medical and/or surgical therapy.

Unfortunately, diagnosis of pediatric SDB is not as straightforward as it is in adult patients. A standardized approach to clinical diagnosis and universal clinical screening protocols is lacking. Clinicians must have a high index of suspicion, especially in high-risk children.

Diagnosis

History

A thorough history is the cornerstone of diagnosis of SDB in children. In general, children with OSAS display similar stereotypical nighttime symptoms as adults with OSAS. These include snoring, gasping for breath, increased respiratory effort, abnormal movements during sleep, witnessed apneas, and restless sleep with or without frequent awakenings. Children may also display several nonspecific daytime symptoms, including mouth breathing, hyponasality, and dysphagia, as well as psychological and behavioral changes including hyperactivity, increased aggression, and poor performance in school. Enuresis is also associated with pediatric SDB. Daytime sleepiness is not a common complaint in affected children.

In an attempt to emphasize early diagnosis and treatment, the American Academy of Pediatrics in 2002 recommended universal screening of children for snoring during routine pediatric care.[1] However, over 9% of the general pediatric population may suffer from habitual snoring, which may occur in the absence of frank OSAS. Moreover, studies have shown that the caregiver's description of the symptoms is not an accurate means to diagnose OSAS.[2] History and physical examination findings correlate poorly with polysomnographic findings.

The clinician must fully evaluate genetic conditions that predispose to oropharyngeal or nasopharyngeal obstruction, creating increased risk for OSAS. Such conditions include Down, Crouzon, and Apert syndromes as well as bilateral choanal atresia. Furthermore, syndromes with retrognathia or micrognathia such as Pierre Robin sequence and Treacher Collins syndrome have been associated with SDB. Finally, conditions that affect tone in the pharynx and upper airway, such as cerebral palsy, can predispose to OSAS that is quite difficult to treat.

Epidemiologic studies have shown that the overall prevalence of pediatric OSAS ranges from 1 to 4%. While it has been thought that prevalence is equal between male and female children, a 2008 systematic review of the literature found that males are more likely to suffer from SDB than females.[3] The incidence is also higher in African Americans than in Caucasians. Finally, obesity has also been associated with an increased incidence of SDB in children and adults (**Table 7.1**).

Physical Examination

The age of a child at presentation is a key consideration when evaluating for SDB, as neonates and infants may have different signs, symptoms, and causes of SDB than older children. Evaluation of a child with possible SDB should begin with an assessment of growth and weight gain. While infants and young children may be more likely to present with poor weight gain or failure to thrive, older children with obstructive sleep apnea (OSA) are more likely to be overweight or obese.

A thorough head and neck examination should be performed to search for the site of airway obstruction. Any signs of syndromes affecting craniofacial anatomy or airway tone should be noted. In addition, the nasal cavity should be examined for inflammation, swelling, or masses, and the posterior nasal cavity should be inspected for choanal stenosis or atresia when suspected. A thorough examination of the nasopharynx may also include an assessment of the adenoid size using nasopharyngoscopy or radiographs.

The oral cavity and oropharynx must also be examined, inspecting for macroglossia as well as palpating the hard

Table 7.1 Relevant Pediatric Obstructive Sleep Apnea History and Physical Examination

Nighttime <ul><li>Snoring</li><li>Gasping for breath or choking during sleep</li><li>Increased respiratory effort</li><li>Witnessed apneas</li><li>Restless sleep with or without frequent awakenings</li><li>Nocturnal enuresis (secondary)</li></ul> **Daytime** <ul><li>Mouth breathing</li><li>Hyponasality</li><li>Dysphagia</li><li>Aggressive behavior or hyperactivity</li><li>Poor school performance</li><li>Excessive daytime sleepiness (less common than in adults)</li></ul>	**General** <ul><li>Blood pressure, height and weight with body mass index</li><li>Obesity or failure to thrive</li><li>Craniofacial alignment—mandible and maxilla position/size</li><li>Adenoid facies</li></ul> **Nasal** <ul><li>External nasal deformity</li><li>Nasal valve (internal and external)</li><li>Inferior turbinates</li><li>Rhinorrhea and nasal edema</li></ul> **Oral cavity** <ul><li>Tonsil size and position (i.e., glossoptosis)</li><li>Modified Mallampati score</li><li>Palate and uvula position</li><li>Dentition and oropharyngeal crowding</li></ul> **Neck** <ul><li>Relative position of the hyoid</li></ul> **Other** <ul><li>Cardiovascular examination</li><li>Chest wall deformity</li><li>Craniofacial or syndromic abnormalities</li></ul>

and soft palate to assess for overt or submucous cleft palate. Tonsillar size is assessed by grading on a 4-point scale with a 0 for tonsils that have been previously removed, 1+ for tonsils within the tonsillar pillars, 2+ for tonsils that protrude just beyond the pillars, 3+ for tonsils that protrude greater than 50% of the way to the midline, and 4+ for tonsils that meet in the midline (**Fig. 7.1**).

A recent systematic review has shown that the association between tonsillar size and obstruction as quantified by polysomnography (PSG) may not be as strong as once suspected.[4] In this study, 20 articles (mean n = 161) were analyzed with 11 supporting a correlation between tonsillar

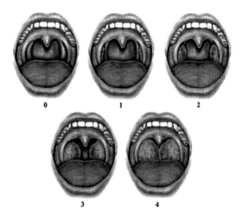

Figure 7.1 Tonsil grading.
Reprinted with permission from: John Wiley and Sons. Friedman M, Ibrahim H, Joseph N. Staging of obstructive sleep apnea/hypopnea syndrome: a guide to appropriate treatment. *The Laryngoscope* 2004;114(3):454–459.

size and obstruction and 9 showing no association. It was the higher quality studies that showed no correlation between tonsil size and OSAS severity. While tonsillar size may be used as a clinical guide, providers must be aware that size may not be the best predictor of OSAS.

PSG

As OSAS has been associated with high body mass index (BMI) score and adenotonsillar hypertrophy in some studies, some clinicians may proceed directly to adenotonsillectomy (AT) in healthy children with signs of SDB and enlarged tonsils on physical examination. However, PSG is considered the gold standard test for diagnosis of OSAS in children.

Commonly referred to as the "sleep study," PSG is the simultaneous electrographic recording of multiple variables during sleep. These parameters include sleep stage, snoring, airflow, respiratory effort, gas exchange, limb position, and limb movement (**Fig. 7.2A–C**). PSG can help distinguish OSAS from other disorders such as primary snoring, narcolepsy, nocturnal seizures, periodic limb movements, and restless leg syndrome. PSG also allows clinicians to stratify the severity of OSAS, and may in fact help identify the children at increased risk for respiratory compromise postoperatively who would benefit from hospital admission.

Unfortunately, there are no validated severity scales for diagnosing mild, moderate, and severe OSAS in children. The current standard research definition recognizes a respiratory disturbance index (RDI) of 1 to <5 events per hour to be mild OSAS, 5 to <10 events per hour as moderate OSAS, and 10 or more events per hour as severe OSAS. However,

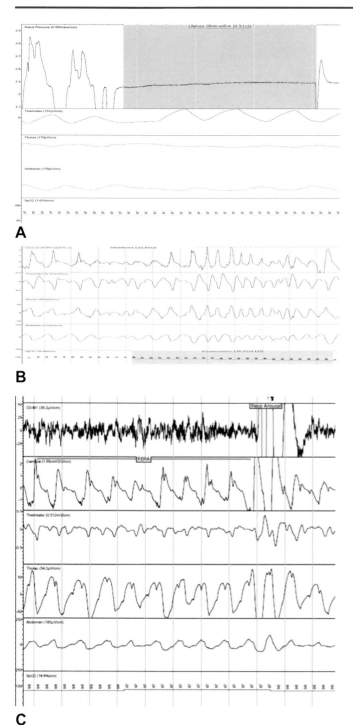

Figure 7.2 (A) Obstructive apnea with cessation of airflow associated with continued respiratory effort; (B) hypopnea with decreased nasal airflow and desaturation; and (C) respiratory event-related arousal with decreased nasal airflow with an arousal.

in the performance and interpretation of PSG studies in children to obtain accurate and reliable results.

A recent review paper has challenged the necessity of PSG for the diagnosis of pediatric OSA.[6] Best practice guidelines proposed by this paper suggest that AT may be performed without PSG in otherwise healthy children with a history consistent with symptoms of SDB and physical examination findings of adenotonsillar hypertrophy. In addition, they propose that preoperative PSG is only needed in children <3 years of age, or when adenotonsillar size is discordant with the degree of airway obstruction.

Due to the difficulties in access to and performance of overnight PSG in children, portable, or "in-home," monitoring devices have been suggested for the diagnosis of pediatric SDB. The American Academy of Sleep Medicine (AASM) updated its guidelines in 2007 to recommend that such in-home studies include measures of airflow, blood oxygenation, and respiratory effort at a minimum. However, in-home testing has not been validated in children.

In 2011, the American Academy of Otolaryngology-Head and Neck Surgery (AAO-HNS) published a clinical practice guideline on use of PSG before tonsillectomy for SDB in children.[7] These guidelines suggest referral for PSG before tonsillectomy for children with high risk factors such as obesity, Down syndrome, craniofacial abnormalities, neuromuscular disorders, sickle cell disease, or mucopolysaccharidoses (MPS). PSG for otherwise healthy children is recommended if the need for surgery is uncertain or if there is a discrepancy between adenoid/tonsil size and SDB symptoms.

In addition, the AAO-HNS advocates communication of PSG results to the anesthesiologist before induction of anesthesia, as the results of PSG can help guide intraoperative decision-making and anesthesia management, and can affect postoperative care plans. For instance, the guidelines suggest postoperative admission for children under the age of 3 or with severe OSAS as defined by an AHI ≥10 or an oxygen saturation nadir <80%. Young age and OSAS severity correlate well with respiratory compromise after adenotonsillectomy that may require intervention.[5]

Finally, the AAO-HNS suggests obtaining in-laboratory 16 channel PSG for children rather than portable monitoring, as the aforementioned AASM guidelines for in-home testing are based on use in adults. PSG for children may be expensive, inconvenient, and unavailable, and is an imperfect gold standard. As such, there has been a search for simpler ways to clinically screen for OSAS such as the OSA-18 quality of life questionnaire, Pediatric Sleep Questionnaire and the Brouillette OSA score. However, each of these has been shown to have poor specificity for OSAS diagnosis.

High-Risk Patients

Childhood obesity, with its rapidly increasing prevalence, is perhaps the most important risk factor for the development of pediatric SDB. In 2007, 16.4% of U.S. children were obese and 31.6% were overweight. As many of these children will be asymptomatic, and are later found to have moderate or

others have advocated that normal breathing may occur up to an apnea–hypopnea index (AHI) of two obstructive events per hour.[5] It is important to note, however, that there are significant differences in the criteria for the performance, scoring, and interpretation of pediatric and adult PSG. As such, it is important that these laboratories have experience even severe OSAS by PSG, routine PSG testing is particularly important for obese children.

A recent review of children undergoing ambulatory surgery at a university medical center found that 36% of obese patients presented for otolaryngologic procedures, most commonly AT, supporting the observation that obesity increases the propensity for airway obstruction.[8] Proposed mechanisms for this include the presence of excess adipose tissue in the upper airway causing distortion and collapse, and neuromotor dysfunction during sleep. Unfortunately, recent studies have shown that 49 to 88% of obese children will have obstructive symptoms even after surgery.[1]

OSAS is also more common in Down syndrome, where as many as 31 to 63% of children may suffer from OSAS.[7] Features of Down syndrome that increase the risk of OSAS are a large tongue, midface hypoplasia, a stocky body habitus, and hypertrophy of not only the adenoids and palatine tonsils but also the lingual tonsils. A recent study showed that 80% of Down syndrome patients in the age group of 4 to 63 months had abnormal PSG results, and caregiver assessments using the Children's Sleep Habits Questionnaire did not predict these abnormalities.[9] Based on these results, it was recommended that all children with Down syndrome be screened for OSAS with a baseline PSG, preferably performed between the ages of 3 and 5. In addition, the American Academy of Pediatrics recommended in 2001 that parents of young children with Down syndrome children be questioned about SDB.

Adenotonsillectomy rarely cures OSAS in children with Down syndrome. A recent study suggests that up to 75% of Down syndrome patients will have an abnormal PSG after surgery. It has been suggested that persistent OSAS is likely from additional areas of anatomic airway obstruction and abnormal neuromotor tone common to these children. A recent study of children less than 2 years old with Down syndrome suggests that some will outgrow their OSAS. In this study, 16 of the 29 patients studied had OSAS, of which 6 were started on continuous positive airway pressure (CPAP) only. Of these, 3 children (50% of the CPAP population

and 19% of the total study population) were found to have no evidence of OSAS on follow-up PSG within the next 10 months.[10] Such resolution has been seen in other young children without Down syndrome.

Other genetic syndromes that predispose children to SDB are the MPS, such as Hunter and Hurler syndromes (**Table 7.2**). Presumably, stereotypic anatomic changes in this patient population such as a short neck, high epiglottis, deep cervical fossa, large tongue, adenotonsillar hypertrophy, and a hypoplastic mandible all contribute to this predisposition toward OSA. Progressive deposition of glycosaminoglycans in the airways contributes to obstruction as well. OSAS has been seen in up to 64% of these patients.[11]

Children with craniosynostosis, as seen in Pfeiffer, Apert, and Crouzon syndromes have SDB in up to 53% of cases. While AT may help those patients with mild craniofacial deformity, OSAS refractory to AT in this group often requires tracheostomy or long-term CPAP. Midface advancement is also a reasonable alternative, with critical objective assessment after surgery. Alternatively, a retrospective analysis of long-term nasopharyngeal airway use in children with a mean age of 5.8 ± 4.1 years showed a significant improvement in oxygen saturations when monitored by PSG.[12]

Obstructive sleep apnea is also more common in children with cleft lip and palate, presumably due to midface hypoplasia and retrognathia, which lead to a narrowed upper airway that may persist even after surgery. In a recent review of 459 patients with nonsyndromic cleft palate/lip, 37.5% had symptoms of SDB while 8.5% had OSAS diagnosed by PSG.[13]

Achondroplasia patients are also at increased risk of OSAS due to characteristic craniofacial anatomy that involves midface hypoplasia, skull enlargement with narrowing of the skull base, and stenosis of the nasal and nasopharyngeal airways. These patients may also experience mixed and central apnea due to brainstem compression secondary to a narrowed foramen magnum. A recent retrospective chart review of children ages 3 to 14 with achondroplasia showed a SDB prevalence of 54.3%.[14] AT was shown to improve

Table 7.2 Conditions Associated with Increased Risk of Sleep Disordered Breathing in Children

• Achondroplasia	• Lymphangioma
• Apert syndrome	• Mucopolysaccharidoses
• Beckwith-Wiedeman syndrome	• Obesity
• Cerebral palsy	• Osteopetrosis
• Choanal stenosis or atresia	• Pierre Robin sequence
• Cleft lip/palate	• Pfeiffer syndrome
• Crouzon syndrome	• Pharyngeal flap surgery
• Down syndrome	• Prader-Willi syndrome
• Goldenhar syndrome/hemifacial microsomia	• Recurrent respiratory papillomatosis (oropharyngeal)
• Hypothyroidism	• Sickle cell disease
• Klippel-Feil syndrome	• Treacher Collins syndrome
• Pfieffer syndrome	

symptoms in the majority of patients as measured by AHI, but 5.3 to 12.3% of patients required some additional form of therapy.

Neuromuscular disorders such as cerebral palsy, muscular dystrophies, as well as spinal muscular atrophy are frequently associated with SDB and OSAS due to hypotonia of the pharyngeal musculature. In one review, 31% of patients with Duchenne muscular dystrophy (DMD) had OSAS diagnosed by PSG when referred for such testing.[15] DMD patients should undergo annual PSG from the time they are wheelchair-bound or when signs of OSAS are seen.

Children with cerebral palsy frequently have OSAS due to decreased neuromuscular control. These children may also have difficulty compensating for airway obstruction during sleep due to a decreased ability to reposition themselves. Unfortunately, these children are also less likely to respond to AT, and are more likely to require additional pharyngeal surgery, CPAP, or even tracheotomy in almost 14% of cases.[16]

Treatment

Nonsurgical Treatment

Dental Appliances and Rapid Maxillary Expansion

In children with OSAS and malocclusion rapid maxillary expansion (RME) can be considered, especially if AT is not indicated or desired by the caregivers or who have persistent symptoms after AT. Fourteen children who underwent RME were found to have reduced snoring as well as a substantial reduction in the AHI.[17] While this report found sustained cure after 24 months, follow-up was not available for all patients, and treatment failures were seen in patients with tonsillar enlargement and/or overweight. Dental appliances are another nonsurgical option for OSAS treatment. The goal of this therapy is to stabilize and increase the oropharyngeal and hypopharyngeal airway spaces. There is limited data to support the use of such appliances in children. In a case–control study, children with mild to moderate OSAS were more likely to have a reduced mandibular length, overbite, and smaller dental arch, in addition to a more superiorly located hyoid bone than healthy controls. In one study, 20 children with OSAS were treated daily with a dental appliance for 6 months showed a mean decrease in the RDI from 7.9 ± 1.8 pretreatment to 3.7 ± 6.8 posttreatment ($p<0.001$).[18] Dental appliances may be efficacious in children, but more data are needed to support this.

Medical Treatment

A 2005 Cochrane review identified two randomized controlled trials of intranasal steroids for children with OSAS.[19] Both studies showed a small but statistically significant decrease in the mean AHI in the treatment group, but cure was not seen in most patients. Leukotriene modifiers have also been studied, with one study of children with mild OSAS showing that a 16-week course of monteleukast

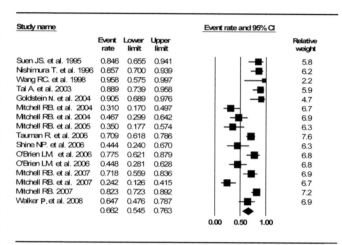

Figure 7.3 Forest plot for success in achieving an apnea–hypopnea index >5 postoperatively.

Source: Friedman M, Wilson MN, Lin HC, Chang HW. Updated systematic review of tonsillectomy and adenoidectomy for treatment of pediatric obstructive sleep apnea/hypopnea syndrome. *Otolaryngol Head Neck Surg* 2009;140(6):800–808, Figure 3.

improved AHI (pretreatment mean 3.0 ± 0.22, posttreatment mean 2.0 ± 0.3, $p = 0.017$) and hypercarbia as well as reducing adenoid size.[20]

Nasal CPAP

Since 2006, nasal CPAP has been approved for use in children older than 7 or weighing more than 40 pounds. As of 2005, there have been at least 2 masks approved by the U.S. Food and Drug Administration for use in children 2 years and older, but there are still none approved for children younger than 2. In addition to problems with mask fit, the masks are often uncomfortable, and compliance is poor (**Fig. 7.3**). A recent analysis of effectiveness and compliance in children 2 to 16 years old found that CPAP reduced RDI and increased oxygen saturation, but 30% of the subjects discontinued the treatment within 6 months.[21] Complications of CPAP include dermatitis, nasal obstruction, and nasal dryness. In a study of children 6 months to 18 years of age using CPAP, 48% had skin injury with erythema and skin necrosis, 68% had global facial flattening, and 37% were found to have maxillary retrusion.[22]

The inability of children to tolerate CPAP has lead researchers to seek other ways to deliver air to these children in a manner that might be more tolerable. One such study showed that children treated with transnasal insufflation (TNI), warm humidified air delivered through a nasal cannula, have reductions in AHI comparable to those treated with CPAP.[23] This method was trialed in 12 children ages 7 to 14, with OSA symptoms ranging from mild to severe. All children received high flow oxygen through a nasal cannula at 20L/min, and had improved oxygen stores and decreased arousals, which decreased the AHI from a baseline mean of 11 +/– 3 to 5 +/– 2 events per hour ($p<0.01$), comparable to that on CPAP in the majority of children. While further evidence is required, it may prove to be an appealing noninvasive alternative in children.

Surgical Treatment

Adenoidectomy

Two studies of adenoidectomy alone for childhood SDB show limited benefits. The first reported on 206 patients followed for 3 to 5 years after adenoidectomy performed for nasal obstruction in 89%, snoring in 88%, and obstructed breathing in 44% of the subjects.[24] Results of this study indicated that 80% of children had an improvement in symptoms postoperatively, but that symptomatic re-growth of the adenoids may occur in as many as 3% of patients. The second study analyzes the incidence of future tonsillectomy or revision adenoidectomy in 48 children who underwent adenoidectomy for obstructive symptoms compared with 52 who had adenoidectomy for nonobstructive reasons.[25] In this study, 38% of children with obstructive symptoms underwent subsequent surgery versus only 19% of those with nonobstructive symptoms. While both of these studies suggest that adenoidectomy alone improves OSA in children, they do not provide a comparison to AT. Additionally, re-growth of adenoids can occur, especially in children who have their adenoids removed before 6 years of age. This results in recurrence of obstructive symptoms and need for revision adenoidectomy.

Adenotonsillectomy

OSAS is the most common indication for AT in the United States. Early complications include bleeding, vomiting, and dehydration due to increased pain on swallowing and poor oral intake. Late complications, which generally occur

within 1 week of the procedure, include delayed bleeding, velopharyngeal insufficiency (VPI), and nasopharyngeal stenosis (NPS). Preoperative evaluation should include assessment of bleeding risk, evaluation of clinical factors associated with postoperative respiratory difficulties, and determination of risk for postoperative hypernasality.

AT has been shown to lead to a complete resolution in symptoms in up to 71% of patients. Multiple studies have shown that the procedure improves quality of life, neurocognitive, and behavioral measures. However, recent evidence suggests that more children are not completely cured of OSAS by AT than previously suspected. A recent review of 578 children who had AT for OSAS showed that 90.1% had an improved AHI, with a mean of 18.2 ± 21.4 preoperatively to 4.1 ± 6.4 postoperatively. Only 27.2% of children had a complete cure of OSAS as defined by an AHI <1 event per hour, while 21.6% had postoperative AHI >5 events per hour.[26] In light of these findings, parents must be counseled that AT may not completely cure the child's obstructive symptoms (**Fig. 7.4**).

Tonsillectomy versus Tonsillotomy

Partial tonsillectomy, intracapsular tonsillectomy, or tonsillotomy has been advocated as a less-morbid alternative to total tonsillectomy, as it reduces tonsillar bulk while preserving the tonsillar capsule and preventing exposure of the pharyngeal musculature. Advocates suggest that tonsillotomy leads to decreased pain and postoperative morbidity than traditional total tonsillectomy, with similar outcomes in terms of snoring and recurrent infections.

In one study, microdebrider intracapsular tonsillectomy was shown to result in efficient removal of tonsil tissue, fewer complications and less pain, in addition to a quicker return to normal diet and activity.[27] Quality of life measures

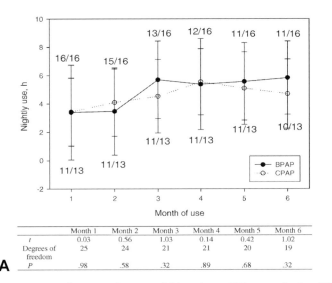

	Month 1	Month 2	Month 3	Month 4	Month 5	Month 6
t	0.03	0.56	1.03	0.14	0.42	1.02
Degrees of freedom	25	24	21	21	20	19
P	.98	.58	.32	.89	.68	.32

A

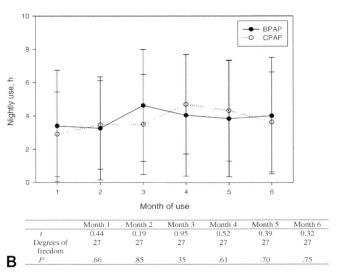

	Month 1	Month 2	Month 3	Month 4	Month 5	Month 6
t	0.44	0.19	0.95	0.52	0.39	0.32
Degrees of freedom	27	27	27	27	27	27
P	.66	.85	.35	.61	.70	.75

B

Figure 7.4   Adherence of CPAP in children shows 30% stopped using CPAP before 6 months.
Source: Marcus CL, Rosen G, Ward SL, et al. Adherence to and effectiveness of positive airway pressure therapy in children with obstructive sleep apnea. *Pediatrics* 2006;117(3):e442–e451, Figure 2a.
BPAP, bilevel positive airway pressure; CPAP, continuous positive airway pressure.

have also been found to improve after tonsillectomy and tonsillotomy.

Most studies comparing tonsillotomy to tonsillectomy only measure outcomes such as postoperative pain, time to return to normal diet and activity, and quality of life. One retrospective study of 33 patients who underwent tonsillotomy and 16 who underwent tonsillectomy compared the procedures in terms of snoring, tonsillar regrowth, recurrent tonsillitis, and recurrent obstruction, and found no statistically significant differences between the two groups.[28]

Nasal Surgery

Nasal obstruction is a known risk factor for sleep-disordered breathing. Nasal obstruction in children can either cause or exacerbate symptoms of OSAS, likely from turbinate hypertrophy. A randomized controlled trial of radiofrequency inferior turbinate ablation showed improved nasal obstruction and increased nasal CPAP compliance.[29] However, turbinate reduction in children remains controversial, as many children with turbinate hypertrophy have benefitted from adenoidectomy alone.

Uvulopalatopharyngoplasty (UPPP)

Some children with complex causes of OSAS, especially those with neurological impairment and craniofacial syndromes, may benefit from UPPP as this procedure addresses posterior oropharyngeal obstruction by the soft palate and lateral pharyngeal walls. However, these studies are limited and subject to selection bias. Most studies of UPPP have been performed in adults, with reported success rates of 30 to 65% when performed alone. Regardless of the technique, the surgeon must be meticulous in both patient selection and technical aspects of surgery to avoid complications such as VPI and NPS.

Lingual Tonsillectomy

While lingual tonsil hypertrophy is uncommon in children, growing evidence suggests that children with Down syndrome and obesity are at increased risk for enlargement of the lingual tonsils.[30] In addition, cases of airway obstruction that resolved after lingual tonsillectomy alone have been reported. A recent series described 26 patients (age range, 3 to 20 years) with persistent OSAS after tonsillectomy who were treated with endoscopic-assisted lingual tonsillectomy. These patients were improved but not cured after this surgery, with reduction of mean RDI from 14.7 to 8.1 after surgery. Lingual tonsillectomy should be performed with caution to avoid pharyngeal scarring. A recent study of lingual tonsillectomy performed as part of multilevel upper airway surgery showed that 8.2% of children developed oropharyngeal stenosis (OPS).[31] Thus, a more conservative, multistep approach may be necessary in children requiring multilevel surgery if they require lingual tonsillectomy.

Tongue Reduction Techniques

Radiofrequency ablation of the tongue base has been shown in adult populations to have moderate ability to improve ESS and RDI with minimal complications. However, this technique has been reported in children only to treat lymphatic and vascular malformations of the tongue.

Other Methods to Address Retroglossal Obstruction

Experience is at best limited for additional procedures that focus on the base of the tongue in children with complex OSAS. Case reports have found decreases in OSAS when children with macroglossia and tongue base hypertrophy were treated with a tongue suspension suture. Tongue reductions can also help treat OSAS in children with macroglossia such as those with Beckwith-Wiedemann syndrome and lymphovascular malformations

Hyoid suspension has also been used to treat obstruction stemming from the base of the tongue although there is very little published pediatric data. Genioglossal advancement (GGA) has been studied in children with OSAS. Adult studies of GGA have shown up to a 70% decrease in RDI, but this procedure was almost always performed simultaneously with other upper airway procedures such as UPPP. A retrospective study of GGA was also performed to determine which patients are likely to benefit most from this procedure. In this study, 28 patients in the age group of 3 to 22 years who had previously undergone GGA to treat OSA were assessed by postoperative PSG. Of them, 17 (61%) were considered successful and 11 (39%) were considered to have failed.[32] Subsequently, the authors analyzed static and dynamic cine MR studies and determined that only relative tongue size and small adenoid size predicted success with GGA.

Children with craniofacial abnormalities may benefit from specific procedures to correct these anatomical deformities. Children with midface hypoplasia may undergo Le Fort osteotomies or midface advancement. Of course, patients must undergo a thorough evaluation of craniofacial anatomy and neuromotor status to determine candidacy for such procedures.

Tracheostomy

Tracheostomy is a definitive treatment for OSAS, as it by definition bypasses virtually all contributing sites of upper airway obstruction. However, high morbidity and complex care issues relegate the role of tracheotomy to treatment of children with complex causes of OSAS that have not responded to more conservative surgical and nonsurgical treatments. It may also be useful in patients with neurologic deficits who have difficulty protecting their own airway, as well as an adjunct procedure before or during craniofacial surgery.

Perioperative Management

AT is one of the most common procedures performed today, and children with SDB are at high risk for complications. AAO-HNS guidelines suggest overnight admission after AT in children less than three years old, and for those with severe OSA (AHI >10, O_2 nadir <80%), as these children are at highest risk for postoperative airway compromise. In addition, admission should be considered in children with more complex medical histories including cardiac complications of OSA, neuromuscular disorders, obesity, failure to thrive, or craniofacial abnormalities,[1] as these patients may be at higher risk of respiratory compromise.

Postoperative analgesia should also be approached with caution, as postoperative opioid administration has been associated with respiratory compromise in OSAS patients. A prospective study of 22 children showed that children with severe OSAS preoperatively (O_2 saturation nadir <85%) required less morphine postoperatively than patients with milder disease, which suggests that recurrent hypoxemia may lead to increased narcotic sensitivity.[33]

Weight Gain Associated with Adenotonsillectomy for Obstructive Sleep Apnea

AT has been associated with weight gain after surgery. As described in the 1990s, weight gain was generally regarded as favorable for children undergoing treatment of OSAS that may have caused failure to thrive. However, later studies suggested that normal weight and even overweight patients showed accelerated weight postoperatively.[34]

A recent large prospective cohort study of 3963 children showed that AT performed before age 7 was associated with obesity at age 8 years (odds ratio of 2.89; confidence interval [CI] 1.74–4.79). Adenoidectomy alone was also associated with obesity, but the association was not as strong (odds ratio 2.19; CI 1.17–4.11).[35] A systematic review of nine studies, including a total of almost 800 children, was performed to study AT as a risk factor for childhood obesity.[36] BMI increased from 5.5 to 8.3%, standardized weight score increased in 46 to 100% of patients, and corrected weight increased in 50 to 75% of the patients after AT. Interestingly, morbidly obese patients (those defined as having weight of 130 to 260% of peers) showed no change postoperatively. While there are limitations to this study, it supports the theory that children gain more weight than normally expected postoperatively, suggesting a link between AT and weight gain.

Another study shows that preschool aged children who underwent AT increase the calories they are consuming daily in the postoperative period, and consume more foods that are high in sugar and fat. Although more data are required, this study suggests a link between AT and increased caloric intake, which could help to explain why children gain weight after the procedure.

Persistent Obstructive Sleep Apnea after Adenotonsillectomy

Although AT is the first line of treatment for pediatric SDB, a significant number of patients will have persistent symptoms. A systematic review by Friedman et al in 2009 showed that only 60 to 66% of children were cured of OSAS after adenotonsillectomy, with cure defined as an AHI <1 and <5.[37] Most children were improved by PSG criteria, but this review focused on otherwise healthy children, where adenotonsillectomy is expected to have the most benefit. Obese children are at even higher risk for persistent OSAS. A meta-analysis showed a complete resolution of PSG parameters in only 10 to 25% of obese children after adenotonsillectomy, as compared with 70 to 80% of normal weight children.[38]

Children with more severe OSAS may be at increased risk for persistent disease following adenotonsillectomy. A study of 79 healthy children undergoing adenotonsillectomy showed that 36% of children with severe preoperative OSAS had persistent PSG abnormalities.[39] Other factors that may place patients at high risk for persistence of disease include chromosomal disorders such as Down syndrome, craniofacial and neuromuscular anomalies, as well as African American race (**Table 7.3**).

Table 7.3 Conditions Associated with Increased Risk of Persistent OSA in Children

Overweight/obesity
Black (African American) or other ethnicity
Craniofacial abnormalities—including Down syndrome
Hypotonia—including cerebral palsy
Severe OSA

OSA, obstructive sleep apnea.

References

1. Section on Pediatric Pulmonology, Subcommittee on Obstructive Sleep Apnea Syndrome. American Academy of Pediatrics. Clinical practice guideline: diagnosis and management of childhood obstructive sleep apnea syndrome. Pediatrics 2002;109(4):704–712

2. Brietzke SE, Katz ES, Roberson DW. Can history and physical examination reliably diagnose pediatric obstructive sleep apnea/hypopnea syndrome? A systematic review of the literature. Otolaryngol Head Neck Surg 2004;131(6):827–832

3. Lumeng JC, Chervin RD. Epidemiology of pediatric obstructive sleep apnea. Proc Am Thorac Soc 2008;5(2):242–252

4. Nolan J, Brietzke SE. Systematic review of pediatric tonsil size and polysomnogram-measured obstructive sleep apnea severity. Otolaryngol Head Neck Surg 2011;144(6):844–850

5. Wilson K, Lakheeram I, Morielli A, Brouillette R, Brown K. Can assessment for obstructive sleep apnea help predict postadenotonsillectomy respiratory complications? Anesthesiology 2002;96(2):313–322

6. Yellon RF. Is polysomnography required prior to tonsillectomy and adenoidectomy for diagnosis of obstructive sleep apnea versus mild sleep disordered breathing in children? Laryngoscope 2010;120(5):868–869

7. Roland PS, Rosenfeld RM, Brooks LJ, et al; American Academy of Otolaryngology–Head and Neck Surgery Foundation. Clinical practice guideline: Polysomnography for sleep-disordered breathing prior to tonsillectomy in children. Otolaryngol Head Neck Surg 2011;145(1, Suppl):S1–S15

8. Olutoye OA, Watcha MF, Andropoulos DB. Pediatric obesity: observed impact in the ambulatory surgery setting. J Natl Med Assoc 2011;103(1):27–30

9. Shott SR, Amin R, Chini B, Heubi C, Hotze S, Akers R. Obstructive sleep apnea: Should all children with Down syndrome be tested? Arch Otolaryngol Head Neck Surg 2006;132(4):432–436

10. Rosen D. Some infants with Down syndrome spontaneously outgrow their obstructive sleep apnea. Clin Pediatr (Phila) 2010;49(11):1068–1071

11. Nashed A, Al-Saleh S, Gibbons J, et al. Sleep-related breathing in children with mucopolysaccharidosis. J Inherit Metab Dis 2009;32(4):544–550

12. Randhawa PS, Ahmed J, Nouraei SR, Wyatt ME. Impact of long-term nasopharyngeal airway on health-related quality of life of children with obstructive sleep apnea caused by syndromic craniosynostosis. J Craniofac Surg 2011;22(1):125–128

13. Hermann NV, Kreiborg S, Darvann TA, Jensen BL, Dahl E, Bolund S. Early craniofacial morphology and growth in children with unoperated isolated cleft palate. Cleft Palate Craniofac J 2002;39(6):604–622

14. Afsharpaiman S, Sillence DO, Sheikhvatan M, Ault JE, Waters K. Respiratory events and obstructive sleep apnea in children with achondroplasia: investigation and treatment outcomes. Sleep Breath 2011;15(4):755–761

15. Suresh S, Wales P, Dakin C, Harris MA, Cooper DG. Sleep-related breathing disorder in Duchenne muscular dystrophy: disease spectrum in the paediatric population. J Paediatr Child Health 2005;41(9-10):500–503

16. Cohen SR, Lefaivre JF, Burstein FD, et al. Surgical treatment of obstructive sleep apnea in neurologically compromised patients. Plast Reconstr Surg 1997;99(3):638–646

17. Villa MP, Malagola C, Pagani J, et al. Rapid maxillary expansion in children with obstructive sleep apnea syndrome: 12-month follow-up. Sleep Med 2007;8(2):128–134

18. Cozza P, Gatto R, Ballanti F, Prete L. Management of obstructive sleep apnoea in children with modified monobloc appliances. Eur J Paediatr Dent 2004;5(1):24–29

19. Kuhle S, Urschitz MS. Anti-inflammatory medications for obstructive sleep apnea in children. Cochrane Database Syst Rev 2011;(1):CD007074

20. Goldbart AD, Goldman JL, Veling MC, Gozal D. Leukotriene modifier therapy for mild sleep-disordered breathing in children. Am J Respir Crit Care Med 2005;172(3):364–370

21. Marcus CL, Rosen G, Ward SL, et al. Adherence to and effectiveness of positive airway pressure therapy in children with obstructive sleep apnea. Pediatrics 2006;117(3):e442–e451

22. Fauroux B, Lavis JF, Nicot F, et al. Facial side effects during noninvasive positive pressure ventilation in children. Intensive Care Med 2005;31(7):965–969

23. McGinley B, Halbower A, Schwartz AR, Smith PL, Patil SP, Schneider H. Effect of a high-flow open nasal cannula system on obstructive sleep apnea in children. Pediatrics 2009;124(1):179–188

24. Joshua B, Bahar G, Sulkes J, Shpitzer T, Raveh E. Adenoidectomy: long-term follow-up. Otolaryngol Head Neck Surg 2006;135(4):576–580

25. Brietzke SE, Kenna M, Katz ES, Mitchell E, Roberson D. Pediatric adenoidectomy: what is the effect of obstructive symptoms on the likelihood of future surgery? Int J Pediatr Otorhinolaryngol 2006;70(8):1467–1472

26. Bhattacharjee R, Kheirandish-Gozal L, Spruyt K, et al. Adenotonsillectomy outcomes in treatment of obstructive sleep apnea in children: a multicenter retrospective study. Am J Respir Crit Care Med 2010;182(5):676–683

27. Koltai PJ, Solares CA, Koempel JA, et al. Intracapsular tonsillar reduction (partial tonsillectomy): reviving a historical procedure for obstructive sleep disordered breathing in children. Otolaryngol Head Neck Surg 2003;129(5):532–538

28. Eviatar E, Kessler A, Shlamkovitch N, Vaiman M, Zilber D, Gavriel H. Tonsillectomy vs. partial tonsillectomy for OSAS in children—10 years post-surgery follow-up. Int J Pediatr Otorhinolaryngol 2009;73(5):637–640

29. Powell NB, Zonato AI, Weaver EM, et al. Radiofrequency treatment of turbinate hypertrophy in subjects using continuous positive airway pressure: a randomized, double-blind, placebo-controlled clinical pilot trial. Laryngoscope 2001;111(10):1783–1790

30. Lin AC, Koltai PJ. Persistent pediatric obstructive sleep apnea and lingual tonsillectomy. Otolaryngol Head Neck Surg 2009;141(1):81–85

31. Prager JD, Hopkins BS, Propst EJ, Shott SR, Cotton RT. Oropharyngeal stenosis: a complication of multilevel, single-stage upper airway surgery in children. Arch Otolaryngol Head Neck Surg 2010;136(11):1111–1115

32. Schaaf WE Jr, Wootten CT, Donnelly LF, Ying J, Shott SR. Findings on MR sleep studies as biomarkers to predict outcome of genioglossus advancement in the treatment of obstructive sleep apnea in children and young adults. AJR Am J Roentgenol 2010;194(5):1204–1209

33. Brown KA, Laferrière A, Lakheeram I, Moss IR. Recurrent hypoxemia in children is associated with increased analgesic sensitivity to opiates. Anesthesiology 2006;105(4):665–669

34. Soultan Z, Wadowski S, Rao M, Kravath RE. Effect of treating obstructive sleep apnea by tonsillectomy and/or adenoidectomy on obesity in children. Arch Pediatr Adolesc Med 1999;153(1):33–37

35. Wijga AH, Scholtens S, Wieringa MH, et al. Adenotonsillectomy and the development of overweight. Pediatrics 2009;123(4):1095–1101

36. Jeyakumar A, Fettman N, Armbrecht ES, Mitchell R. A systematic review of adenotonsillectomy as a risk factor for childhood obesity. Otolaryngol Head Neck Surg 2011;144(2):154–158

37. Friedman M, Wilson MN, Lin HC, Chang HW. Updated systematic review of tonsillectomy and adenoidectomy for treatment of pediatric obstructive sleep apnea/hypopnea syndrome. Otolaryngol Head Neck Surg 2009;140(6):800–808

38. Costa DJ, Mitchell RB. Adenotonsillectomy for obstructive sleep apnea in obese children: a meta-analysis. Otolaryngol Head Neck Surg 2009;140(4):455–460

39. Mitchell RB. Adenotonsillectomy for obstructive sleep apnea in children: outcome evaluated by pre- and postoperative polysomnography. Laryngoscope 2007;117(10):1844–1854

8 Pediatric Sinusitis

Yaniv Ebner and Max M. April

Sinusitis is defined as inflammation of the mucosa of one or more paranasal sinuses. When it is acute it is often of viral etiology as part of rhinosinusitis (e.g., in the common cold).

Uncomplicated viral rhinosinusitis is a self-limited infection which spontaneously resolves in 7 to 10 days. Approximately 6 to 13% of viral rhinosinusitis episodes are complicated by acute bacterial rhinosinusitis (ABRS) and only in those cases should an antibiotic be prescribed.

Chronic sinusitis is usually caused by a persistent bacterial infection of the sinuses which fails to resolve due to other associated diseases such as allergy, chronic adenoiditis, immunodeficiency, gastroesophageal reflux disease (GERD), cystic fibrosis (CF), and anatomical abnormalities. Rarely, the etiology might be fungal.

Both acute and chronic sinusitis impairs the patient's quality of life and rarely can progress to an orbital infection endangering vision, or intracranial infection that might result in neurological sequelae or death.

Embryology and Anatomy

The paranasal sinuses evaginate from the nasal cavity and their development is directly linked to the development of the skull and to dentition[1]. The ethmoid and maxillary sinuses are the first to develop in the embryo by the 9th week of gestation. By 1 year of age, the maxillary sinus extends laterally beneath the orbit and elongates posteriorly to approach the periapical region of the first molar. By the 8th year of life, the floor of the maxillary sinus reaches the level of the hard palate. The maxillary sinuses have ostia located superiorly on their medial walls, requiring mucociliary activity for drainage of secretions from the sinus into the nose. The size ratio between the ethmoid and maxillary sinus regions in infants is 2:1 as oppose to 4:5 in adults.[1]

The sphenoid sinus pneumatization of the sphenoid bone begins by 4 years of age and reaches its permanent size by the age of 12 years. Its permanent shape develops during adolescence.[1] The frontal sinuses are the last to develop, starting to pneumatize the frontal bone at about 4 years of age and continue to develop up to late adolescence. The development of the frontal sinuses is variable among individuals, with 80% having bilateral frontal sinuses, about 18% having unilateral frontal sinus hypoplasia, and the remainder with agenesis of the frontal sinuses.

Definitions

Rhinosinusitis is defined as an inflammation of the mucosal lining of the nasal cavity associated with one or more of the paranasal sinuses.[2] Such inflammation occurs commonly during a viral upper respiratory tract infection (URI; common cold). If a secondary bacterial infection is present in the sinuses then the state becomes *bacterial rhinosinusitis* (BRS).[3] BRS is further classified according to duration and recurrence.[2] *Acute bacterial rhinosinusitis* (ABRS) is when symptoms completely resolve in less than 30 days; in *subacute BRS* symptoms completely resolve in ≥30 and <90 days; and in *recurrent BRS* there are at least three episodes of <30 days duration separated by intervals of ≥10 days without symptoms in a 6-month period, or at least four such episodes in a 12-month period.

Chronic sinusitis is defined as a persistence of symptoms (cough, rhinorrhea, nasal obstruction) that last >90 days. *Chronic paranasal inflammation* may be noninfectious in etiology (e.g., allergy, CF, gastroesophageal reflux, exposure to environmental pollutants[2]) or infectious (e.g., bacterial or fungal).

Acute Sinusitis

Young children experience an average of six to eight colds per year. Viral URI in infants and children up to 3 years old is complicated by the development of a secondary bacterial sinusitis in 6 to 8% of those in home care setting and in 10 to 13% of those in group or day care setting.[4] There are no evidence-based data about the prevalence of this complication in children older than 3 years. In temperate climates, ABRS is more common during the autumn and winter seasons.[5] The high prevalence of viral URI in the pediatric population and hence ABRS makes it a very common disease with substantial burden on the patients, caregivers and medical services.

Pathogenesis

To keep normal physiology of the paranasal sinuses, several elements must be preserved: the sinuses should be sterile and in case of bacterial contamination, it should be transient. Bacteria that colonize the mucosa of the nasal cavity and nasopharynx may spread to the adjacent mucosa of the sinuses. Factors that might contribute to sinus bacterial contamination are excessive pressure gradient between the nasal cavity and the sinus during sniffing, sneezing, or blowing the nose resulting in influx of colonized secretions from the nasal cavity into the sinuses. Another suggested mechanism for anaerobe growth in the sinus is decreased partial pressure of oxygen. The predominant pathogens of ABRS are *Streptococcus pneumoniae, Haemophilus influenzae* (nontypable), and *Moraxella catarrhalis.*[6]

Proper mucociliary clearance is crucial to remove contaminating bacteria from the sinus and may be altered due to either mucous viscosity (e.g., in CF and asthma) or ciliary dysfunction. Failure to continuously clear the sinuses would result in bacterial accumulation and infection.

Clearance of the contaminated content of the sinus may be also interfered by obstruction of the ostia. Congestion and edema of the sinonasal mucosa due to viral URI or allergic rhinitis may result in narrowing and obstruction of the sinus ostia that would impair effective drainage.[7] Sinus drainage route may be also affected by anatomic abnormalities such as Haller cell, lateralization of the uncinate process, polyps or masses, concha bullosa, paradoxical concha, septal deviation, nasal foreign body (e.g., nasogastric tube), and craniofacial anomalies.

Children with immunoglobulin (Ig) G subclass immunodeficiency, impaired polysaccharide responsiveness, and selective IgA deficiency are prone to recurrent respiratory infections, usually sinusitis, otitis, or bronchitis.[8]

Diagnosis

The differentiation between uncomplicated viral URI and ABRS is challenging and is made by the length and severity of symptoms.[3] Physical findings and imaging manifestations are similar between the viral and bacterial diseases and thus are not reliable in differentiating between the two. Viral URI should be suspected to be complicated and become an ABRS when nasal symptoms, cough, or both worsen on the sixth or seventh day or persist for more than 10 days without improvement.[2,3]

Nasal symptoms may include discharge, which may be anterior or posterior and of any quality (serous, mucoid, or purulent), and nasal congestion and obstruction. In ABRS, there is a persistent daytime cough (either productive or dry) which is usually worse at night.

ABRS may be diagnosed also when symptoms persist for less than 10 days but are severe at onset. As opposed to viral URI that may present with low-grade fever for less than 48 hours, severe symptoms of ABRS are defined as combination of high fever (at least 39°C) and concurrent purulent nasal discharge for at least three to four consecutive days in a child who appears ill.[2] Facial pain and headache are less common in young children and are not required for the diagnosis of ABRS in a pediatric patient.[9] Halitosis may be reported by the parents as well. Findings on physical examination are similar to those in an uncomplicated viral URI.

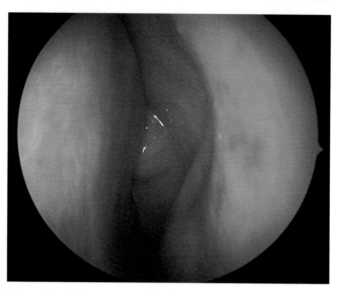

Figure 8.1   Endoscopic view of middle concha with sinusitis findings.

Anterior rhinoscopy may be remarkable for erythematous and congested turbinates as well as discharge. Postnasal drip may be present on oropharyngeal examination.[2] Maxillary and frontal sinus tenderness, elicited with percussion or direct pressure, is infrequent in young children.[10]

Flexible fiberoptic nasal endoscopy is feasible in any age when using a small diameter pediatric endoscope and may show drainage from the osteomeatal complex (**Fig. 8.1**) or sphenoethmoidal recess and can verify the diagnosis.[11] Imaging studies are not recommended as part of the workup of pediatric ABRS and cannot differentiate between viral URI and ABRS.[2] When orbital or intracranial complications of ABRS are suspected then contrast-enhanced computed tomography (CT) scan should be obtained.

Reliable cultures cannot be obtained routinely in children. Although sinus aspiration with a culture that yields ≥10^4 colony-forming units/mL of a significant pathogen is the gold standard for diagnosis of ABRS and specifying the pathogen,[2] it cannot be performed routinely in children in the office setting. Sinus aspiration should be kept to complicated cases (including immunocompromised hosts). Cultures obtained from the throat, nasopharynx, and even the middle meatus are unreliable.[9,12,13]

Treatment

About 50 to 60% of children with ABRS will improve gradually without the use of antibiotics.

There are several objectives of treatment of ABRS with antibiotics. First, adequate antibiotic treatment fosters rapid recovery.[14] The recovery of 20 to 30% of children with ABRS is delayed substantially compared with children who receive appropriate antibiotics.[2] The second objective of antimicrobial treatment is the prevention of suppurative complications,[2] although its effectiveness in doing so has not been adequately studied. The third objective of antibiotic treatment is to minimize exacerbation of asthma.[2,14]

The most common pathogen in children with ABRS is *S. pneumoniae* accounting for approximately 30% of cases, followed by *H. influenzae* and *M. catarrhalis,* each of which are recovered in about 20% cases. *S. pyogenes* accounts for 2 to 5% and anaerobes for 2 to 5%. The maxillary sinus aspirate is found to be sterile in about 30% of pediatric ABRS. Approximately 25% of *S. pneumoniae* are not susceptible to penicillin through alterations in the penicillin-binding proteins; approximately 50% of those are highly resistant to penicillin, and the remaining 50% are intermediate in resistance. Many isolates of *H. influenzae* (35 to 50%) and *M. catarrhalis* (55 to 100%) are β-lactamase-producing and resistant to penicillin.[15]

For treatment to be effective the antibiotic should have an appropriate bacterial coverage against the common pathogens. The probability of resistant pathogen should be evaluated. Dosage and length of treatment period should be sufficient.

Antibiotics are routinely administered via the oral route. For uncomplicated ABRS that is of mild to moderate severity, with no risk factors for bacterial resistance such as attendance in day care, and without antibiotic treatment in the preceding 90 days, the first line of treatment is amoxicillin (45 to 90 mg/kg/d in two divided doses).[16] In case of increased likelihood of microbial resistance (e.g., antibiotic treatment in the preceding 90 days, or attendance in day care), amoxicillin–clavulanate is recommended with dosage of 80 to 90 mg/kg/d of amoxicillin component in two divided doses. Other treatment options are with cephalosporins which are usually safe in children with mild allergic reaction (e.g., mild rash) to penicillins. Patients with severe allergic reaction to penicillins (e.g., severe rash, angioedema, anaphylaxis), should be treated with macrolides such as clarithromycin or azithromycin. Patients with type 1 hypersensitivity reactions to penicillin who are known to be infected with penicillin-resistant pneumococci can be treated with clindamycin.[2]

In more complicated cases (e.g., severe symptoms, immunodeficient patient, and potential orbital or intracranial complications), hospitalization for intravenous antibiotic therapy is recommended. Regimens options include cefotaxime or ceftriaxone.

Antibiotic therapy should last 10 to 14 days or be continued until the patient is symptom-free for 7 days.[2]

Symptoms are expected to improve within 48 to 72 hours.[14] In children who do not respond to amoxicillin, antibiotic therapy may be changed to either high-dose amoxicillin–clavulanate or a cephalosporin. If these regimens fail, CT should be considered to confirm the diagnosis and intravenous (IV) ceftriaxone or cefotaxime may be tried. Sinus aspiration may be indicated to obtain cultures and antibiotics sensitivities. If cultures cannot be obtained, the addition of vancomycin with or without metronidazole may be indicated.

Adjunctive Therapy

Saline nasal irrigation, decongestants (topical or systemic), antihistamines, and intranasal corticosteroids are widely used as adjuncts to antibiotics in the treatment of ABRS.

Decongestants may reduce tissue edema, improve ostial drainage, and provide symptomatic relief.[17] However, these benefits may be offset by an increased viscosity of secretions and decreased blood flow to the nasal mucosa, which may impair delivery of antibiotics to the sinuses. Similarly, antihistamines have the potential to dry secretions and impair sinus drainage.

A Cochrane review was conducted in 2010 to address the controversy about the efficacy of these adjuncts in children with ABRS.[18] This evidence-based review found no evidence supporting the use of saline irrigation, decongestants, or antihistamines in children with ABRS. Furthermore, there is growing evidence from observational studies and from randomized trials of these medications in children with other URIs, which shows that the use of antihistamines and decongestants can lead to significant adverse events, especially in young children. Accordingly, the use of these medications was not recommended. Saline irrigation in general is well-tolerated, although there is no data to support its efficacy.[18]

Intranasal corticosteroids theoretically may decrease inflammation of the mucous membranes which contributes to obstruction of the ostia and impaired mucociliary clearance. According to the available data, intranasal budesonide has a modest effect on cough and nasal discharge, but the effect is noted only during the second week of therapy.[19] Given this late marginal effect, the use of intranasal corticosteroids in children with ABRS does not seem to be beneficial.

Complications of ABRS

ABRS, if left untreated, may spread bacterial infection to adjacent structures and cause serious orbital or intracranial complications, which can also be the presenting manifestation.

The orbit is the most common site of extension of rhinosinusitis. Ethmoid sinusitis may spread through the thin lamina papyracea or through congenital, surgical, or traumatic dehiscences. Infection may also spread through the anterior and posterior ethmoid neurovascular foramina and the valveless veins. Orbital extension of ethmoid sinusitis is the most common cause of unilateral proptosis in children.[20] A commonly used classification of orbital complications was introduced by Chandler in 1970[21]:

Chandler Classification

I. Preseptal Cellulitis

Impeded venous and lymphatic drainage from the obstructed sinus may result in inflammatory edema anterior to the

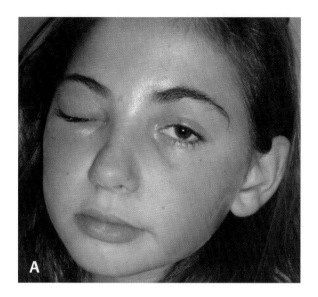

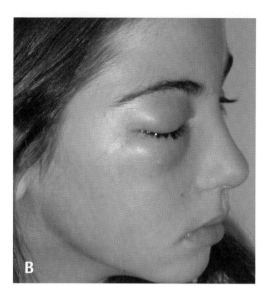

Figure 8.2 Preseptal cellulitis. (A) Anterior view and (B) lateral view. *Printed with permission.*

orbital septum. Manifestations are eyelid swelling, erythema, and tenderness (**Fig. 8.2A, B**). Visual acuity, pupillary reaction, extraocular motility, and intraocular pressure are normal. A CT scan is usually unnecessary. Treatment includes broad-spectrum antibiotics which may be oral in mild cases with ensured follow-up. Admission for IV antibiotics and close observation is usually recommended under 3 years of age. Additional recommendations are head elevation, warm packs, and management of the underlying cause.[22]

II. Postseptal Orbital Cellulitis

This is defined as diffuse orbital infection and inflammation confined to the bony wall of the orbit and without abscess formation. The findings are eyelid edema and erythema, mild proptosis, and chemosis. Motility may be limited but visual acuity is not impaired. The patient should be admitted for IV antibiotic treatment and an ophthalmology consultation is warranted for daily assessments of visual acuity and color vision, pupillary reaction, and extraocular motility. A CT scan of the sinuses and orbits is required as well. Indications for surgical drainage of the sinuses are the following:

1. Visual acuity of 20/60 (or worse) or other severe orbital complications on initial evaluation.
2. Progression of orbital signs and symptoms despite therapy.
3. Lack of improvement within 48 hours despite medical therapy.[23]

III. Subperiosteal Abscess

Ethmoid sinusitis may spread through the lamina papyracea to the adjacent orbit and cause an orbital subperiosteal abscess (SPA), which is usually superomedial or inferomedial. An SPA can expand rapidly and may lead to blindness by compromising optic nerve function.

An SPA should be suspected when a patient who has orbital cellulitis develops worsening proptosis and gaze restriction. It can also be the presenting symptom. Ophthalmologic evaluation is essential if an SPA is suspected. A loss of red–green perception may happen before the deterioration of visual acuity. A contrast-enhanced sinus CT is required to verify the diagnosis and to assess its severity. Findings are a ring-enhanced lesion or air–fluid level in the extraconal space, displacement and enlargement of the medial rectus muscle and proptosis (**Figs. 8.3** and **8.4**).

Treatment consists of the immediate administration of IV antibiotics with the potential need for surgical

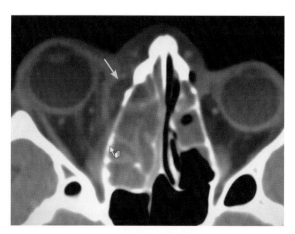

Figure 8.3 Computed tomography axial scan of ethmoiditis with right side subperiosteal abscess (arrow).

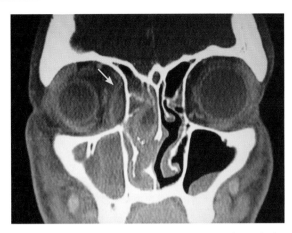

Figure 8.4   Computed tomography scan (coronal view) showing lateralization of the right globe due to subperiosteal abscess (arrow).

intervention. Criteria for medical management of medial SPA are the following[24]:

1. Normal vision, pupil, and retina.
2. No ophthalmoplegia.
3. Intraocular pressure of less than 20 mm Hg.
4. Proptosis of 5 mm or less.
5. Abscess width of 4 mm or less.

Surgical treatment for SPA includes transnasal endoscopy that involves ethmoidectomy, skeletonizing of the lamina papyracea, and drainage of the orbital collection by penetrating the lamina papyracea. When location of the abscess precludes a transnasal endoscopic approach, an external approach via a Lynch incision might be warranted. Transnasal and external approaches can be combined for maximal access and exposure.

IV. Orbital Abscess

When infection breaches the orbital periosteum and orbital phlegmon organizes into a pus collection, an orbital abscess forms. Symptoms and signs include marked proptosis, chemosis, complete ophthalmoplegia, and visual impairment. Orbital abscess carries a risk for progression to irreversible blindness. A CT scan is required and will show areas of cavitation that appear radiolucent.

Surgical drainage is mandatory and includes the involved sinuses and the orbital abscess. As opposed to SPA drainage, in the case of orbital abscess the periorbita must be incised to access the orbital content. Drainage of an intraconal abscess is best achieved through a transnasal endoscopic approach combined with external orbital approach.

V. Cavernous Sinus Thrombosis

Infection from the sinuses and the orbit can spread to the cavernous sinus. Routes of spread include free anastomosis, valveless venous system as well as the superior and inferior ophthalmic veins which all drain into the cavernous sinus

posteriorly. The hallmark of cavernous sinus thrombosis is a progression of symptoms to the opposite eye. Physical examination is remarkable for rapidly progressive chemosis and ophthalmoplegia, severe retinal engorgement, fever, and prostration. The patient condition may progress to loss of vision, meningitis, and death. Carotid thrombosis may follow and result in concomitant strokes, subdural empyema, and brain abscess.

Imaging studies include CT scan and magnetic resonance imaging using flow parameters and magnetic resonance venography.

Treatment of cavernous sinus thrombosis should include high-dose IV antibiotics that cross the blood–brain barrier for 3 to 4 weeks or for 6 to 8 weeks if an intracranial complication is evident. In addition, surgical drainage of the affected sinuses is required. The role of anticoagulation in the treatment of cavernous sinus thrombosis is controversial.

Intracranial complications are less frequent than orbital complications and are seen more with frontal or sphenoidal sinusitis. Intracranial spread of the infection should be suspected when a change in neurological or mental status is evident. Other symptoms and signs are high fever, severe headache, nausea and vomiting, seizures and signs of increased intracranial pressure. Neurological and/or neurosurgical consultation is warranted in case a patient with sinusitis develops one of the above issues. Intracranial complications include meningitis, epidural abscess, subdural empyema (**Figs. 8.5** and **8.6A, B**), and brain abscess. Frontal sinusitis may spread to the sinus bony walls and result in an osteomyelitis of the anterior and/or posterior tables. This may result in a frontal bone SPA and forehead cellulitis (Pott's puffy tumor).[25]

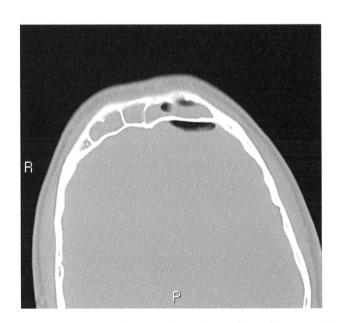

Figure 8.5   Computed tomography axial scan of frontal sinusitis with subdural empyema.

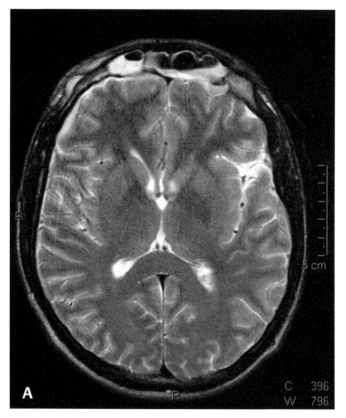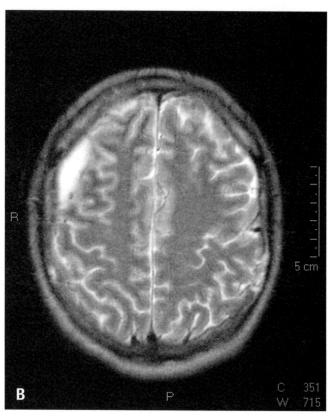

Figure 8.6 (A) Magnetic resonance image T2 axial view of frontal sinusitis associated with subdural empyema and (B) Magnetic resonance image T2 axial superior section showing subdural empyema.

Chronic Sinusitis

Chronic rhinosinusitis (CRS) is an inflammation of the sinuses that endures for more than 3 months despite treatment. This ailment is associated with significant decrement of quality of life.[26]

Pathogenesis

Pediatric CRS histopathology shows a different inflammatory response from the adult form that may attest to a different pathophysiologic pathway.[28] The etiology of CRS is derived from interactions among local host factors, systemic host factors, and environmental factors:

Anatomic abnormalities (e.g., septal deviation, conch bullosa, and Haller cells) might be a contributing factor to CRS but are uncommon in children. If the structural abnormality is obvious this might lead to earlier surgical intervention. Enlarged adenoid may have no relationship to increased incidence of CRS according to recent studies.[29,30]

The causal relationship of allergic rhinitis and asthma to CRS is unclear. The "united airway theory" suggests that allergic rhinitis, asthma, and CRS are all manifestations of inflammation of a continuous airway and lie in the spectrum of symptoms rather than as distinct disease entities. Although it was suggested that up to 70% of children with CRS also have allergic rhinitis,[31] one study has shown an incidence of allergies in pediatric CRS patients similar to that of the general population at approximately 30%.[32] Asthma has been reported to predispose to CRS.[33]

GERD has been implicated as a cause of nasal mucosal chronic inflammatory changes and as predisposing factor in CRS.[34] A high prevalence of GERD (63%) was found in children with medically refractory CRS.[35]

Impaired mucociliary clearance secondary to CF or, less commonly, to primary ciliary dyskinesia or Kartagener syndrome increases the risk to CRS as well as its severity.[36] Such patients may benefit from a more prompt surgical intervention.

Sinonasal symptoms correlate with the quantity of bacterial colonization in the adenoid.[37] The adenoid pad in pediatric CRS patients has been shown to be covered with a biofilm of bacteria that may be resistant to antibiotics and may provide a reservoir of bacteria in patients with CRS.

Diagnosis

Diagnosis of CRS in children is challenging given the high prevalence of recurrent URIs and perennial allergic rhinitis in this population. Symptoms in the pediatric population can be age dependent. In younger patients the objective witnessed signs are usually described by the parents. An infant might express pain and discomfort only as irritability. Chronic cough is a very common presenting symptom in pediatric CRS. Nasal discharge and nasal obstruction may also be reported. Older children can give a more detailed and localized description of their subjective symptoms, such as nasal congestion, otalgia, facial pressure or pain, or hyposmia.

Physical Examination

Rhinoscopy with an otoscope is used to examine the nose for signs of mucosal inflammation such as congestion, erythema, crusting, and mucopurulent discharge. This method of examination in children is often limited to the anterior nose, especially when the turbinates are congested. To fully evaluate the nasal cavity flexible endoscopy is required. A mixture of topical anesthetic (e.g., lidocaine) and a sympathomimetic drug (e.g., oxymethazolone) is used topically in the nasal cavity before examination. Cocaine is usually avoided due to side effects. A pediatric flexible fiberoptic endoscope is lubricated and inserted into the nasal cavity. The middle meatus and sphenoethmoidal recess are evaluated for obstruction and discharge. The nasopharynx can be evaluated for adenoid inflammation and size.

Imaging is usually done when either complications of sinusitis are suspected or for evaluation of the extent of the disease and the patient anatomy before planned sinus surgery. The imaging study of choice is CT. It has been proven to have both high sensitivity and specificity.[27] Plain radiographs tend to be less reliable. The potential risk of exposing a pediatric patient to radiation should be considered when ordering a CT scan.

Treatment

Initial treatment of pediatric CRS should be medical. An exception may be considered when there is an obvious anatomic obstruction or in a patient with CF or mucociliary dyskinesia.

Medical Therapy

Broad-spectrum antibiotics that cover the polymicrobial nature of CRS should be given for a long-term treatment of 3 to 6 weeks.[38] Ideally, the choice of antibiotic is based on culture susceptibility results. Practically it is challenging to acquire a reliable culture from the pediatric patient in the office setting. The first line of therapy is usually amoxicillin–clavulanic acid 90 mg/kg/d in divided doses every 12 hours with meals. For the treatment of methicillin-resistant *Staphylococcus aureus*, a combination of clindamycin and trimethoprim–sulfamethoxazole is an option. In patients with polyps such as in CF and "triad asthma syndrome," *Pseudomonas aeruginosa* is prevalent. Those patients may be treated with fluoroquinolones such as levofloxacin or a combination of ciprofloxacin plus metronidazole.

When oral antibiotic treatment fails, a long-term intravenous antibiotic course may be considered as an alternative to surgery.[39] The role of fungal infection in pediatric CRS remains unclear, as fungi can colonize the sinuses without clinical significance.[40]

Nasal steroid sprays are commonly used with the logic of decreasing the inflammation and improving the edema and mucociliary clearance. This practice is not supported by randomized controlled clinical trials and a review of the literature concluded a probable, modest benefit from topical intranasal steroid use.[41] At present, there is no evidence-based support to the benefit of other adjunct therapies such as oral antihistamines, mucolytic agents, oral steroids, and nasal saline irrigation.

Reflux was found to be prevalent in pediatric CRS patients resistant to medical treatment with antireflux therapy improving the symptoms in most of those patients.[35] Exposure of the patient to second-hand smoke was shown to decrease the efficacy of CRS treatment and thus it should be avoided.

Surgical Treatment

When long-term medical treatment fails, surgery should be considered. Surgery is performed in a stepwise approach and has been shown to improve symptoms significantly. Parents should be informed that a complete cure is not always possible.

Adenoidectomy

Adenoidectomy with or without antral lavage is recommended as first-line surgery. The adenoid may provide a reservoir of pathogenic bacteria and the presence of a biofilm may decrease the efficacy of antibiotics to clear the infection.[37] To remove this reservoir an adenoidectomy may be required and has been reported to be effective in alleviating pediatric CRS in up to 70% of cases. Antral lavage performed at the time of adenoidectomy can improve the results of the surgery to as high as 88%.[42] Patients with asthma or a high Lund-Mackay CT score are less likely to benefit from adenoidectomy alone, and in this patient population adenoidectomy should be combined with functional endoscopic sinus surgery (FESS).[43]

FESS

In those cases when adenoidectomy with antral lavage fails, FESS is the second line in surgical treatment algorithm. In patients with a small or minimal adenoid pad, FESS can be considered as first-line intervention. FESS is considered a safe intervention in the pediatric population in regard to midfacial growth[44] and results in improvement of symptoms in 80 to 100% of patients.[43] Complication rates from surgery are low and include orbital injury, cerebrospinal fluid leak, nasolacrimal duct injury, and bleeding.

Preoperative CT scan of the sinuses is essential to give the surgeon "a road map" of the nasosinusal complex and to detect structural variants or abnormalities that might increase the risk of injuring adjacent structures. In pediatric patients it is important to have a current scan due to the ongoing change in size and shape of the sinuses during the development of the child.

Surgical intervention is usually conservative and a maxillary antrostomy and anterior ethmoidectomy is sufficient in most cases.[45] A deviated septum or a concha bullosa, if present, may be addressed as well. Image guidance may be helpful for complicated cases involving the frontal sinus, sphenoid sinus, orbit, or skull base.[46] Postoperative saline irrigation may prevent crusting and facilitate the re-mucosalization but the compliance is expected to be low in a young pediatric patient. A "second look" endoscopy and debridement has been shown not to affect the clinical outcome and is not routinely preformed.[47]

Special consideration should be taken with CRS patients who have an underlying disease process that interferes with physiologic mucociliary clearance (e.g., ciliary dyskinesia, Kartagener syndrome, CF). The CRS of this group of patients is difficult to treat and often requires revision surgeries.[48] In addition, those patients might not benefit from "functional" sinus surgery of the natural ostia and a gravity-based drainage surgery should be considered.

Immunocompromised patients are susceptible to opportunistic infections as well as severe intraorbital and intracranial complications from rhinosinusitis. Thus, FESS should be considered even in an acute setting in case of failure of an aggressive medical therapy. FESS should be offered early to pediatric patients with allergic fungal sinusitis in whom medical therapy alone is less effective. The treatment of those patients should be comprehensive and include nasal steroids, saline irrigation, and immunotherapy for fungal allergy.[49]

References

1. Wolf G, Anderhuber W, Kuhn F. Development of the paranasal sinuses in children: implications for paranasal sinus surgery. Ann Otol Rhinol Laryngol 1993;102(9):705–711

2. American Academy of Pediatrics. Subcommittee on Management of Sinusitis and Committee on Quality Improvement. Clinical practice guideline: management of sinusitis. Pediatrics 2001;108(3):798–808

3. Meltzer EO, Hamilos DL, Hadley JA, et al. Rhinosinusitis: Establishing definitions for clinical research and patient care. Otolaryngol Head Neck Surg 2004;131(6, Suppl):S1–S62

4. Wald ER, Guerra N, Byers C. Upper respiratory tract infections in young children: duration of and frequency of complications. Pediatrics 1991;87(2):129–133

5. Van Buchem FL, Peeters MF, Knottnerus JA. Maxillary sinusitis in children. Clin Otolaryngol Allied Sci 1992;17(1):49–53

6. Wald ER. Microbiology of acute and chronic sinusitis in children and adults. Am J Med Sci 1998;316(1):13–20

7. Carson JL, Collier AM, Hu SS. Acquired ciliary defects in nasal epithelium of children with acute viral upper respiratory infections. N Engl J Med 1985;312(8):463–468

8. Stiehm ER. The four most common pediatric immunodeficiencies. J Immunotoxicol 2008;5(2):227–234

9. Wald ER, et al. Acute maxillary sinusitis in children. N Engl J Med 1981;304(13):749–754

10. Fireman P. Diagnosis of sinusitis in children: emphasis on the history and physical examination. J Allergy Clin Immunol 1992;90(3 Pt 2):433–436

11. Berger G, Berger RL. The contribution of flexible endoscopy for diagnosis of acute bacterial rhinosinusitis. Eur Arch Otorhinolaryngol 2011;268(2):235–240

12. Slavin RG, Spector SL, Bernstein IL, et al. The diagnosis and management of sinusitis: a practice parameter update. J Allergy Clin Immunol 2005;116(6, Suppl):S13–S47

13. Gordts F, Abu Nasser I, Clement PA, Pierard D, Kaufman L. Bacteriology of the middle meatus in children. Int J Pediatr Otorhinolaryngol 1999;48(2):163–167

14. Wald ER, Nash D, Eickhoff J. Effectiveness of amoxicillin/clavulanate potassium in the treatment of acute bacterial sinusitis in children. Pediatrics 2009;124(1):9–15

15. Brook I. Current issues in the management of acute bacterial sinusitis in children. Int J Pediatr Otorhinolaryngol 2007;71(11):1653–1661

16. Anon JB, Jacobs MR, Poole MD, et al. Antimicrobial treatment guidelines for acute bacterial rhinosinusitis. Otolaryngol Head Neck Surg 2004; 130(1, Suppl):1–45

17. Leung AK, Kellner JD. Acute sinusitis in children: diagnosis and management. J Pediatr Health Care 2004;18(2):72–76

18. Shaikh N, Wald ER, Pi M. Decongestants, antihistamines and nasal irrigation for acute sinusitis in children. Cochrane Database Syst Rev 2010;(12):CD007909

19. Barlan IB, Erkan E, Bakir M, Berrak S, Başaran MM. Intranasal budesonide spray as an adjunct to oral antibiotic therapy for acute sinusitis in children. Ann Allergy Asthma Immunol 1997;78(6):598–601

20. Osguthorpe JD, Hochman M. Inflammatory sinus diseases affecting the orbit. Otolaryngol Clin North Am 1993;26(4):657–671

21. Chandler JR, Langenbrunner DJ, Stevens ER. The pathogenesis of orbital complications in acute sinusitis. Laryngoscope 1970;80(9):1414–1428

22. Donahue SP, Schwartz G. Preseptal and orbital cellulitis in childhood. A changing microbiologic spectrum. Ophthalmology 1998;105(10):1902–1905; discussion 1905–1906

23. Younis RT, Lazar RH, Bustillo A, Anand VK. Orbital infection as a complication of sinusitis: are diagnostic and treatment trends changing? Ear Nose Throat J 2002;81(11):771–775

24. Oxford LE, McClay J. Medical and surgical management of subperiosteal orbital abscess secondary to acute sinusitis in children. Int J Pediatr Otorhinolaryngol 2006;70(11):1853–1861

25. Bambakidis NC, Cohen AR. Intracranial complications of frontal sinusitis in children: Pott's puffy tumor revisited. Pediatr Neurosurg 2001;35(2):82–89

26. Cunningham JM, Chiu EJ, Landgraf JM, Gliklich RE. The health impact of chronic recurrent rhinosinusitis in children. Arch Otolaryngol Head Neck Surg 2000;126(11):1363–1368

27. Bhattacharyya N, Jones DT, Hill M, Shapiro NL. The diagnostic accuracy of computed tomography in pediatric chronic rhinosinusitis. Arch Otolaryngol Head Neck Surg 2004;130(9):1029–1032

28. Berger G, Kogan T, Paker M, Berger-Achituv S, Ebner Y. Pediatric

chronic rhinosinusitis histopathology: differences and similarities with the adult form. Otolaryngol Head Neck Surg 2011; 144(1): 85–90

29. Tuncer U, Aydogan B, Soylu L, Simsek M, Akcali C, Kucukcan A. Chronic rhinosinusitis and adenoid hypertrophy in children. Am J Otolaryngol 2004;25(1):5–10

30. Bercin AS, Ural A, Kutluhan A, Yurttaş V. Relationship between sinusitis and adenoid size in pediatric age group. Ann Otol Rhinol Laryngol 2007;116(7):550–553

31. Furukawa CT. The role of allergy in sinusitis in children. J Allergy Clin Immunol 1992;90(3 Pt 2):515–517

32. Leo G, Piacentini E, Incorvaia C, Consonni D, Frati F. Chronic rhinosinusitis and allergy. Pediatr Allergy Immunol 2007;18 (Suppl 18):19–21

33. Tosca MA, Riccio AM, Marseglia GL, et al. Nasal endoscopy in asthmatic children: assessment of rhinosinusitis and adenoiditis incidence, correlations with cytology and microbiology. Clin Exp Allergy 2001;31(4):609–615

34. Bothwell MR, Parsons DS, Talbot A, Barbero GJ, Wilder B. Outcome of reflux therapy on pediatric chronic sinusitis. Otolaryngol Head Neck Surg 1999;121(3):255–262

35. Phipps CD, Wood WE, Gibson WS, Cochran WJ. Gastroesophageal reflux contributing to chronic sinus disease in children: a prospective analysis. Arch Otolaryngol Head Neck Surg 2000; 126(7):831–836

36. Babinski D, Trawinska-Bartnicka M. Rhinosinusitis in cystic fibrosis: not a simple story. Int J Pediatr Otorhinolaryngol 2008;72(5):619–624

37. Shin KS, Cho SH, Kim KR, et al. The role of adenoids in pediatric rhinosinusitis. Int J Pediatr Otorhinolaryngol 2008;72(11):1643–1650

38. Clement PA, Bluestone CD, Gordts F, et al. Management of rhinosinusitis in children. Int J Pediatr Otorhinolaryngol 1999;49 (Suppl 1):S95–S100

39. Don DM, Yellon RF, Casselbrant ML, Bluestone CD. Efficacy of a stepwise protocol that includes intravenous antibiotic therapy for the management of chronic sinusitis in children and adolescents. Arch Otolaryngol Head Neck Surg 2001;127(9):1093–1098

40. Ponikau JU, Sherris DA, Kern EB, et al. The diagnosis and incidence of allergic fungal sinusitis. Mayo Clin Proc 1999;74(9):877–884

41. Fiocchi A, Sarratud T, Bouygue GR, Ghiglioni D, Bernardo L, Terracciano L. Topical treatment of rhinosinusitis. Pediatr Allergy Immunol 2007;18(Suppl 18):62–67

42. Ramadan HH, Cost JL. Outcome of adenoidectomy versus adenoidectomy with maxillary sinus wash for chronic rhinosinusitis in children. Laryngoscope 2008;118(5):871–873

43. Ramadan HH. Surgical management of chronic sinusitis in children. Laryngoscope 2004;114(12):2103–2109

44. Bothwell MR, Piccirillo JF, Lusk RP, Ridenour BD. Long-term outcome of facial growth after functional endoscopic sinus surgery. Otolaryngol Head Neck Surg 2002;126(6):628–634

45. Sobol SE, Samadi DS, Kazahaya K, Tom LW. Trends in the management of pediatric chronic sinusitis: survey of the American Society of Pediatric Otolaryngology. Laryngoscope 2005;115(1):78–80

46. Parikh SR, Cuellar H, Sadoughi B, Aroniadis O, Fried MP et al. Indications for image-guidance in pediatric sinonasal surgery. Int J Pediatr Otorhinolaryngol 2009;73(3):351–356

47. Younis RT. The pros and cons of second-look sinonasal endoscopy after endoscopic sinus surgery in children. Arch Otolaryngol Head Neck Surg 2005;131(3):267–269

48. Ramadan HH. Revision endoscopic sinus surgery in children: surgical causes of failure. Laryngoscope 2009;119(6):1214–1217

49. Campbell JM, Graham M, Gray HC, Bower C, Blaiss MS, Jones SM. Allergic fungal sinusitis in children. Ann Allergy Asthma Immunol 2006;96(2):286–290

9 Allergic Rhinitis in Children

Andrea Ellen Nath and Fuad M. Baroody

Allergic rhinitis is a manifestation of the hypersensitivity of the nasal mucosa to foreign substances mediated through immunoglobulin (Ig) E antibodies. It usually manifests with nasal and eye symptoms, which include sneezing, runny nose, stuffy nose, itching of the nose, throat and ears, as well as eye tearing, redness, and itching. Because eye manifestations are often present, the disease is more commonly referred to as allergic rhinoconjunctivitis (AR). AR is the most common chronic condition in children and is most prevalent during school age. It is estimated to affect anywhere between 25 and 40% of the pediatric population in the United States with the highest incidence in the 13 to 14 year age group.[1] During childhood, males are affected more often than females, but this gender distribution equalizes in adulthood. Most patients with AR develop symptoms before 20 years of age, with seasonal rhinitis rarely seen in children less than 2 years of age. This reflects the need for low exposure over a period of time to generate sensitization and clinical symptoms. Both a family history of allergy and a diagnosis of asthma increase the likelihood of developing AR.

Burden of Disease

Several studies have demonstrated significant impairment of quality of life in patients with AR and this applies to both generic and disease-specific measures. Disease-specific tools are more sensitive to change, with the rhinoconjunctivitis quality-of-life questionnaire developed by Juniper and colleagues being the most commonly used.[2] There are modifications of this questionnaire that are used for perennial rhinitis in adolescents (12 to17 years old) and children (6 to 12 years old). AR also affects the emotional well-being, productivity, cognitive functioning, and school performance of affected children and adolescents. In a survey of 35,757 U.S. households—the Pediatric Allergies in America survey—subjects with nasal allergy between 4 and 17 years of age were targeted with various questionnaires aimed at their own as well as their parents' perceptions of the effects of nasal allergies on daily life.[3] The responses were compared between children with and without allergies. A significantly lower percentage of children with nasal allergies were rated as having excellent health by their parents (43%) as compared with parents of children without allergies (59%). Similarly, lower proportions of children with allergies were described as "happy," "calm and peaceful," having "lots of energy," and being "full of life" as compared with children without allergies. When looking at missed school or day care in the past

12 months because of allergies, health reasons, or both, the absenteeism rate was similar in children with and without nasal allergies. However, the proportion of children with diminished performance while at school as assessed by the parents was significantly higher in children with nasal allergies (40%) as compared with their nonallergic peers (11%). The parents of children with allergies also reported a 30% decrease in their children's productivity at school and at home when allergy symptoms were at their worst. When asked about effects of nasal allergies on sleep, parents of children with nasal allergies were twice more likely to describe sleep problems in their children as compared with the parents of children without allergies. Thus, when comparing children with nasal allergies to those without allergies, higher proportions of the children with allergies were reported to have difficulty falling asleep (32 vs. 12%), waking up during the night (26 vs. 8%), and lack of a good night's sleep (29 vs. 12%). The reported sleep disturbances associated with allergic rhinitis probably contribute to the significant negative impact of the disease on the quality of life of affected children.

In addition to the emotional and physical sequelae of the disease, AR imparts a significant economic burden related to the above sequelae, with direct costs to patients and insurance providers, and indirect costs that include absenteeism and decreased productivity. It is therefore estimated that the total economic burden of AR in children in the United States may be higher than US$ 5 billion a year.

Pathophysiology

AR is caused by an IgE-mediated hypersensitivity reaction that involves one or more allergens. The events involve a series of cellular and physiologic reactions that can be summarized as follows.[4] During the initial stage of the disease, low-dose exposure of the antigen over a prolonged period of time leads to the production of specific IgE antibodies and *sensitization*. Antigen that is deposited on the nasal mucosa is taken up by antigen presenting cells such as macrophages, dendritic cells, and Langerhans cells. These cells partially degrade the antigen and the by-products are then presented to T-helper (TH) cells in the context of class II major histocompatibility complex molecules. Interleukin (IL)-1-activated TH cells then secrete cytokines, which promote other cells involved in the immune response. TH cells have varying phenotypes, the most common of which are differentiated by cytokine secretion. TH1 CD4+ cells secrete interferon-γ and play a major role in intracellular pathogen clearance and delayed-type hypersensitivity. TH2

75

CD4+ cells are important in allergic reactions, secreting IL-4, IL-5 and IL-13, which are involved in the production of IgE and recruitment and survival of eosinophils at the sites of allergic reactions. Antigen-specific IgE then attaches to mast cells and basophils, sensitizing the nasal mucosa.

On repeated exposure to the allergen to which the individual is now sensitized, the IgE antibodies on the surface of mast cells and basophils act as receptors for the allergen and resultant cross-linking of the IgE receptors by antigen leads to the release of preformed (histamine and tryptase) and newly synthesized (leukotrienes, prostaglandins, platelet-activating factor, bradykinin, cytokines) inflammatory mediators (**Fig. 9.1**). The released mediators stimulate nerves, glands, and blood vessels and lead to the typical symptoms of AR namely, pruritus, sneezing, rhinorrhea, and nasal congestion. This sequence of events, referred to as the *early phase response*, has been supported by actual measurement of these mediators in nasal secretions during seasonal allergic disease and nasal allergen provocation experiments.

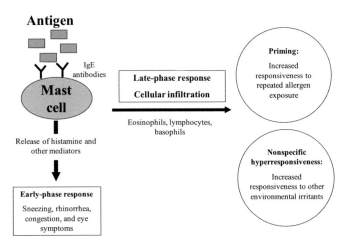

Figure 9.1 Schematic of the pathophysiologic events in allergic rhinitis. Cross-linking of immunoglobulin E receptors on the surface of mast cells by allergen in a sensitized individual leads to the release of mediators and the early phase allergic response. This is followed by cellular recruitment into the nasal mucosa and the late phase response. As a result of increased inflammation, the nasal mucosa becomes more responsive to repeated allergen exposure (priming) as well as to nonspecific environmental stimuli (nonspecific hyperresponsiveness).

The nasal response to allergen also leads to the stimulation of *nasal reflexes* by the inflammatory substances released during the early phase response. This leads to an amplification of the nasal response by the generation of a nasonasal reflex that is secretory in nature and mediated by the parasympathetic nervous system. Furthermore, these reflexes lead to the propagation of the allergic response to distant organs such as the eyes and the paranasal sinuses. In addition to the parasympathetic nervous system, several neuropeptides have been identified within the nasal mucosa in patients with AR and are thought to contribute to these reflexes.

Hours after the early phase response, there is a recurrence of nasal symptoms as well as the influx of inflammatory cells, notably eosinophils, into the nasal mucosa and nasal secretions, a phenomenon referred to as the *late phase response*. The levels of several cytokines including IL-4, IL-5, granulocyte-macrophage–colony-stimulating factors, IL-3, and IL-2 have been reported to increase within the nasal mucosa after allergen exposure. These cytokines are instrumental in orchestrating the allergic inflammatory response and are known to stimulate IgE production by plasma cells, as well as the recruitment and survival of inflammatory cells from the peripheral circulation into the nasal mucosa. Again, these processes are well documented by the recovery of these cytokines and inflammatory cells in allergic patients during seasonal disease as well as after experimental allergen provocation.

The above-described allergic inflammation results in a state of heightened responsiveness of the nasal mucosa. This translates into increased reaction to repeated allergen exposure, a phenomenon referred to as *priming*, as well as increased responsiveness to nonallergenic stimuli, such as histamine or methacholine, referred to as *nonspecific hyperresponsiveness*. Clinically, patients demonstrate worsening of symptoms as the allergy season progresses related to increased responsiveness to lower amounts of allergen related to priming. Patients can also exhibit an increased reaction after exposure to strong odors, pollution, or cigarette smoke during the allergy season, an example of nonspecific hyperresponsiveness.

Clinical Manifestations

Allergic rhinitis is often underdiagnosed in children due to their inability to communicate the duration of symptoms and subtle signs of allergic rhinitis. The most common symptoms of allergic rhinitis are recurrent episodes of sneezing, pruritus, rhinorrhea, nasal congestion, and watery and itchy eyes. Less common symptoms include itchy throat, itchy ears, and postnasal drip. When a large cohort of children with allergic rhinitis and their parents were surveyed, the reported frequency of nasal allergy symptoms during the worst month in the past year were quite similar between the parents and the children and were in descending frequency of occurrence: nasal congestion, repeated sneezing, runny nose, watering eyes, postnasal drip, red/itching eyes, nasal itching, dry cough, awakened/unable to sleep, headache, facial pain, and ear pain.[3] The following symptoms were reported as most bothersome: nasal congestion (highest proportion), headache, runny nose, repeated sneezing, red/itching eyes, dry cough, postnasal drip, watering eyes, ear pain, nasal itching, and facial pain (lowest proportion). Therefore, it is clear that nasal congestion is the most common and also the most bothersome symptom of allergic rhinitis in children.

The disease has been classified differently in different guidelines and practice parameters. It is labeled as seasonal (symptoms occurring during specific seasons, e.g., spring [in patients sensitized to grasses and trees] and fall [in patients sensitized to ragweed]), perennial (symptoms occur continuously such as in individuals sensitized to indoor allergens [dust mite, indoor molds, and pets]), or episodic, a new category described in the most recent American guidelines (symptoms elicited by sporadic exposures to allergens [e.g., a cat-allergic individual who occasionally visits relatives who have a cat in the house]).[5] In an international set of guidelines developed in Europe under the auspices of the World Health Organization, the Allergic Rhinitis and its Impact on Asthma guidelines, allergic rhinitis is classified based more on duration and severity of symptoms.[6] In these guidelines, allergic rhinitis is classified as intermittent (symptoms occurring less than 4 days a week *or* less than 4 weeks a year) or persistent (symptoms occurring more than 4 days per week *and* for more than 4 weeks in a year). Additionally the rhinitis is described as mild (the patient has normal sleep, daily activities, sport, leisure, work and school, and no troublesome symptoms) or moderate to severe (the patient has abnormal sleep, impairment of daily activities, sport, leisure, problems caused at work or school, and troublesome symptoms).

The clinician should establish the pattern and timing of allergic symptoms as well as assess the severity and interference with daily activities. Timing of symptoms during different seasons, or after exposure to certain pets, gives the physician an idea of the potential sensitizations of each particular patient. Perennial sensitization is a little more difficult to detect from history taking, but chronicity of symptoms may indicate perennial AR. History should also be elicited about home and school environmental exposures, as well as the effectiveness of any previous allergy therapy.

Physical Examination

A complete ear, nose, and throat examination is required for children suspected of AR. Children with allergic rhinitis often exhibit the "allergic salute" in which the child uses their palm to rub the nose in an upward direction. Resorting to this behavior repetitively can lead to a supratip nasal crease. The patients will also demonstrate "allergic shiners" which are dark circles under the eyes related to venous congestion as a sequelae of chronic nasal obstruction (**Fig. 9.2**). Mouth breathing is a common symptom, especially in children who also have concomitant adenoid hypertrophy. Anterior rhinoscopy using the largest speculum of the otoscope or a nasal speculum is very useful in evaluating the inferior, and possibly, the middle turbinates. A pale nasal mucosal color is often very suggestive, though not pathognomonic, of allergic rhinitis, and children with allergies typically have clear, thin nasal drainage (**Fig. 9.3**). It is also important to evaluate the nasal septum for deviations that could be the source of fixed nasal obstruction and could exacerbate congestion in patients with coexisting allergic rhinitis. Nasal endoscopy can also be performed in the

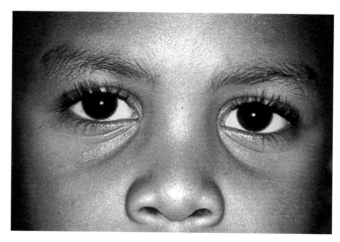

Figure 9.2 Allergic shiners, a usual sequelae of chronic nasal obstruction in a child with allergic rhinitis.

Source: http://www.peds.ufl.edu/PEDS2/research/debusk/pages/page4_02.html. Printed with permission from the Department of Pediatrics, University of Florida.

cooperative and willing child/adolescent. This examination allows the appreciation of all the changes seen with anterior rhinoscopy and adds a thorough evaluation of the middle meatus for signs of sinusitis or nasal polyposis, an appreciation of possible posterior septal abnormalities, and a good look at both posterior choanae and the adenoids. Examination of the oral cavity yields important information about possible postnasal drainage and the size of the tonsils which could contribute to upper airway obstruction, especially during nighttime.

Diagnostic Testing for Allergic Rhinitis

The most common diagnostic tools available are skin testing and in vitro testing for serum-specific IgE antibodies. Skin testing is performed by placing the allergen on the skin either intradermally or via a prick and observing for a reaction, which usually involves a wheal and flare in the sensitized subject (**Fig. 9.4**). A negative control consists of the diluent for the allergen extracts and a positive control is usually histamine, and both are placed on the skin in similar fashion as the allergens. Severity of the reaction is usually graded by comparison to the negative and positive controls. Most practitioners use prick testing routinely and reserve intradermal testing for the patient who tests negative to prick testing but has a very suggestive history. Skin testing is not reliable in individuals who have taken antihistamines or have certain skin sensitivity conditions such as dermatographism. Antihistamines have to be stopped (different periods for the different agents) before testing. Furthermore, some children are not amenable to multiple skin pricks. The risk of an anaphylactic reaction during testing is real but fortunately rare if appropriate recommended concentrations of allergens are used. In vitro testing for serum levels of IgE antibodies measure both total IgE levels as well as allergen-specific IgE levels.

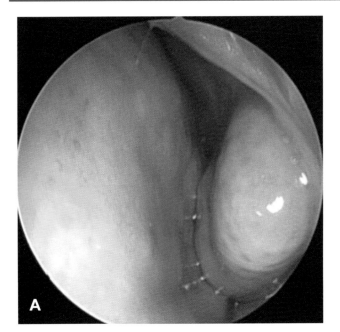
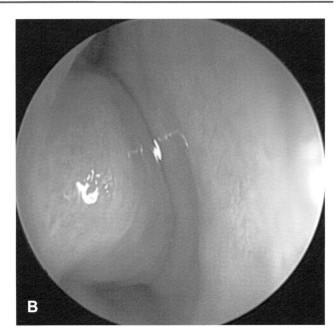

Figure 9.3 Congested, pale, edematous nasal mucosa of a patient with allergic rhinitis. The inferior turbinates touch the nasal septum bilaterally (A) left nasal cavity and (B) right nasal cavity compromising the nasal airway.

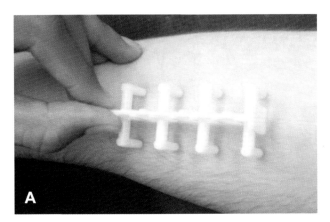
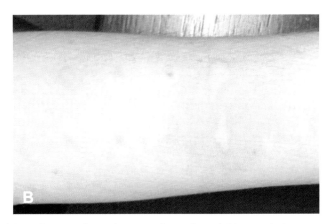

Figure 9.4 Example of a positive skin-prick test in an allergic subject. (A) Application of a multipronged intradermal skin test device on a patient's forearm. (B) Test results interpreted 15 minutes after application of allergens. In this instance, the positive control (histamine) is depicted in the upper row all the way to the left and shows a positive wheal and minimal flare, the negative control (diluent for the allergen extracts) is depicted in the lower row all the way to the left and is negative. Two positive reactions are depicted in the upper and lower rows all the way to the right and show distinctly positive wheal and flare responses which are larger than that produced by histamine. The two allergens were tree and dust mite in this case.

Radioallergosorbent test (RAST) is the most commonly used assay. While in vitro testing is less specific than skin testing, it is better tolerated (involves only one blood draw) and is not affected by medication intake, or skin conditions. Results of in vitro testing are usually available within 1 to 2 weeks whereas skin test results are apparent within 15 minutes. Total IgE levels are elevated in 30 to 40% of individuals with allergic rhinitis and a positive test alone does not confirm the diagnosis. Patients must have both a positive history as well as a positive test result. Choice of the technique used for allergy testing depends on the location of the practice, training of the practitioner and availability of facilities for the different types of tests.

Comorbid Conditions and Allergic Rhinitis

Several respiratory and airway conditions can affect children with allergic rhinitis. In the Pediatric Allergies in America survey, the children with nasal allergies were 2.8-fold more likely to have headaches, 7-fold more likely to have face pain/pressure, 11-fold more likely to report sinus problems, and 2.5 to 3-fold more likely to snore every day or on most days.[3] Furthermore, children with allergic rhinitis were threefold more likely to have an asthma diagnosis and four times more likely to have had asthma in the past 12 months compared with their nonallergic counterparts.

Other studies have supported these findings. In fact, asthma is far more common in patients with allergic rhinitis than in those without, with as many as 50% of allergic rhinitis patients having asthma.[7] Sinusitis and rhinitis also often coexist and are usually referred to as rhinosinusitis. Allergic rhinitis is a risk factor for acute rhinosinusitis across all age groups. The inflammatory response associated with allergic rhinitis contributes to edema and impairment of sinus drainage and may be a contributing factor in as many as 30% of young adult patients with acute rhinosinusitis.[8] Allergic rhinitis also commonly coexists with recurrent or chronic rhinosinusitis with 25 to 84% of patients with rhinosinusitis having concomitant allergic rhinitis.[9]

Acute otitis media and otitis media with effusion (OME) are among the most common problems of childhood. Several clinical studies have evaluated the association between allergic rhinitis and OME, with one series demonstrating a 21% prevalence of OME in unselected schoolchildren with allergic rhinitis[10] and another finding a 50% prevalence of allergic rhinitis in children with OME.[11] In one study of 209 children with a history of chronic or recurrent otitis media who had been referred to a multidisciplinary "glue ear/allergy" clinic, allergic rhinitis was confirmed in 89%, asthma in 36%, and eczema in 24%.[12] Skin tests were positive to one or more of eight common inhalant allergens in 57% of children, and, among those undergoing serum testing, peripheral eosinophilia was documented in 40% and an elevated serum IgE in 28%. Although there is a clear possibility of referral bias in this specialty population, the high frequency of allergy is notable. Furthermore, analysis of middle ear effusions and mucosal biopsies from atopic subjects with allergic rhinitis has demonstrated a pattern of inflammatory mediators not seen in nonatopic children, with significantly higher levels of eosinophil activity markers, mast cell products, and cytokines.

A link has also been postulated between adenoid hypertrophy and allergy via inflammation of the nasal mucosa, which is in direct proximity to the adenoids. A study found that the incidence of adenoid hypertrophy was almost twofold higher in children with allergic disease (allergic rhinitis, bronchial asthma, or atopic dermatitis) when compared with nonallergic controls (40 vs. 22%).[13] Among those children with allergic disease, the incidence of adenoid hypertrophy was higher in children with allergic rhinitis, alone or coexisting with bronchial asthma (71%) compared with those children who had bronchial asthma alone (25%). The authors speculate that ongoing nasal inflammation from allergy could contribute to adenoid hypertrophy. Patients with allergic disorders of the upper airway often have significant sleep disturbances. While the mechanisms are not fully understood, congestion in the nose is presumed to be a key factor. Several epidemiologic studies have shown that allergic rhinitis is a risk factor for obstructive sleep apnea syndrome (OSAS) in children.[14] In a group of children presenting to the sleep laboratory for the evaluation of symptoms of OSAS by polysomnogram,

36% had a positive RAST test. Furthermore, a significantly higher proportion of allergic children had an abnormal polysomnogram (57%) compared with nonallergic children (40%).[15] It is therefore clear from these descriptive studies that allergic inflammation of the nose seems to be associated with similar inflammatory processes in other parts of the upper and lower airways. The effects that link these disease processes have been speculated to be related to multiple mechanisms including direct contiguity of the involved organs, systemic allergic inflammation, and neural reflexes.

Treatment of Allergic Rhinitis

Avoidance

Avoidance of allergens is beneficial but difficult to achieve to a significant degree, especially in the case of environmental allergens. For indoor allergens, avoidance is probably more practical. A Cochrane review found that use of high-efficiency particulate air filters, acaricides, mattress covers, and hot-water laundering to eliminate allergens significantly reduced symptoms of perennial allergic rhinitis.[16] In another study, Morgan and colleagues evaluated the effect of environmental control on asthma symptoms in children where specific allergens were important in the genesis of these symptoms. The authors instituted interventions targeted at both indoor allergens and environmental tobacco smoke. They found that reductions in the environmental load of dust mite and cockroach allergens were proportional to a reduction in wheezing and significantly correlated with reduced complications of asthma.[17]

Antihistamines

Antihistamines block the action of released histamine and are known to effectively control sneezing, itching, rhinorrhea, and eye symptoms. These agents are not as effective in helping nasal congestion. First-generation antihistamines (diphenhydramine, hydroxyzine, chlorpheniramine, brompheniramine, and clemastine) are lipophilic and cross the blood–brain barrier, thus leading to the notable side effect of sedation. They also have anticholinergic side effects which can lead to drying of secretions. Indeed, in a study evaluating learning scores in schoolchildren, allergic children receiving placebo were found to have lower scores than normal nonallergic children, suggesting a deleterious effect of allergic rhinitis on learning ability.[18] When the allergic children received diphenhydramine, the sedating antihistamine for 2 weeks, their learning scores became even worse than the group on placebo and were significantly lower than nonallergic controls. In contrast, loratadine, a nonsedating agent, resulted in an improvement of learning scores that were not different from those of the control nonallergic group. To avoid such side effects, second-generation antihistamines were developed (**Table 9.1**). They have reduced or absent anticholinergic side effects and do not lead to significant sedation, as they do not cross the blood–brain barrier. These agents are available in liquid form, and many are approved for use in children as young as 6 months of age. They have relatively rapid absorption and onset of action (within hours) and the longer half-life of the second-generation drugs allows once daily administration. Multiple clinical studies in children have documented the efficacy and safety of these drugs in allergic rhinitis. Intranasal antihistamines are also available for use in children (**Table 9.1**). Azelastine, a phthalazinone derivative, is available for the treatment of allergic rhinitis. Its efficacy is comparable to other antihistamines, and it might be more effective than oral antihistamines for nasal congestion. It is usually given twice daily, and can cause somnolence. Taste alteration may occur immediately after use with an incidence as high as 20%. Olopatadine hydrochloride (0.6%) has been shown to be safe and effective for the treatment of seasonal allergic rhinitis and is usually administered twice

daily. The most commonly reported adverse reaction is bitter taste, and the incidence of somnolence is minimally higher than placebo vehicle.

Decongestants

Topical as well as systemic decongestants act to cause vascular constriction and reduce the nasal blood supply by alpha-adrenergic stimulation. Prolonged use of topical agents can lead to rebound nasal congestion, also known as rhinitis medicamentosa. Therefore their use should be limited to situations where severe allergic nasal congestion precludes the administration of other intranasal medications. In these cases, a short 3- to 5-day course of intranasal decongestants is used in conjunction with other intranasal agents (steroids, antihistamines) to facilitate access to the nasal mucosa. Oral decongestants are less effective than their intranasal

Table 9.1 Newer Generation Antihistamines

Chemical Name	Trade Name	Formulation	Dose/Pediatric
Intranasal			
Azelastine hydrochloride spray	Astelin	Nasal solution 0.1%, 137 µg/spray	≥12 y: 2 sprays/nostril BID
Olopatadine hydrochloride spray	Patanase	Nasal solution 0.6%, 2.77 µg/spray	≥12 y: 2 sprays/nostril BID
Oral			
Cetirizine hydrochloride	Zyrtec	Tabs: 5, 10 mg Tabs (chewable): 5, 10 mg Syrup: 5 mg/5 mL Solution: 5 mg/5 mL	• 6–12 mo: 2.5 mg QD • 12–23 mo: 2.5 mg QD up to 2.5 mg BID • 2–5 y: 2.5 mg/d up to 5 mg QD • 6–11 y: 5–10 mg QD • ≥12 y: 5–10 mg QD
Desloratadine	Clarinex	Tabs: 5 mg Syrup: 0.5 mg/mL Reditabs: 2.5, 5 mg (rapidly disintegrating tabs)	• 6–11 mo: 1 mg QD • 1–5 y: 1.25 mg QD • 6–11 y: 2.5 mg QD • ≥12 y: 5 mg QD
Fexofenadine hydrochloride	Allegra	Suspension: 6 mg/mL Tablet: 30, 60, 180 mg Reditabs: 30 mg Caps: 60 mg	• 6 mo–<2 y: 15 mg BID • 2–11 y: 30 mg BID • ≥12 y: 60 mg BID or 180 mg QD
Loratadine	Claritin	Tabs: 10 mg Syrup: 1 mg/mL Reditabs: 10 mg (rapidly disintegrating tabs) Chewable tabs: 5 mg	• 2–5 y: 5 mg QD • 6–11 y: 10 mg QD • ≥12 y: 10 mg QD
	Claritin D 12 hour	Extended release tabs: 5 mg loratadine, 120 mg pseudoephedrine sulfate	≥12 y: One tab BID
	Claritin D 24 hour	Extended release tabs: 10 mg loratadine, 240 mg pseudoephedrine sulfate	≥12 y: One tab QD
Levocetirizine dihydrochloride	Xyzal	Solution: 0.5 mg/mL Tab: 5 mg	• 6 mo–5 y: 1.25 mg QD • 6–11 y: 2.5 mg QD • ≥12 y: 5 mg QD

y, years; BID, twice daily; mo, months; QD, once daily; d, day(s).

counterparts, but do not cause rebound nasal congestion. Pseudoephedrine hydrochloride and phenylephrine are the most commonly used. Pseudoephedrine-containing decongestant products are now sold behind the counter in U.S. pharmacies because of the use of this medication in the illicit manufacture of methamphetamine. They are used most frequently in combination preparations with antihistamines (pseudoephedrine), or over the counter in cough and cold products in combination with analgesics and antitussives. Phenylephrine is another over-the-counter decongestant, also used in combination products. A recent meta-analysis showed lack of efficacy of phenylephrine on both objective and subjective measures of nasal congestion compared with placebo.[19] In addition, their most common side effects are insomnia and irritability, which can be seen in as many as 25% of patients.

Anticholinergics

These agents are useful in the control of rhinorrhea associated with allergic rhinitis and have no therapeutic efficacy on any of the other symptoms of the disease. Ipratropium bromide is available for intranasal administration and lacks the systemic effects of atropine. It is used in patients with allergic rhinitis who continue to have significant symptoms of rhinorrhea despite maximal therapy with other agents.

Cromolyn Sodium

Cromolyn sodium is a mast cell stabilizer and is available over the counter as a 4% solution for intranasal use in allergic rhinitis. It has been shown to be helpful for sneezing, itching, and rhinorrhea but not as effective for nasal obstruction. It does not cross the blood–brain barrier and is unlikely to cause sedation. It is noted to be safe in children and pregnant women but the need for frequent dosing reduces compliance and makes this agent less attractive as a therapeutic choice.

Leukotriene Modifiers

Because leukotrienes are generated in allergic rhinitis, the effects of inhibitors of the 5-lipoxygenase pathway and leukotriene receptor antagonists have been investigated. By far, the most commonly used agent in this category is montelukast which is approved in the United States for the treatment of seasonal and perennial allergic rhinitis in children as young as 6 months of age. Montelukast has repeatedly been shown to be more effective than placebo and equally effective as antihistamines for all ocular and nasal symptoms of allergic rhinitis, including congestion, rhinorrhea, and sneezing. Some, but not all, studies examining the combination of montelukast with an antihistamine (loratadine, desloratadine, cetirizine) have shown synergistic benefit.[20,21]

Intranasal Steroids

Intranasal steroids are considered the most effective treatment for allergic rhinitis, based, in large part, on their potent anti-inflammatory effects. In natural exposure as well as nasal allergen challenge studies, treatment with intranasal steroids inhibits symptoms, mediator release, T helper cell type 2 (Th2) cytokine expression, inflammatory cellular influx (notably eosinophils) into nasal secretions and the nasal mucosa, as well as hyperresponsiveness to allergen and nonspecific stimuli. These agents have been shown to be superior to both antihistamines and leukotriene receptor antagonists in the control of the symptoms of allergic rhinitis.[22,23] Most guidelines suggest the use of these agents as first line in moderate-to-severe disease and even in some cases of mild allergic rhinitis. Efficacy begins at 7 to 8 hours after administration and starting these agents a few days before the start of the season has been recommended.

The principal side effect of intranasal steroids is local nasal irritation and epistaxis which occur in 5 to 10% of patients and septal perforations, although rare, have been reported. Biopsy specimens from the nasal mucosa of patients with perennial rhinitis who had been treated with such agents for 1 year showed no evidence of atrophy or epithelial injury. In the pediatric age group, studies looking at objective reproducible measures of growth (stadiometry or knemometry) and hypothalamic pituitary axis suppression after administration of intranasal steroids for periods up to 1 year, failed to show any adverse effects of the newer agents compared with placebo.[24,25] Studies following intraocular pressure in patients on long-term intranasal steroids have failed to show a significant increase in intraocular pressure or the incidence of glaucoma compared with placebo.[26] Based on these reassuring results, mometasone furoate and fluticasone furoate are approved by the U.S. Food and Drug Administration (FDA) for use starting at 2 years of age and fluticasone propionate starting at 4 years of age. Available agents and age of administration are listed in **Table 9.2**.

Systemic Steroids

The role of systemic steroids in the treatment of AR is limited. Steroid pulses may be useful to help wean patients from topical decongestant use in cases of rhinitis medicamentosa. They can also be useful in cases of severe nasal congestion, given in 3- to 5-day courses, to enhance the penetration of concomitantly administered intranasal steroids.

Immunotherapy

Immunotherapy is allergen-specific repeated administration of increasing doses of antigen extract, either subcutaneously or sublingually, in an attempt to reduce a patients' immunologic response. Immunotherapy is usually reserved for patients who have not responded to maximal multifaceted pharmacologic treatment.

Subcutaneous Immunotherapy

Subcutaneous immunotherapy (SCIT), which has been used for decades, alters the immune response with suppression of immediate and late allergic reactions, as a consequence of

Table 9.2   Commonly Used Intranasal Steroid Preparations

Chemical Name	Trade Name	Formulation	Dose/Actuation	Recommended Dosage
Triamcinolone acetonide	Nasacort	Propellant, aqueous	55 µg	<ul><li>2–5 y: 1 spray/nostril (110 µg daily)</li><li>6–11 y: 2 sprays/nostril QD (220 µg daily)</li><li>≥12 y: 2 sprays/nostril QD-BID (220–440 µg daily)</li></ul>
Budesonide	Rhinocort	Propellant	32 µg	≥6 y: 2 sprays/nostril BID or 4 sprays/nostril in the morning (256 µg daily)
Flunisolide	Nasalide Nasarel	0.025% solution	25 µg	<ul><li>6–14 y: 1 spray/nostril TID (150 µg daily)</li><li>2 sprays/nostril BID(200 µg daily)</li><li>≥14 y: 2 sprays/nostril BID/TID (200/300 µg daily)</li></ul>
Fluticasone propionate	Flonase	0.05% nasal spray (aqueous)	50 µg	4 y–adolescents: 1 spray/nostril QD (100 µg daily) Adults: 2 sprays/nostril QD (200 µg daily)
Mometasone furoate	Nasonex	Aqueous	50 µg	<ul><li>2–11 y: 1 spray/nostril daily (100 µg daily)</li><li>≥12 years: 2 sprays/nostril once daily (200 µg daily)</li></ul>
Ciclesonide	Omnaris	Suspension	50 µg	<ul><li>2–11 y: 1–2 sprays daily divided per nostril</li><li>≥12 y: 2 sprays/nostril daily (200 µg daily)</li></ul>
Fluticasone furoate	Veramyst	Suspension	27.5 µg	<ul><li>2–11 y: 1 spray/nostril daily (can increase to 2 sprays/nostril daily (110 µg/daily)</li><li>>11 y: 2 sprays/nostril daily (110 µg daily)</li></ul>

y, years; QD, once daily; BID, twice daily; TID, thrice daily.

suppression of infiltration of effector cells and subsequent mediator release. An immune deviation of allergen-specific T-cell responses from a Th2-biased in favor of a protective Th1-biased response has been observed. This seems to occur as a local immune event and has been associated variably with decreases in Th2 and increases in Th1 cytokines detectable in the periphery.[27] More recently, it has been proposed that successful immunotherapy modifies the T-cell response to allergen through the induction of regulatory mechanisms, mostly regulatory T cells and their inhibitory cytokines IL-10 and transforming growth factor-beta (TGF-β). Support for this hypothesis comes in part from the description of populations of induced T-regulatory cells following SCIT and by the fact that allergen immunotherapy has been associated with upregulation of IL-10 and, variably, with increased TGF-β expression. Furthermore, local increases in IL-10–positive cells have been demonstrated within the nasal mucosa following SCIT.

As far as the humoral immune response is concerned, following an initial early increase in allergen-specific IgE concentrations during the updosing phase, SCIT results in blunting of seasonal increases in IgE and a long-term gradual reduction in serum allergen-specific IgE levels. On the other hand, SCIT is associated with marked and sustained increases in allergen-specific IgG1 and IgG4 antibodies and a more modest increase in serum allergen-specific IgA concentrations. The IgG antibodies produced after SCIT, specifically IgG4, possess blocking activity as evidenced by several studies. In one study, IgG and IgA antibodies from nasal washings of patients on SCIT were able to inhibit histamine release in vitro and in another, IgG4 antibodies produced following treatment blocked allergen-induced, IgE-dependent histamine release by basophils. Improvement of symptoms with SCIT starts within 12 weeks of initiation of therapy. A series of injections with increasing doses of allergen(s) over several months is followed by maintenance therapy that is typically administered for 3 to 5 years. There is ample evidence to support the clinical efficacy of this treatment modality for the symptoms of allergic rhinitis. In a meta-analysis which reviewed 1111 publications, 51 satisfied inclusion criteria and involved 2871 participants,[28] there were no fatalities of SCIT, and active treatment resulted in a significant positive effect, compared with controls using outcomes of reduced symptom scores and use of rescue medications. Other studies have demonstrated a beneficial effect on quality of life. In addition to its beneficial clinical effects, SCIT has shown to be effective in the prevention of subsequent asthma in allergic children. In a study of 205 birch or grass allergic children 6 to 14 years of age treated with either SCIT or control, active treatment resulted in a significant improvement of symptoms and a significantly lower rate of asthma than the control group at the 2-year follow-up.[29] In another smaller study, SCIT for 3 years resulted in a significant reduction in the development of new skin test sensitizations and the prevalence of seasonal asthma 12 years after therapy. Furthermore, SCIT is the only treatment of allergic rhinitis that has been shown to affect the natural history of the disease, with persisting clinical and immunological benefits several years after discontinuation of therapy.[30] Despite its beneficial effects, SCIT involves systemic administration of allergen and has been associated with side effects, the worst of which are anaphylaxis and potentially death. In a review of the safety and efficacy of SCIT, epinephrine administration was required in 0.13% (19 of 14,085) injections, but no fatalities were seen.[28] Other reviews suggest an incidence of fatal reactions from SCIT of 1 per 2.5 million injections or 3.4 deaths per year.

Sublingual Immunotherapy

Because of the potential significant side effects of SCIT and the inconveniences of administration, sublingual immunotherapy (SLIT) has gained widespread attention over the past two decades. SLIT involves sublingual placement of small doses of the offending allergen. This route of administration is thought to limit side effects while maintaining benefits secondary to mucosal penetration. The majority of trials related to SLIT have been performed in Europe, and the

therapy has not yet been approved by the FDA for clinical use in the United States. A meta-analysis of SLIT in children with AR which included 10 studies and 577 patients, demonstrated the clinical efficacy of SLIT with reduction in symptoms and medication use compared with untreated control patients.[31] In a larger review of SLIT in adults and children with AR, 49 trials were included in a meta-analysis (2333 patients on SLIT and 2256 patients on placebo).[32] The analysis again showed a significant reduction in symptoms and medication requirements in the actively treated subjects. None of the trials reported severe systemic reactions or anaphylaxis and none of the systemic reactions required the use of epinephrine.

Typical side effects of this therapy that have been reported are local oral (oral itching and swelling) and gastrointestinal reactions. Nonetheless, there have been isolated reports of more severe systemic reactions with SLIT, the most significant of which is a single report of anaphylaxis after SLIT.[33] It is noteworthy that this patient had interrupted maintenance therapy for 3 weeks and then took a dose six times larger than the maintenance dose which precipitated the event.[33]

Like SCIT, SLIT has been shown to lead to positive immunologic effects and to modify the course of disease in children with rhinitis, conjunctivitis, and asthma. It can be administered for a limited period of time before and during a specific allergy season or on a year-round basis for perennial and multiple seasonal allergies. It carries the distinct advantage of being administered outside a doctor's office.

Conclusion

Allergic rhinitis is a common disease in children, and has significant signs and symptoms that affect the quality of life as well as their ability to concentrate and learn effectively in school. Available therapies are safe and effective and lead to an improvement in both symptoms and quality of life. These therapies range from environmental controls to pharmacologic therapy to immunotherapy. Clinical suspicion supplemented by specific diagnostic testing can identify the children who require allergy management.

References

1. Collins JG. Prevalence of Selected Chronic Conditions: United States, 1990–92. Hyattsville, MD: US Department of Health and Human Services Publication 97–1522, National Center for Health Statistics; 1997;1–89
2. Juniper EF, Howland WC, Roberts NB, Thompson AK, King DR. Measuring quality of life in children with rhinoconjunctivitis. J Allergy Clin Immunol 1998;101(2 Pt 1):163–170
3. Meltzer EO, Blaiss MS, Derebery MJ, et al. Burden of allergic rhinitis: results from the Pediatric Allergies in America survey. J Allergy Clin Immunol 2009;124(3, Suppl)S43–S70
4. Baroody FM, Naclerio RM. Immunology of the upper airway and pathophysiology and treatment of allergic rhinitis. In: Flint PW, Haughey BH, Lund VJ, et al, eds. Otolaryngology-Head and Neck Surgery. 5th ed. Vol. 1. Philadelphia, PA: Mosby Elsevier; 2010:597–623
5. Wallace DV, Dykewicz MS, Bernstein DI, et al; Joint Task Force on Practice; American Academy of Allergy; Asthma & Immunology; American College of Allergy; Asthma and Immunology; Joint Council of Allergy, Asthma and Immunology. The diagnosis and management of rhinitis: an updated practice parameter. J Allergy Clin Immunol 2008;122(2, Suppl):S1–S84
6. Bousquet J, Khaltaev N, Cruz AA, et al; World Health Organization; GA(2)LEN; AllerGen. Allergic Rhinitis and its Impact on Asthma (ARIA) 2008 update (in collaboration with the World Health

Organization, GA(2)LEN and AllerGen). Allergy 2008;63(Suppl 86): 8–160

7. Meltzer EO. The relationships of rhinitis and asthma. Allergy Asthma Proc 2005;26(5):336–340

8. Savolainen S. Allergy in patients with acute maxillary sinusitis. Allergy 1989;44(2):116–122

9. Steinke JW, Borish L. The role of allergy in chronic rhinosinusitis. Immunol Allergy Clin North Am 2004;24(1):45–57

10. Luong A, Roland PS. The link between allergic rhinitis and chronic otitis media with effusion in atopic patients. Otolaryngol Clin North Am 2008;41(2):311–323, vi

11. Tomonaga K, Kurono Y, Mogi G. The role of nasal allergy in otitis media with effusion. A clinical study. Acta Otolaryngol Suppl 1988;458:41–47

12. Alles R, Parikh A, Hawk L, Darby Y, Romero JN, Scadding G. The prevalence of atopic disorders in children with chronic otitis media with effusion. Pediatr Allergy Immunol 2001;12(2):102–106

13. Modrzynski M, Zawisza E. An analysis of the incidence of adenoid hypertrophy in allergic children. Int J Pediatr Otorhinolaryngol 2007;71(5):713–719

14. Ng DK, Chan CH, Hwang GY, Chow PY, Kwok KL. A review of the roles of allergic rhinitis in childhood obstructive sleep apnea syndrome. Allergy Asthma Proc 2006;27(3):240–242

15. McColley SA, Carroll JL, Curtis S, Loughlin GM, Sampson HA. High prevalence of allergic sensitization in children with habitual snoring and obstructive sleep apnea. Chest 1997;111(1):170–173

16. Sheikh A, Hurwitz B. House dust mite avoidance measures for perennial allergic rhinitis. Cochrane Database Syst Rev 2001;4(4):CD001563

17. Morgan WJ, Crain EF, Gruchalla RS, et al; Inner-City Asthma Study Group. Results of a home-based environmental intervention among urban children with asthma. N Engl J Med 2004;351(11):1068–1080

18. Vuurman EF, van Veggel LM, Uiterwijk MM, Leutner D, O'Hanlon JF. Seasonal allergic rhinitis and antihistamine effects on children's learning. Ann Allergy 1993;71(2):121–126

19. Hatton RC, Winterstein AG, McKelvey RP, Shuster J, Hendeles L. Efficacy and safety of oral phenylephrine: systematic review and meta-analysis. Ann Pharmacother 2007;41(3):381–390

20. Meltzer EO, Malmstrom K, Lu S, et al. Concomitant montelukast and loratadine as treatment for seasonal allergic rhinitis: a randomized, placebo-controlled clinical trial. J Allergy Clin Immunol 2000;105(5):917–922

21. Ciebiada M, Górska-Ciebiada M, DuBuske LM, Górski P. Montelukast with desloratadine or levocetirizine for the treatment of persistent allergic rhinitis. Ann Allergy Asthma Immunol 2006;97(5):664–671

22. Weiner JM, Abramson MJ, Puy RM. Intranasal corticosteroids versus oral H1 receptor antagonists in allergic rhinitis: systematic review of randomised controlled trials. BMJ 1998;317(7173):1624–1629

23. Wilson AM, O'Byrne PM, Parameswaran K. Leukotriene receptor antagonists for allergic rhinitis: a systematic review and meta-analysis. Am J Med 2004;116(5):338–344

24. Allen DB, Meltzer EO, Lemanske RF Jr, et al. No growth suppression in children treated with the maximum recommended dose of fluticasone propionate aqueous nasal spray for one year. Allergy Asthma Proc 2002;23(6):407–413

25. Schenkel EJ, Skoner DP, Bronsky EA, et al. Absence of growth retardation in children with perennial allergic rhinitis after one year of treatment with mometasone furoate aqueous nasal spray. Pediatrics 2000;105(2):E22

26. Ozkaya E, Ozsutcu M, Mete F. Lack of ocular side effects after 2 years of topical steroids for allergic rhinitis. J Pediatr Ophthalmol Strabismus 2011;48(5):311–317

27. James LK, Durham SR. Update on mechanisms of allergen injection immunotherapy. Clin Exp Allergy 2008;38(7):1074–1088

28. Calderon MA, Alves B, Jacobson M, Hurwitz B, Sheikh A, Durham S. Allergen injection immunotherapy for seasonal allergic rhinitis. Cochrane Database Syst Rev 2007;(1):CD001936

29. Niggemann B, Jacobsen L, Dreborg S, et al; PAT Investigator Group. Five-year follow-up on the PAT study: specific immunotherapy and long-term prevention of asthma in children. Allergy 2006;61(7):855–859

30. Durham SR, Walker SM, Varga EM, et al. Long-term clinical efficacy of grass-pollen immunotherapy. N Engl J Med 1999;341(7):468–475

31. Penagos M, Compalati E, Tarantini F, et al. Efficacy of sublingual immunotherapy in the treatment of allergic rhinitis in pediatric patients 3 to 18 years of age: a meta-analysis of randomized, placebo-controlled, double-blind trials. Ann Allergy Asthma Immunol 2006;97(2):141–148

32. Radulovic S, Calderon MA, Wilson D, Durham S. Sublingual immunotherapy for allergic rhinitis. Cochrane Database Syst Rev 2010;(12):CD002893

33. Blazowski L. Anaphylactic shock because of sublingual immunotherapy overdose during third year of maintenance dose. Allergy 2008;63(3):374

SECTION III: Aerodigestive and Voice Disorders

10 Anesthesia for Pediatric Otolaryngology

Rosalie F. Tassone and Timothy B. McDonald

Children who present to the hospital for otolaryngology procedures and operations frequently require anesthesia to tolerate procedures and operations that would otherwise be extremely uncomfortable and painful. Consultation with a pediatric anesthesiologist is important for the comprehensive care of the pediatric patient. This chapter is divided into three sections: preoperative evaluation, intraoperative management, and postoperative care. Each section will highlight the concerns of the anesthesiologist for the care of the pediatric patient.

Preoperative Evaluation

The preoperative evaluation allows the anesthesiologist to integrate the patient's medical history, physical status, and planned procedure into an anesthetic management plan tailored to the patient's perioperative course. Identification of areas of concern in the patient with a complex medical history facilitates discussion and planning of postoperative disposition, such as the need for postoperative intensive care. Additionally, anesthetic consultation and evaluation before the day of surgery may also increase operating room efficiency and decreased cancellations on the day of surgery, although not all children need a preoperative evaluation.[1]

The American Society of Anesthesiologists (ASA) has created a physical status classification system, based on the severity of the patient's systemic disease (**Table 10.1**). For example, the assessment of the otherwise healthy child (ASA 1) for a routine operation such as placement of bilateral myringotomy tubes may not warrant a separate trip to the anesthesiologist. However, if this child has a complex medical history such as concomitant congenital heart disease or a bleeding disorder (ASA 3 or 4), preoperative evaluation would be helpful in the planning of the intraoperative management, which may be far from routine.

The preoperative assessment includes taking a thorough medical history to assess any associated medical problems that might affect the anesthetic or surgical outcome. Of keen interest to the pediatric anesthesiologist is a history of problems associated with anesthesia in the child or the child's family, such as malignant hyperthermia (MH), latex allergy or allergies to anesthetic medications.

Identification and medical optimization of chronic conditions, such as a history of premature birth, reactive airway disease, systemic disease, bleeding disorders, developmental delay, or acute conditions such as in the child with an active upper respiratory tract infection may occur at the preoperative evaluation. Also, workup of additional associated concerns can be scheduled and performed before the day of surgery, such as the assessment of a potentially unstable cervical spine in the child with Trisomy 21 or the preoperative assessment of a bleeding disorder.[2]

Premature Neonates

Neonates who are born prematurely (<37 weeks of gestation) are at risk for increased apnea and bradycardia after general anesthesia.[2,3] Neonates born prematurely, who

Table 10.1 ASA Physical Status Classification System

ASA Physical Status	Description
ASA Physical Status 1 (ASA 1)	A normal healthy patient
ASA Physical Status 2 (ASA 2)	A patient with mild systemic disease
ASA Physical Status 3 (ASA 3)	A patient with severe systemic disease
ASA Physical Status 4 (ASA 4)	A patient with severe systemic disease that is a constant threat to life
ASA Physical Status 5 (ASA 5)	A moribund patient who is not expected to survive without the operation
ASA Physical Status 6 (ASA 6)	A declared brain-dead patient whose organs are being removed for donor purposes

Additionally, if the surgery is an emergency, the physical status classification is followed by "E" (for emergency).

are under 60 weeks postgestational age should be admitted to the hospital for postoperative apnea and bradycardia monitoring overnight after administering sedatives or general anesthesia. Likewise, full-term newborns are at increased risk of apnea and bradycardia for the first 4 weeks of life and should be admitted to the hospital for overnight observation as well.[2,4]

Upper Respiratory Tract Infection

In general, pediatric patients have a higher incidence of respiratory events than adults, and the child with an active respiratory tract infection is at an even higher increased risk for respiratory-related anesthetic complications such as laryngospasm, bronchospasm, and hypoxemia.[2] Classically it has been shown that the risk of respiratory complications decreases 4 to 6 weeks after an upper respiratory tract infection has resolved;[2] however, it sometimes can be difficult to schedule a child's procedure at a time when the child is not actively ill. Preoperative assessment can be helpful in creating a plan where the child may be at the least risk for complications from an upper respiratory tract infection and maximum benefit from the surgery. Some sources suggest that a shorter time after an upper respiratory tract infection has resolved might be acceptable, with careful assessment and caution.[2,5]

Obstructive Sleep Apnea

Children with long-standing obstructive sleep apnea may develop significant cor pulmonale or pulmonary hypertension. Postoperatively they are at risk for perioperative hypoxemia and acute right heart failure.[2] These children are also exquisitely more sensitive to sedatives and narcotics.[6,7] It is postulated that this may likely be a result of upregulation of mu-receptors in the brainstem, where an increased respiratory sensitivity to fentanyl has been shown after recurrent hypoxia in a rat model.[8]

Mediastinal Masses

Masses in the neck may sometimes be associated with extension of the mass into the mediastinum. If a mediastinal mass is suspected, a preoperative work-up including imaging studies is prudent to help plan for the anesthetic induction and intraoperative care. Patients with an anterior mediastinal mass are at increased risk of cardiopulmonary compromise and, possibly, arrest on induction of anesthesia. The planning of appropriate personnel and equipment, such as flexible fiberoptic scopes, invasive lines, and possible cardiopulmonary bypass, may be necessary for the care of these patients.[9]

Physical Examination

A physical examination of the patient is an important step in preoperative assessment. Observation of the general well-being and demeanor of the patient can yield a sense as to how the child might separate from the parents. It has been shown that children who are anxious before surgery require more pain medication postoperatively and may exhibit maladaptive behavioral changes postoperatively as well.[10,11] Parental anxiety has also been shown to influence the pediatric patient's anxiety.[11] Counseling the patient and family at a time before the surgery may be helpful in alleviating perioperative anxiety.

Vital signs, including temperature, may also indicate presence of systemic disease. Examination of the airway includes use of the Mallampati classification (**Fig. 10.1**), which has been shown to predict the ease of intubation, and is based on the visibility of the base of uvula, faucial pillars, and the soft palate. Scoring may be done with or without phonation. A high Mallampati score (class 4) is associated with more difficult intubation, and an increased severity of obstructive sleep apnea.[12,13]

In addition to the Mallampati classification of the airway, the anesthesiologist will also assess airway abnormalities that may be present such as masses, tracheal deviation, absent structures, range of motion of the head and neck, and thyromental distance.

Intraoperative Management

General Considerations

Preprocedure Debriefing

The patient presenting for pediatric otolaryngology surgery has much to gain from all members of the operating room team, by taking advantage of a preprocedure debriefing.[14] Even the relatively routine pediatric otolaryngology case will involve some degree of airway sharing, some mindfulness related to room configuration, need for special airway equipment considerations, and decisions about medication management for maintaining anesthesia, pain control, and prophylaxis against postoperative nausea and vomiting (PONV).

The debriefing also provides for special consideration about the availability of special airway equipment, implant devices (such as cochlear implants), appropriate room

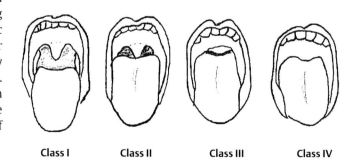

Class I   Class II   Class III   Class IV

Figure 10.1 Mallampati classification. Class I: Full visibility of the tonsils, uvula, and soft palate in the airway. Class II: Visibility of hard and soft palate, and upper portion of the tonsils and uvula. Class III: Soft and hard palate, and base of the uvula are visible. Class IV: Only the hard palate is visible.

configuration, plans for use of a facial nerve monitor (and, therefore, avoidance of long-acting paralytic agents), potential risk of fire, and other special needs of the patient and surgeon.[14] During this time, the otolaryngologist and anesthesia provider should agree on whether a preformed or atypical size endotracheal tube may also be needed for the case.

Nitrous Oxide

With the propensity of nitrous oxide to accumulate and cause increased pressure in closed mucosa-lined spaces, the otolaryngologist and anesthesia provider should also discuss the use of nitrous oxide on a case-by-case basis.[15] This is especially true for pediatric otolaryngology cases involving middle ear surgery. In addition, operating personnel should remain mindful of the fact that nitrous oxide supports combustion and should assure to some degree that oxygen is minimized when there is a measurable risk of fire in any otolaryngology case.[16]

Difficult Airway

Failure to appropriately manage a difficult airway of a child in respiratory distress or one who is deeply anesthetized and cannot be mask ventilated or intubated remains a significant source of potentially preventable patient harm. Preoperative preparation includes a detailed assessment and search for signs, symptoms, anatomical predictors, and syndrome associations that might suggest the potential of less than straightforward airway management.

While assembling and preparing the appropriate equipment for cases that may involve difficult airway management, consideration of the ASA difficult airway algorithm may prove useful. The algorithm contemplates a list of potential equipment for the team to consider that includes, but is not limited to, appropriate masks, a variety of laryngoscope blades with and without optics, endotracheal tubes, fiberoptic scopes and screens, laryngeal mask airways, jet ventilation methodologies, boogie use, and surgical tracheostomy/cricothyrotomy sets.[17]

Unlike cooperative adults and older adolescent patients, securing the difficult airway in the fully awake child can prove extremely challenging.[18] Therefore, most pediatric difficult airway cases proceed with a decision to provide some sedation or anesthetic. Here, effective communication between the otolaryngologist and anesthesia provider becomes paramount. In general, attempts are made to provide adequate sedation/anesthesia while maintaining spontaneous ventilation. This approach allows for "waking up the child" in the event airway management difficulties ensue.

Foreign Body Aspiration

Basically, two anesthetic approaches exist for retrieving an aspirated foreign body in a child: (1) deeply anesthetized, spontaneously breathing method and (2) controlled ventila-

tion and brief paralysis. Of course, the goal is to provide the surgeon with optimal conditions to safely retrieve the entire foreign body with minimal complications. Each approach has its own advantages and disadvantages.

The spontaneously breathing approach decreases the likelihood that the anesthesia provider will force the foreign body more deeply in the trachea or bronchus with the administration of positive pressure ventilation. The downside to this approach may include a significantly increased time for induction of a deep plane of anesthesia and the increased likelihood of patient movement during laryngoscopy and bronchoscopy if the depth of anesthesia is inadequate.

The paralyzed, controlled ventilation approach decreases the likelihood of any movement and, for at least a brief time, provides the surgeon with the optimal circumstance of an anesthetized patient with full muscle relaxation. The downside to this approach rests with the possibility that the foreign body will not be retrievable as intact during the period of apnea once laryngoscopy ensues. In this case, the anesthesia provider may need to provide positive pressure ventilation to maintain adequate oxygenation while potentially forcing the foreign body deeper into the airway.

Ultimately, either approach may be reasonable, based upon the individual facts and presentation of the case. Effective communication between the otolaryngologist and anesthesia provider is essential before and during the procedure.

Airway Laser Surgery

In addition to usual challenges of sharing the child's airway between the surgeon and the anesthesiologist, two specific issues related to the use of laser include reducing the risk of airway fire and the preparation for the possible need for jet ventilation or insufflation techniques.

The fire triangle in the airway consists of (1) an ignition source, in this case, the laser; (2) fuel (endotracheal tube); and (3) oxidizing agent (oxygen or nitrous oxide). Reducing the risk of airway fire involves the use of fire-resistant endotracheal tubes and the minimization of an oxidizing-rich environment with avoidance of nitrous oxide and the blending of oxygen and air to the lowest possible fraction of inspired oxygen while still maintaining adequate blood oxygen levels.[19]

During use of a laser during airway surgery, all personnel in the operating room must be prepared to immediately extinguish an airway fire, reduce the flow of oxidizing gases, and determine the need for removal and possible replacement of the endotracheal tube. In the microscope-assisted laser procedures, ventilation during moments without an endotracheal tube in place can take place with Venturi jet ventilation or with a spontaneous breathing child. If Venturi jet ventilation is employed, the team must recognize the possibility for the known complications of pneumomediastinum, pneumothorax, and pneumopericardium. Minimizing the amount of force generated by the jet ventilator can minimize the likelihood of these complications. In addition, the surgeon must take special care to ensure that the tip of the jet ventilation apparatus is appropriately "aimed" at the lumen of the trachea.

Malignant Hyperthermia

Malignant hyperthermia (MH) is a hypermetabolic state triggered by exposure to any of the potent inhalation agents and/or succinylcholine.[20] The key diagnostic features of MH are muscle rigidity, unexplained increase in exhaled carbon dioxide, acidosis, hyperthermia, hyperkalemia, and rhabdomyolysis.[20] The incidence ranges from 1:10,000 to 1:100,000 anesthetic exposures while the genetic prevalence appears to be approximately 1:3000 persons. Often, the earliest manifestations of MH during a surgical procedure include an unexplained increase in exhaled carbon dioxide and tachycardia.[20] These signs may be accompanied by muscular rigidity. In the event the diagnosis of MH is made, this becomes an operating room emergency that will require large numbers of personnel to assist. The steps for the management of MH are shown in **Table 10.2**.[21]

With prompt identification and appropriate treatment, the mortality has dropped from 80% in the 1970s to less than 5% at present. Genetic counseling is appropriate following a documented case of MH in a family member.[20]

Postoperative Care

After the conclusion of surgery and anesthesia, the pediatric patient has time to recover in the postanesthesia care unit (PACU). This is a time and place where monitoring patients is still important as it is a time of transition to recovery. This section will review some of the common issues in the PACU.

Pain Control

Adequate control of pain is one of the most fundamental concerns for care of the postoperative patient. Effective

pain control is beneficial at multiple levels as it reduces morbidity and mortality, encourages earlier mobilization and faster recovery.[4] Assessment of pain should be done at regular intervals so that a patient has adequate pain relief without being oversedated. Medications given intraoperatively for pain relief should be incorporated into the postoperative pain relief regimen. It is important to understand the pharmacokinetics of pharmacodynamics of medications given intraoperatively and postoperatively such that the patient does not develop inadequate pain relief or oversedation once discharged.

Several classes of drugs can be used for treatment of postoperative pain (**Table 10.3**). Frequently, nonopioid analgesics, such as acetaminophen, may be administered preoperatively by mouth or intraoperatively per rectum. Other nonopioid analgesics such that the nonsteroidal anti-inflammatory drugs (NSAIDs) may be given orally (aspirin, ibuprofen, naproxen, diclofenac) or intravenously (ketorolac). Although a retrospective review of pediatric patients who underwent tonsillectomy with or without adenoidectomy revealed no significant frequency of postoperative hemorrhage in patients who received ketorolac,[22] a quantitative systematic review of NSAIDs and the risk of operative site bleeding after tonsillectomy noted that of four bleeding end points (intraoperative blood loss, postoperative bleeding, hospital admission, and reoperation because of bleeding), only reoperation happened significantly more often with NSAIDs.[23] Thus, use of this class of drugs should be discussed with the surgeon before administration as many otolaryngologists prefer avoiding this class of drugs for certain procedures.

Narcotics are another class of drugs that may be useful in obtaining pain relief for children. Based on the age of the child and nature of the surgery, narcotics may be a good choice for pain control. Fentanyl, morphine, and hydromorphone have all been used to control pain intraoperatively and postoperatively. It is important to note that with these agents, respiratory depression may occur, especially in the patient with a history of obstructive sleep apnea. These patients have been shown to be more sensitive to this class of drugs[6,7] and smaller doses can sometimes yield adequate effect. Support of the airway and use of opioid antagonists may be necessary in cases where respiratory depression occurs. It is important to note that opioid antagonists, such as naloxone, are not devoid of complications themselves. Complications including flash pulmonary edema have been reported.[24] Overnight monitoring of the patient with a history of obstructive sleep apnea who also receives narcotics postoperatively may sometimes be necessary.

Codeine is an oral narcotic often prescribed for postoperative pain relief. Codeine is converted to its active metabolite, morphine, by the highly polymorphic CYP2D6 pathway of the cytochrome P4502D6 system. It should be noted that fatalities and life-threatening respiratory depression have been reported in patients identified as

Table 10.2 Management of Malignant Hyperthermia

1.	Discontinue triggering agents
2.	Discontinue surgery whenever possible
3.	Hyperventilate
4.	Administer the first intravenous dose of dantrolene (2.5 mg/kg)
5.	Begin cooling methods
6.	Treat hyperkalemia—consider insulin and glucose
7.	Obtain laboratory tests to ascertain degree of metabolic derangement
8.	Maintain adequate urine output
9.	Assess and treat for rhabdomyolysis

Table 10.3 Commonly Used Pharmacologic Agents for Pain Relief

Drug	Route	Usual Dose (mg/kg)
Acetaminophen	PO	10–20
Acetaminophen	PR	20
Ibuprofen	PO	10–20
Codeine	PO	0.5–1
Ketorolac	IV/IM	0.5
Fentanyl	IV	0.5–1
Morphine	IV	0.02–0.05

PO, per os (by mouth); PR, per rectum; IV, intravenous; IM, intramuscular.

ultra-rapid metabolizers.[25] Judicious use of codeine and other opioids that use the CYP2D6 pathway should be exercised in children with sleep apnea syndrome. These adverse outcomes may be avoided by CYP2D6 genetic testing before prescribing.[26] Genetic testing at this time is not commercially available.

Complications

Airway Obstruction

Airway obstruction is one of the most common concerns in the postoperative patient after airway surgery. Many perioperative factors made contribution to the development of postoperative airway obstruction. These include a history of sleep apnea or central apnea, anatomic narrowing of the airway, laryngospasm, bronchospasm, administration of narcotics, mechanical causes, and severe bleeding. Severe airway obstruction may lead to sudden pulmonary edema, secondary to strong negative-pressure inspiratory force against a closed glottis. Pink frothy secretions may be seen if the case is severe enough. Treatment consists of relief of the obstruction, with consideration of endotracheal intubation, supplemental oxygen administration, continuous positive airway pressure, and potential administration of diuretics.

Emergence Agitation

Emergence agitation is common in the pediatric population, and occurs in approximately18 to 80% of children undergoing anesthesia.[27] It is most common in children who present for short procedures under general anesthesia with inhalation agents, and its mechanism remains unclear. It can increase the distress of health care providers and families, expose the child to potential injury, and delay

recovery after anesthesia.[27] Treatments for emergence agitation range from allowing the child to settle in time without medication to pharmacologic intervention with benzodiazepines, narcotics, propofol or dexmedetomidine. Alternative techniques such as acupuncture have also been shown to be helpful.[28]

Postoperative Nausea and Vomiting

Preoperative nausea and vomiting (PONV) is common in children undergoing otolaryngology procedures, and has been reported to be as high as 50 to 89% posttonsillectomy.[29] It is troublesome to patients and families, and is known to delay discharge. Some of the risk factors include age older than 3 years, surgery lasting longer than 30 minutes, or a patient or family history of PONV.[29,30] Prophylaxis administration of one or more agents including dexamethasone, 5-hydroxy-tryptamine-3 antagonists, droperidol, or promethazine is recommended.[31] Dexamethasone has also been shown to be effective in reducing PONV as well as decreasing swelling, improving oral intake, and decreasing postoperative pain.[32]

Conclusion

The anesthetic management of the child undergoing otolaryngology procedures ranges from the straight forward and mask induction and myringotomy tube placement to the very complex neck exploration and reconstruction in a child with comorbidities and potentially difficult airway. Consultation and collaborative planning between the surgeon and anesthesiologist to create a comprehensive and thoughtful perioperative plan is important in the care of the pediatric patient, all with the goal, as Keats described, of "a sleep full of sweet dreams, and health, and quiet breathing."

References

1. Wittkugel EP, Varughese AM. Pediatric preoperative evaluation–a new paradigm. Int Anesthesiol Clin 2006;44(1):141–158
2. Maxwell LG, Yaster M. Perioperative management issues in pediatric patients. Anesthesiol Clin North America 2000;18(3):601–632
3. Welborn LG, Greenspun JC. Anesthesia and apnea. Perioperative considerations in the former preterm infant. Pediatr Clin North Am 1994;41(1):181–198
4. Coté CJ, Zaslavsky A, Downes JJ, et al. Postoperative apnea in former preterm infants after inguinal herniorrhaphy. A combined analysis. Anesthesiology 1995;82(4):809–822
5. Tait AR, Malviya S. Anesthesia for the child with an upper respiratory tract infection: still a dilemma? Anesth Analg 2005;100(1):59–65
6. Brown KA, Laferrière A, Lakheeram I, Moss IR. Recurrent hypoxemia in children is associated with increased analgesic sensitivity to opiates. Anesthesiology 2006;105(4):665–669
7. Brown KA, Laferrière A, Moss IR. Recurrent hypoxemia in young children with obstructive sleep apnea is associated with reduced opioid requirement for analgesia. Anesthesiology. 2004;100(4):806–810; discussion 5A
8. Moss IR, Brown KA, Laferrière A. Recurrent hypoxia in rats during development increases subsequent respiratory sensitivity to fentanyl. Anesthesiology 2006;105(4):715–718
9. Frey TK, Chopra A, Lin RJ, et al. A child with anterior mediastinal mass supported with veno-arterial extracorporeal membrane oxygenation. Pediatr Crit Care Med 2006;7(5):479–481
10. Kotiniemi LH, Ryhänen PT, Valanne J, Jokela R, Mustonen A, Poukkula E. Postoperative symptoms at home following day-case surgery in children: a multicentre survey of 551 children. Anaesthesia 1997;52(10):963–969
11. Kain ZN, Caldwell-Andrews AA, Mayes LC, et al. Family-centered preparation for surgery improves perioperative outcomes in children: a randomized controlled trial. Anesthesiology 2007;106(1):65–74
12. Mallampati SR, Gatt SP, Gugino LD, et al. A clinical sign to predict difficult tracheal intubation: a prospective study. Can Anaesth Soc J 1985;32(4):429–434
13. Nuckton TJ, Glidden DV, Browner WS, Claman DM. Physical examination: Mallampati score as an independent predictor of obstructive sleep apnea. Sleep 2006;29(7):903–908
14. Haynes AB, Weiser TG, Berry WR, et al; Safe Surgery Saves Lives Study Group. A surgical safety checklist to reduce morbidity and mortality in a global population. N Engl J Med 2009;360(5):491–499
15. Hohlrieder M, Keller C, Brimacombe J, et al. Middle ear pressure changes during anesthesia with or without nitrous oxide are similar among airway devices. Anesth Analg 2006;102(1):319–321
16. Neuman GG, Sidebotham G, Negoianu E, et al. Laparoscopy explosion hazards with nitrous oxide. Anesthesiology 1993;78(5):875–879
17. Amathieu R, Combes X, Abdi W, et al. An algorithm for difficult airway management, modified for modern optical devices (Airtraq laryngoscope; LMACTrach™): a 2-year prospective validation in patients for elective abdominal, gynecologic, and thyroid surgery. Anesthesiology 2011;114(1):25–33
18. Fiadjoe J, Stricker P. Pediatric difficult airway management: current devices and techniques. Anesthesiol Clin 2009;27(2):185–195
19. Corvetto MA, Hobbs GW, Taekman JM. Fire in the operating room. Simul Healthc 2011; 6(6):356–359
20. Hopkins PM. Malignant hyperthermia: advances in clinical management and diagnosis. Br J Anaesth 2000;85(1):118–128
21. Larach MG, Localio AR, Allen GC, et al. A clinical grading scale to predict malignant hyperthermia susceptibility. Anesthesiology 1994;80(4):771–779
22. Agrawal A, Gerson CR, Seligman I, Dsida RM. Postoperative hemorrhage after tonsillectomy: use of ketorolac tromethamine. Otolaryngol Head Neck Surg 1999;120(3):335–339
23. Møiniche S, Rømsing J, Dahl JB, Tramèr MR. Nonsteroidal antiinflammatory drugs and the risk of operative site bleeding after tonsillectomy: a quantitative systematic review. Anesth Analg 2003;96(1):68–77
24. Horng HC, Ho MT, Huang CH, Yeh CC, Cherng CH. Negative pressure pulmonary edema following naloxone administration in a patient with fentanyl-induced respiratory depression. Acta Anaesthesiol Taiwan 2010;48(3):155–157
25. Kelly LE, Rieder M, van den Anker J, et al. More codeine fatalities after tonsillectomy in North American children. Pediatrics 2012;129(5):e1343-e1347
26. Sadhasivam S, Myer Lii CM. Preventing opioid-related deaths in children undergoing surgery. Pain Med 2012;13(7):982-983, doi 10.1111/j.1526-4637.2012.01419.x
27. Vlajkovic GP, Sindjelic RP. Emergence delirium in children: many questions, few answers. Anesth Analg 2007;104(1):84–91
28. Lin YC, Tassone RF, Jahng S, et al. Acupuncture management of pain and emergence agitation in children after bilateral myringotomy and tympanostomy tube insertion. Paediatr Anaesth 2009;19(11):1096–1101
29. Collins CE, Everett LL. Challenges in pediatric ambulatory anesthesia: kids are different. Anesthesiol Clin 2010;28(2):315–328
30. Eberhart LH, Geldner G, Kranke P, et al. The development and validation of a risk score to predict the probability of postoperative vomiting in pediatric patients. Anesth Analg 2004;99(6):1630–1637
31. Gan T.J., Meyer T., Apfel C.C., et al. Consensus guidelines for managing postoperative nausea and vomiting. Anesth Analg 2003;97(1):62–71
32. Cardwell M, Siviter G, Smith A. Non-steroidal anti-inflammatory drugs and perioperative bleeding in paediatric tonsillectomy. Cochrane Database Syst Rev 2005;(2):CD003591

11 Tracheostomy in Children

Roy Rajan and Emily F. Boss

Tracheotomy is defined as the creation of an opening in the neck into the trachea, bypassing the larynx for air circulation. The term derives from the Greek word *tome* meaning "a cutting." *Tracheostomy* refers to the semi-permanent or permanent physical opening between the trachea and the skin. The two terms are often used interchangeably, and likely the semantic difference is negligible. Whereas tracheotomy defines the physical operation itself, tracheostomy is typically used to describe the general procedure and circumstance and will be used as such throughout this chapter.

Nicholas Habicot is credited for performing the first successful pediatric tracheotomy in the 16th century on a child who had tracheal compression secondary to swallowed coins lodged in the cervical esophagus.[1] While tracheostomy was performed most often in the remote past to relieve upper airway obstruction in children who had acute infection, prolonged mechanical ventilation is now the most common indication.[2] Subglottic stenosis and bilateral vocal cord paralysis are other common indications for tracheostomy. Modern advances in neonatal and pediatric care including vaccination, use of soft polyvinyl chloride endotracheal tubes, and improved education in airway management have contributed to an increase in survival of premature infants without a need for tracheostomy. Today, the decision to perform tracheostomy in a child is generally dictated by the anticipation of long-term cardiopulmonary compromise due to chronic ventilatory or cardiac insufficiency, or by the presence of a fixed upper airway obstruction that is unlikely to resolve for a significant period of time or is not amenable to early surgical treatment.

The mortality related to pediatric tracheostomy is estimated to be as high as 3.6% of the cases, and overall morbidity from this procedure ranges from 22 to 77%.[3] While the morbidity associated with tracheostomy has generally decreased, tracheostomy is associated with higher mortality in children than in adults.[4] This disparity is partly due to anatomical differences, as children have shorter necks, higher extension of pleura, more pliable tracheal cartilage, as well as decreased pulmonary reserve.

In addition to complications specifically related to the operative procedure, children with tracheostomy can experience tube dislodgement, tracheal stenosis, mucous plugging of the tracheostomy tube, dysphagia, and speech dysfunction. Children, compared with adults, are less often able to signal for help in the event of tube obstruction. These factors, as well as the special care considerations for children with long-term tracheostomy, focus the need for multidisciplinary involvement in the decision to perform tracheostomy in a

child. Preoperative counseling and postoperative education and care for the child and family are an essential part of this process.

Indications

Prolonged mechanical ventilation due to respiratory disease or neuromuscular compromise in the neonate is currently the most common indication for pediatric tracheostomy. Anatomic or functional upper airway obstruction is also a common indication for tracheostomy in children. Finally, children with chronic neurological impairment may require tracheostomy to assist with ventilation, decrease risk of chronic aspiration, and facilitate pulmonary toilet.[5]

Tracheostomy is often recommended for children, most commonly neonates, who require *prolonged ventilation* due to chronic lung disease (bronchopulmonary dysplasia) or conditions associated with congenital or acquired neurologic, pulmonary, or cardiovascular anomalies. In adults, tracheostomy is typically performed within two weeks of intubation to avoid more permanent laryngeal trauma. In contrast, many infants tolerate intubation for weeks to months without adverse laryngeal effects, and therefore the term "prolonged intubation" is not well-defined in the pediatric population. In recent decades, advances in endotracheal tube materials and attention to correct sizing of endotracheal tubes for the pediatric airway, have allowed extubation of many infants without airway sequelae. In general, tracheostomy is considered when weaning from mechanical ventilation is unlikely and attempts at extubation have failed.

Upper airway obstruction is a broad indication for tracheostomy in children. Airway obstruction from diphtheria and epiglottitis, historically common indications for tracheostomy, have disappeared due to widespread vaccination against diphtheria and *Haemophilus influenzae* type B. Causes of upper airway obstruction in children that may require tracheotomy include subglottic stenosis, bilateral vocal cord paralysis, congenital airway malformations, and neoplasms. Children with craniofacial syndromes may require tracheostomy for relief of airway obstruction due to micrognathia, glossoptosis, macroglossia, or oropharyngeal/nasopharyngeal crowding, or to facilitate airway management at the time of reconstructive surgery. Children with upper airway neoplasms such as subglottic hemangiomas or recurrent respiratory papillomatosis (RRP) occasionally require tracheostomy for severe obstruction not amenable to other treatments. In cases of RRP, tracheostomy is avoided if at all possible because of concern about distal dissemination of papillomas to the tracheobronchial tree or pulmonary parenchyma, but this procedure may be unavoidable with extensive or refractory disease causing life-threatening airway obstruction.[6]

Finally, children with neurological impairment may benefit from tracheostomy to relieve dynamic upper airway obstruction from pharyngeal hypotonia, assist with ventilation, help manage chronic aspiration, and most significantly, to facilitate *pulmonary toilet*. Children with neurological impairment have often experienced multiple hospital admissions for recurrent pneumonia, and most are fed via gastrostomy to reduce the risk of aspiration. These children tend to have a lower probability of decannulation and have a higher mortality following hospital discharge.[7] Neurological conditions in children requiring tracheostomy include cerebral palsy, encephalopathy, muscular dystrophy, and traumatic brain injury.

Operative Considerations

Tube Selection

The proper choice of a tracheostomy tube is dictated both by the indication for the procedure and by the age and weight of the child. Tubes are made of metal, polyvinyl chloride, or silicone, the latter two being more popular in recent years due to increased pliability and less adherence by secretions (**Fig. 11.1**). Metal tracheostomy tubes can facilitate endoscopic laser airway surgery, but long-term use in children is rarely seen. Both diameter and length should be considered when choosing a tracheostomy tube. If the diameter is too large, the tracheal mucosa can be damaged due to pressure, with development of granulation, scarring, and even tracheal

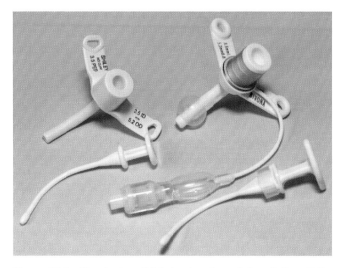

Figure 11.1 Standard pediatric tracheostomy tubes. Left, a Shiley 3.5 pediatric cuffless tube (inner diameter 3.5 mm, length 40 mm). Right, a Bivona 3.5 neonatal cuffed tube (inner diameter 3.5 mm, length 34 mm).
Reprinted with permission from: Elsevier. Boss EF. Pediatric tracheostomy. Operative Techniques in Otolaryngology – Head and Neck Surgery 2009; 20(4):212–217.

stenosis. If the diameter is too small, ventilation may be inadequate because of leak around the tracheostomy tube, and mucous plugging may also occur if a tube is too small for clearance of secretions with cough and suctioning.

Tube length is also an important consideration. Ideally the tip of the tracheostomy tube should rest 8 to 20 mm above the carina. Pediatric tracheostomy tubes are available in neonatal or pediatric sizes which differ in length by 8 to 10 mm. In children with airway pathology such as tracheomalacia, tracheal stenosis, or obesity, tracheostomy tubes with customized lengths may be necessary to safely bypass obstructing lesions.

Pediatric tracheostomy tubes are available with and without cuffs. Ventilators may be adjusted to minimize hypoventilation and excessive air leak around a cuffless tube. Cuffed tracheostomy tubes are sometimes useful to provide ventilation when increased inspiratory pressures are required, but these tubes may be associated with a higher risk of tracheal stenosis or pressure ulceration if the cuff pressure is not closely monitored.[8] Cuffed tubes may also be more difficult to change in young children, although tubes with low-profile "tight-to-shaft" cuffs have improved this problem.

In general, the tracheostomy tube with the smallest lumen that will maintain adequate ventilation without excessive plugging is selected. Tube size is typically determined based on the weight and age of the child, but may also be determined by an age-based formula (**Table 11.1**).[9] As children grow, the size of the tube should be appropriately adjusted to allow adequate respiration and minimize mucous plugging.

Standard Operative Technique

In most cases, tracheostomy is performed under controlled circumstances with the child intubated under general anesthesia. Urgent tracheotomy in a young child without a secured airway is fraught with disaster. An appropriately sized tracheostomy tube is selected, as well as a smaller tracheostomy tube and uncuffed endotracheal tube, for use in the event of difficult insertion.

Although there are many variations in operative technique, most surgeons approach the procedure in a fairly standard manner.[10] The child is positioned with neck extended and the head stabilized. Nasogastric tubes are removed, as the presence of a stiff esophageal tube may complicate palpation of the trachea in small neonates. Local anesthetic is often infiltrated for hemostasis and anesthesia, along a planned horizontal skin incision approximately one-third distance between the cricoid cartilage and the sternal notch. Orientation of the incision varies by surgeon preference; while the more commonly used horizontal skin incision leaves a more cosmetically sensitive scar, a vertical skin incision allows for ease of retraction of soft tissue during the procedure.[10] Subcutaneous fat is removed or reflected and the cervical fascia is identified. The strap muscles are separated in the midline along the midline raphe to the

Table 11.1   Tracheostomy Tube Sizing in Children

Tube size (inner diameter) based on child age and weight[a]	
Infants <1 kg	2.5 mm
Infants 1–2.5 kg	3 mm
Term infants (0–6 mo)	3–3.5 mm
Term infants 6–12 mo	3.5–4 mm
Infants 1–2 y	4–4.5 mm
Children > 2 y	(Age in years + 16)/4
Formulaic prediction of tube size in children[b]	
Inner diameter (mm)	Outer diameter (mm)
Age (y)/3 + 3.5	Age (y)/3 + 5.5

[a]*Adapted from:* Wetmore RF. Tracheotomy. In: Bluestone CD, Stool SE, Alper CM, et al., eds. *Pediatric Otolaryngology*. Philadelphia: Saunders; 2003:1583–1598.

[b]*Adapted from*: Behl S, Watt J. W. Prediction of tracheostomy tube size for pediatric long-term ventilation: an audit of children with spinal cord injury. *Br J Anaesth* 2005;94(1):88–91.

mo, month(s); y, year(s).

thyroid isthmus, which may need to be divided or reflected inferiorly. Care should be taken to avoid aggressive dissection inferiorly or laterally to preserve the integrity of the pleura and prevent vascular injury.

Once the laryngotracheal cartilage is clearly exposed, vertically oriented "stay" sutures are placed on both sides of the midline of tracheal rings 2 to 4 (**Fig. 11.2**). These sutures can help provide traction during the procedure and help identify the tracheotomy lumen should there be accidental decannulation. The lateral retractors can then often be removed, and the trachea is incised vertically at rings 2 to 4 to enter the airway. A vertical incision has been shown in some studies to have less risk of suprastomal collapse or stenosis than other tracheal incisions.[11] If electrocautery is used during the procedure, the inspired oxygen concentration in the anesthesia circuit should be reduced to avoid airway fire.[12] With the tracheal lumen well exposed by gentle retraction on the stay sutures, the endotracheal tube is withdrawn under direct view until it lies just proximal to the tracheal incision, and the tracheostomy tube is gently inserted with an obturator. Following connection of the circuit, forceful ventilation is avoided until proper tracheostomy position is confirmed by presence of breath sounds, chest inflation, and end-tidal CO_2 on monitors. The tube is usually secured with circumferential cloth neck ties placed and tied with the neck is flexed. Skin sutures, or a combination of sutures and trach ties, are less commonly used.[10] Stay sutures are clearly labeled "right" and "left" and secured to the chest. Flexible tracheobronchoscopy may be performed to confirm appropriate positioning of the tracheostomy tube proximal to the carina.

The stay sutures are left in place until the first tracheostomy tube change, usually at 5 to 7 days after the procedure. The sutures can help provide traction and identify the tracheotomy should there be a decannulation. A chest radiograph may be obtained to check the tube position and identify pneumothorax, but the need for routine postoperative chest films has recently been questioned for asymptomatic patients.[13]

Alternative Techniques

Because of the complexity of the pediatric anatomy and the potentially severe complications of tube dislodgement in children, several variations in tracheotomy technique have

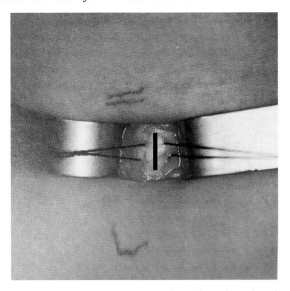

Figure 11.2 Stay sutures (3–0) are placed lateral to the planned incision site through the second and third tracheal cartilages in preparation for vertical tracheotomy incision.

been described. To avoid inadvertent dissection lateral to the trachea and neurovascular injury, Pereira and Weinstock propose bronchoscopy-assisted neonatal tracheostomy.[14] This technique involves rigid bronchoscopy to define the trachea with placement of an angiocatheter in the midline of the trachea just inferior to the first tracheal ring. A guidewire is passed through it and grasped from within the bronchoscope. The wire is then used to elevate the surgically exposed trachea and guide operative dissection.

Several variations of tracheal incision and stomal creation have also been proposed to limit postoperative accidental decannulation, tracheal stenosis, or anterior tracheal wall collapse. As opposed to a vertical tracheal incision with stay sutures, some surgeons make a horizontal incision in the trachea with creation of an inferior cartilage flap sutured to the skin as initially described by Bjork[15] (**Fig. 11.3**). An "H"-type, or double Bjork flap, may further minimize risk of accidental decannulation, but is associated with greater incidence of suprastomal collapse.[16] Tracheotomy techniques with extensive tracheal flaps may be unwise in infants and neonates, in whom tracheal diameters are small. Koltai proposed a "starplasty," which is created with a cruciate incision in the skin and trachea. The tracheostomy cartilage flaps are then affixed to the skin flaps with sutures to create a formal stoma (**Fig. 11.4**).[17] Another method of fashioning a more permanent stoma is the use of maturation sutures from the anterior wall of the trachea to the surrounding skin flaps.[18] These stoma maturation procedures may increase the incidence of persistent tracheocutaneous fistula after decannulation.[2]

Percutaneous tracheotomy has become common in the adult population. It is a procedure which can be performed

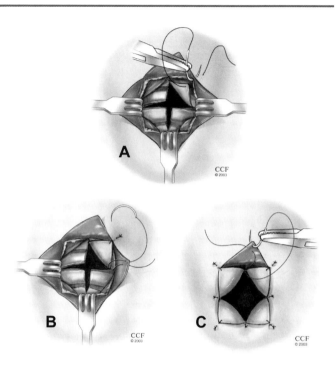

Figure 11.4 Starplasty tracheostoma modification. (A) Corner of trachea is sutured to diagonal skin. (B) Skin is sutured to trachea circumferentially. (C) Final configuration.
Reprinted with permission from: Elsevier. Solares CA, Krakovitz P, Hirose K, Koltai PJ. Starplasty: revisiting a tracheostomy technique. *Otolaryngology – Head and Neck Surgery* 2004;131(5):717–722.

quickly in the intensive care unit setting without the need for operation room personnel or associated costs. The rate of infection with percutaneous tracheotomy is also significantly less than with open techniques in adults.[19] The technique has been described in some older children with comparable complication rates to open procedures. Candidates for this procedure must be carefully selected as anatomical obscuration of landmarks such as from morbid obesity or goiter may be contraindications. Experience with the technique is also key to avoiding complications. The technique uses a Seldinger technique to dilate a tracheal opening over a guidewire with visualization from a bronchoscope at the end of an endotracheal tube in the subglottis. Application of percutaneous tracheotomy in children is still novice, and as such it is not recommended in neonates and very young children.

Complications

Complications of tracheostomy in children, both early and delayed, are outlined in **Table 11.2**. More common complications are discussed below.

Tracheostomy may result in *hemorrhage* during or after surgery. The rate of postoperative bleeding is approximately 5 to 7%.[2] The thyroid isthmus is a common site for intraoperative bleeding and is usually controlled with electrocautery or suture ligation. Early postoperative hemorrhage may arise from raw mucosal surfaces either from suctioning

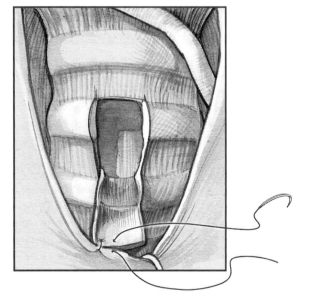

Figure 11.3 Bjork flap tracheostoma modification.
Reprinted with permission from: Elsevier. Scurry Jr WC, McGinn JD. Operative tracheotomy. *Operative Techniques in Otolaryngology – Head and Neck Surgery* 2007;18(2):85–89.

Table 11.2 Early and Delayed Complications of Tracheotomy

Early	Delayed
• Hemorrhage	• Hemorrhage, tracheo-innominate fistula
• Accidental decannulation	• Accidental decannulation
• Mucous plugging	• Mucous plugging
• Subcutaneous emphysema	• Tracheoesophageal fistula
• Pneumothorax/pneumomediastinum	• Tracheitis/stomal infections
• Recurrent laryngeal nerve injury	• Granulation tissue/granuloma
• Esophageal injury	• Subglottic/tracheal stenosis
• Tracheitis/stomal infections	• Tracheomalacia
• Airway fires	

the trachea or from dissected soft tissues in the neck. This bleeding is usually limited and resolves without aggressive management, but control with hemostatic agents or temporary packing around the tracheostomy tube may be necessary.

With long-term tracheotomy, the tip of the tube may erode through the tracheal wall and create a communication between the trachea and innominate artery. This rare phenomenon of *tracheo-innominate fistula* can produce a massive hemorrhage and is usually fatal. A small sentinel bleed may be the first sign of this phenomenon in up to one-third of patients, but a massive hemorrhage is more common.[20] Suspicion of tracheo-innominate fistula in a patient with unusual tracheal bleeding may warrant further investigation, including bronchoscopy, computed tomographic angiography, or formal arteriography.

Pneumomediastinum and *pneumothorax* are complications seen most commonly in the early postoperative period, and their incidence ranges from 4 to 43%.[2] In infants, the apex of the lung can extend into the root of the neck. Midline dissection and attention to avoid inferior dissection may prevent violation of the pleura. A postoperative chest radiograph can be used to exclude or diagnose pneumothorax.

Mucous plugging with tube obstruction is the most common complication of tracheostomy with an incidence of 14 to 72%.[2] Mucous plugging is more common in premature infants and newborns due to the smaller size of the tracheostomy tubes. This complication can be severe and may even lead to arrest and death. Saline should be gently instilled within the tracheostomy tube, and the tube should be suctioned at regular intervals according to the individual needs of the child. Medical management of increased or changed tracheal secretions may be necessary. Routine upsizing of tracheostomy tube according to age, humidification, and regularly scheduled tube changes also are key steps in preventing tube obstruction.

Accidental decannulation is a feared complication and is the second most common complication following tracheostomy. In the immediate postoperative period, accidental decannulation is particularly worrisome as the tracheotomy site and tract are not mature and established. For this

reason, young children are usually observed postoperatively in the intensive care unit for 5 to 7 days until the first tracheostomy tube change. A false passage can mistakenly be created during emergent reinsertion. Proper use of the stay sutures, visualization, and an orderly approach are the best ways to prevent false entry. Care providers must not forget that endotracheal intubation from above may often be the best way of securing the airway after accidental decannulation. Early tube dislodgement should be prevented as possible by carefully securing the tracheostomy with appropriately tight ties (one fingerbreadth between the tie and neck) or sutures that are directly observed on a daily basis after surgery. Bjork flap modification, starplasty, and other stomaplasty techniques have been proposed to allow easy tube replacement should there be dislodgement. Two spare tracheostomy tubes (one of a smaller size) and a small clamp should be available at the bedside at all times. Neonatal tubes are more likely to dislodge accidentally because of the shorter tube length. Once the stoma has matured, the tube is easier to safely reinsert, though dislodged tubes should be replaced as soon as possible to prevent stomal stenosis and closure. Delayed dislodgement becomes more of a risk as the child develops the dexterity to remove the tracheostomy tube. Despite these precautions, tube dislodgement and blockage remain the most important late complications and are responsible for a mortality rate of 1 to 2%.

Children with tracheostomy are susceptible to stomal or pulmonary *infections*. Aseptic suctioning and site cleaning should be employed as possible to prevent infection. A Humi-Vent™ (Hudson/Teleflex, Durham, North Carolina, United States) may also help filter pathogens and prevent respiratory irritation from decreased ciliary activity and inspissated secretions.[21] Topical, inhaled, and/or systemic antibiotics may be necessary depending on the symptoms and signs of infection.

Tracheal mucosal *granulation* or suprastomal *granuloma/fibroma* formation is reported in 30 to 40% of children with tracheostomy (**Fig. 11.5**).[22] Granulation tissue refers to the pink, friable healing tissue whereas granulomas/fibromas represent the more thickened and indurated respiratory mucosa. The most common cause of granulation tissue

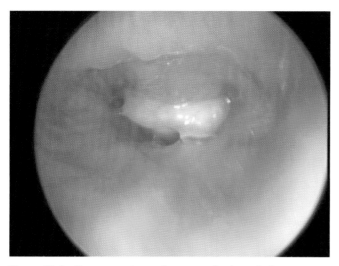

Figure 11.5 Suprastomal granuloma completely occluding suprastomal airway leading to impaired phonation and inability to decannulate.

is either trauma at the distal tip of the tracheostomy tube or excessive suctioning. Granulation can lead to bleeding or partial tube occlusion. Suprastomal granuloma, tissue on the anterior tracheal wall proximal to the stomal site, can be problematic when voice is diminished or when decannulation is being attempted. Formation is likely due to several factors, most significantly tube movement and irritation. These lesions can be removed endoscopically using microlaryngeal instruments, lasers, or microdebriders, or they can be excised through the stoma using open techniques.

Suprastomal collapse and *tracheal stenosis* may result from local chondritis and weakening of cartilage.[23] Suprastomal collapse is more common in younger children. Removal of a cartilaginous window at the time of initial tracheotomy may contribute to stomal narrowing or collapse. Fry et al demonstrated that tracheal stenosis is less common in the setting of vertical tracheotomy incision when compared with other methods.[24]

Persistent tracheocutaneous fistula after decannulation occurs in 19 to 65% of children.[2] Stomal maturation techniques may affect the incidence of fistula following decannulation.[23] Young age at tracheotomy and longer durations of tracheotomy use seem to be the most significant factors contributing to fistula. Treatment involves either excision of the epithelialized tract with closure of the defect, or excision of the tract with allowed secondary healing. The risk of *subcutaneous emphysema* and pneumothorax from postoperative air leak needs to be considered during surgical decision-making,

Airway fires are rare complications of tracheostomy. According to a recent survey of otolaryngologists, 18% of operating room fires were attributed to tracheostomy.[12] The electrosurgical unit was attributed as the cause when supplemental oxygen was in use.

Additional Considerations

Tracheostomy affects *speech and language* development in those with and without neurological disorders. Factors associated with speech and language delay in neurodevelopmentally normal children include young age at time of the tracheostomy and longer duration of the tracheostomy before decannulation. Children who experience long periods of aphonia during critical periods of language development (birth to 3 years) are known to be at risk for delayed communication skills. Thus, early decannulation improves the likelihood for normal speech and language development.[25] Children with tracheostomy should be encouraged to learn to temporarily and safely occlude their stomas to create sound. Early intervention with a speech and language pathologist (SLP) is important in developing the most effective way of verbal communication for the individual patient. A one-way speaking valve (Passy-Muir) is an effective tool both in facilitation of verbal communication as well as intermediary to capping. The child is assessed for alertness; cognition to follow directions; the absence of thick, copious secretions; and the ability to move air through the glottis before using the valve.[26] Any use of speech valve or tube cap should be monitored by a capable adult due to the obstruction created from capping.

Additionally, the presence of a tracheostomy may produce difficulties with swallowing and feeding. Inhibition of laryngeal reflexes, pressure, or interruption of the strap musculature, reduction of laryngeal elevation, poor coordination of breathing and swallowing, and pressure in the esophagus from the tube or tube cuff may all contribute to aspiration and dysphagia in children with tracheostomy. Tracheostomy may also impede generation of adequate subglottic pressure for the child to adequately cough out secretions. Some studies have shown speaking valves can improve swallowing by increasing subglottic pressure.[27] SLP evaluation can be helpful in determining appropriateness of oral feeding and necessary modifications.

Successful *decannulation* depends on significant improvement or resolution of the primary underlying disorder for which the tracheostomy was originally placed. Secondary anatomic abnormalities that may impede respiration such as suprastomal collapse or granuloma must also be ruled out and treated. Prescott suggested that the most common reason for failure of decannulation is peristomal pathology including tracheal granuloma, suprastomal collapse, stomal tracheomalacia, and stenosis.[28] Microlaryngoscopy and bronchoscopy are routinely used to evaluate the airway for any contributing factors to decannulation failure. The frequency of these evaluations after tracheostomy placement has not reached universal consensus.[5] Reconstructive procedures may be necessary to facilitate decannulation. Capped polysomnography evaluation or monitored intensive care unit stays with downsized capped tracheotomy tubes are means of evaluating readiness to decannulate.[29] The creation of fenestrations in a capped tracheostomy has also been proposed to get a more accurate measure of tracheostomy-independent breathing.[22] There is a 2 to 5% risk of decannulation failure when attempted, often related to dynamic airway problems.[30]

Summary

Tracheostomy in children is most commonly indicated for prolonged ventilation, upper airway obstruction, or pulmonary toilet in the setting of neurological disease. The technical aspects of tracheotomy in children are unique, as the airway and neck anatomy differs from adults and complications are potentially severe. The postoperative care issues are substantial. Tracheostomy impacts voice, language development, and swallowing in children. Decannulation, following assessment for peristomal sequelae and controlled capping trials, is often achieved when the indications for tracheotomy have been successfully treated or have resolved. A multidisciplinary approach to care of the child with tracheostomy may promote positive long-term functional outcomes.

References

1. Frost EA. Tracing the tracheostomy. Ann Otol Rhinol Laryngol 1976;85(5 Pt 1):618–624

2. Kremer B, Botos-Kremer AI, Eckel HE, Schlöndorff G. Indications, complications, and surgical techniques for pediatric tracheostomies—an update. J Pediatr Surg 2002;37(11):1556–1562

3. Carr MM, Poje CP, Kingston L, Kielma D, Heard C. Complications in pediatric tracheostomies. Laryngoscope 2001;111(11 Pt 1):1925–1928

4. Durbin CG Jr. Early complications of tracheostomy. Respir Care 2005;50(4):511–515

5. Kraft S, Patel S, Sykes K, Nicklaus P, Gratny L, Wei JL. Practice patterns after tracheotomy in infants younger than 2 Years. Arch Otolaryngol Head Neck Surg 2011;137(7):670–674

6. Shapiro AM, Rimell FL, Shoemaker D, Pou A, Stool SE. Tracheotomy in children with juvenile-onset recurrent respiratory papillomatosis: the Children's Hospital of Pittsburgh experience. Ann Otol Rhinol Laryngol 1996;105(1):1–5

7. Dursun O, Ozel D. Early and long-term outcome after tracheostomy in children. Pediatr Int 2011;53(2):202–206

8. Arola MK, Puhakka H, Mäkelä P. Healing of lesions caused by cuffed tracheostomy tubes and their late sequelae; a follow-up study. Acta Anaesthesiol Scand 1980;24(3):169–177

9. Wetmore RF. Tracheotomy. In: Blustone CD, Stool SE, Alpert CM, et al., eds. Pediatric Otolaryngology. Philadelphia: Saunders; 2003:1583–1598

10. Ruggiero FP, Carr MM. Infant tracheotomy: results of a survey regarding technique. Arch Otolaryngol Head Neck Surg 2008;134(3):263–267

11. Fraga JC, Souza JC, Kruel J. Pediatric tracheostomy. J Pediatr (Rio J) 2009;85(2):97–103

12. Smith LP, Roy S. Operating room fires in otolaryngology: risk factors and prevention. Am J Otolaryngol 2011;32(2):109–114

13. Genther DJ, Thorne MC. Utility of routine postoperative chest radiography in pediatric tracheostomy. Int J Pediatr Otorhinolaryngol 2010;74(12):1397–1400

14. Pereira KD, Weinstock YE. Bronchoscopy assisted neonatal tracheostomy (BANT): a new technique. Int J Pediatr Otorhinolaryngol 2007;71(2):211–215

15. Bjork VO. Partial resection of the only remaining lung with aid of respirator treatment. J Thorac Cardiovasc Surg 1960;39:179–188

16. Antón-Pacheco JL, Villafruela M, López M, García G, Luna C, Martínez A. Surgical management of severe suprastomal cricotracheal collapse complicating pediatric tracheostomy. Int J Pediatr Otorhinolaryngol 2008;72(2):179–183

17. Koltai PJ. Starplasty: a new technique of pediatric tracheotomy. Arch Otolaryngol Head Neck Surg 1998;124(10):1105–1111

18. Craig MF, Bajaj Y, Hartley BE. Maturation sutures for the paediatric tracheostomy—an extra safety measure. J Laryngol Otol 2005;119(12):985–987

19. Friedman Y, Fildes J, Mizock B, et al. Comparison of percutaneous and surgical tracheostomies. Chest 1996;110(2):480–485

20. Gelman JJ, Aro M, Weiss SM. Tracheo-innominate artery fistula. J Am Coll Surg 1994;179(5):626–634

21. Oberwaldner B, Eber E. Tracheostomy care in the home. Paediatr Respir Rev 2006;7(3):185–190

22. Merritt RM, Bent JP, Smith RJ. Suprastomal granulation tissue and pediatric tracheotomy decannulation. Laryngoscope 1997;107(7):868–871

23. Colman KL, Mandell DL, Simons JP. Impact of stoma maturation on pediatric tracheostomy-related complications. Arch Otolaryngol Head Neck Surg 2010;136(5):471–474

24. Fry TL, Jones RO, Fischer ND, Pillsbury HC. Comparisons of tracheostomy incisions in a pediatric model. Ann Otol Rhinol Laryngol 1985;94(5 Pt 1):450–453

25. Jiang D, Morrison GA. The influence of long-term tracheostomy on speech and language development in children. Int J Pediatr Otorhinolaryngol 2003;67(Suppl 1):S217–S220

26. Baumgartner CA, Bewyer E, Bruner D. Management of communication and swallowing in intensive care: the role of the speech pathologist. AACN Adv Crit Care 2008;19(4):433–443

27. Eibling DE, Gross RD. Subglottic air pressure: a key component of swallowing efficiency. Ann Otol Rhinol Laryngol 1996;105(4):253–258

28. Prescott CA. Peristomal complications of paediatric tracheostomy. Int J Pediatr Otorhinolaryngol 1992;23(2):141–149

29. Tunkel DE, McColley SA, Baroody FM, Marcus CL, Carroll JL, Loughlin GM. Polysomnography in the evaluation of readiness for decannulation in children. Arch Otolaryngol Head Neck Surg 1996;122(7):721–724

30. O'Connor HH, White AC. Tracheostomy decannulation. Respir Care 2010;55(8):1076–1081

12 Pediatric Esophageal and Swallowing Disorders

J. Paul Willging

Disorders of feeding and swallowing are being recognized more frequently both in healthy infants and young children as well as in children with concomitant airway disease. This chapter describes esophageal anatomy and the physiology of swallowing, as well as the diseases and anatomic lesions that can cause swallowing dysfunction. Common disorders, such as gastroesophageal reflux, and less common disease, such as eosinophilic esophagitis, are outlined. The role of the otolaryngologist in diagnosis and treatment of dysphagia and esophageal disease is emphasized, particularly with the use of endoscopic evaluation of swallowing. Readers should note the common association of airway disease with disorders of swallowing.

Esophageal Anatomy

The esophagus is a conduit connecting the hypopharynx and the stomach. It is predominantly a left-sided structure. It has circular muscle fibers surrounding the lumen, with an outer layer of longitudinally oriented muscle fibers. It has no serosal layer. A combination of voluntary and involuntary muscle tissue is present in the esophagus. The striated muscle is located superiorly, with smooth muscle located in the distal half.

The upper esophageal sphincter (UES) is composed of striated muscle from both the cricopharyngeus and the inferior pharyngeal constrictor muscles. Tonic contraction prevents material in the esophagus from refluxing into the hypopharynx, thus reducing aspiration risk. The UES also prevents the unintentional passage of air from the pharynx into the stomach during respiration.

The UES relaxes in coordination with bolus transfer into the pharynx for swallowing. The tonic contraction within the UES is inhibited during the act of swallowing, and due to the attachment of the cricopharyngeus muscle to the cricoid plate, the UES is actively opened when the larynx elevates with swallowing. The neural control of the events associated with swallowing occurs in the brainstem.

The lower esophageal sphincter (LES) is also under tonic control, and prevents the reflux of gastric contents into the esophagus. The LES relaxes in response to neural inhibition of the muscle, triggered by transit of food material with distension of the lower esophagus.

Tracheoesophageal Fistula with Esophageal Atresia

This congenital anomaly is seen in 1 in 3000 live births.[1] The most common variant of this anomaly, accounting for 85% of cases, involves an atretic upper pouch of the esophagus with the distal stump of the esophagus connecting to the posterior tracheal wall. Classic theory suggests they develop as a result of incomplete separation of the respiratory and digestive division of the foregut anlage. The primitive foregut is divided into an anterior airway and posterior esophagus by the medial advancement of the lateral foregut grooves. Failure of the two grooves to fuse in the midline leads to the development of a tracheoesophageal fistula (TEF). Abnormal directional growth of these grooves leads to esophageal atresia (EA).[2] An alternate explanation for the development of these disorders suggests that insufficient blood supply to the developing esophagus may lead to areas of necrosis and development of an atretic segment. A TEF would develop from abnormal fusion of the developing trachea and esophagus due to abnormally directed growth vectors.[3]

Infants with EA are identified early in life secondary to the feeding and respiratory difficulties that develop. Coughing, choking, and pneumonia are often seen in patients with EA, as the overflow of contents from the nonpatent upper esophageal segment can be aspirated. Gastric distension with positive pressure ventilation with a mask or endotracheal tube is seen with a TEF. The presence of EA or a TEF should prompt investigation for other associated anomalies as 50% of patients will have other abnormalities such as congenital heart disease (20%); gastrointestinal (13%); genitourinary (10%); musculoskeletal (9%); or facial anomalies (5%).[4]

Esophageal Motility Disorders

Cricopharyngeal achalasia (CPA) is characterized by failure of the UES to relax in response to propulsion of a bolus through the pharynx. The cricopharyngeus muscle may be hypertrophic or may demonstrate fibrosis. The lack of relaxation can be demonstrated on contrast radiographic studies of the esophagus as a cricopharyngeal bar protruding into the lumen of the UES segment of the esophagus during swallowing. CPA causes pharyngeal dysphagia. Treatment may include dilation treatments. Botulinum toxin injections may also provide temporary resolution of symptoms. Cricopharyngeal myotomy is a definitive treatment. In all children with CPA, an evaluation for an Arnold-Chiari malformation must be obtained due to their common association.[5] A common presenting symptom of patients with CPA is choking associated with feeding. The child will often shift their diet preferences away from foods of increased texture toward liquids and pureed materials.

Achalasia of the LES presents as a slowly progressive dysphagia for solids and liquids. This is an uncommon cause of dysphagia in children, most commonly affecting middle-aged adults. The proximal esophagus dilates, and a progressive narrowing of the lower esophagus creates the classic "bird-beak" deformity seen on radiographic studies. Similar to CPA, serial dilation procedures and botulinum toxin injections are effective treatments to temporize the condition. Longitudinal myotomy of the distal 2 cm of the esophagus and 2 cm of the anterior gastric wall down to the submucosa (modified Heller procedure) is generally definitive treatment for the condition.[6]

Gastroesophageal Reflux

Gastroesophageal reflux disease (GERD) is the most common esophageal disorder in children. Gastroesophageal reflux occurs when gastric contents pass retrograde from the stomach into the esophagus. Physiologic reflux occurs in normal individuals with episodes occurring infrequently and associated with rapid clearance of the refluxate from the esophagus. Physiologic reflux causes no irritation to the esophageal mucosa. When the esophageal mucosa is exposed to an increasing frequency of reflux events, or the duration of acid exposure within the esophagus increases with each reflux event, the mucosa becomes inflamed. Chronic inflammation of the esophageal mucosa by reflux is a hallmark of GERD. In children, GERD may have a host of manifestations, including irritability, failure to thrive, food refusal, cough, dysphagia, stridor, hoarseness, bronchospasm, recurrent pneumonia, and apnea. Clinically apparent regurgitate episodes need not be present with GERD.

Reflux events are normally cleared from the esophagus. Saliva and secretions produced by mucus glands within the esophagus neutralize gastric acid. The peristaltic action within the esophagus clears gastric secretions from the esophagus protecting the lining of the esophagus from the inflammatory actions of the reflux material. No single symptom or symptom complex is diagnostic of GERD. Clinical suspicion may lead to specific testing to determine the presence/severity of gastroesophageal reflux.

Tests for GERD

Esophageal pH Monitoring

Intraluminal pH is monitored and recorded continuously for 24 hours.[7] The length of time the esophagus is exposed to a pH less than 4 is determined. The number of episodes of acidic reflux is determined, and the number of reflux episodes lasting more than 5 minutes is determined. The probe is positioned within 3 cm of the LES for accurate recordings. To increase the sensitivity of the study, a second sensor can be positioned at the UES to assess the number of reflux events ascending to the level of the pharynx. Such pH monitoring can detect only acidic events reaching the level of the sensor. The volume of the reflux event cannot be determined. Gastric contents that have been buffered to a neutral pH by foods, bile, or medications do not trigger the sensor as an event. Esophageal pH monitoring is useful for evaluating the effectiveness of anti-acid and antisecretory therapies for gastroesophageal reflux.

Combined Multiple and Intraluminal Impedance with pH Monitoring

A probe that measures a change in the impedance between pairs of electrodes allows a determination of the presence of liquid, air, or solids in the esophagus passing the probe.[8] Multiple pairs of electrodes allow a reflux event to be followed as it ascends the esophagus and again as it is cleared from the esophagus. A pH sensor is incorporated into the sleeve of the sensor to allow a determination of the acidic or neutral nature of the reflux event.

Impedance monitoring provides significantly more information regarding reflux events than does a pH probe study. Antegrade and retrograde flow through the esophagus can be measured. Acidic and pH neutral reflux events can be identified. The height of a single event can be followed and the rate of clearance from the esophagus defined.

Contrast Radiographic Studies

The upper gastrointestinal radiographic study is useful in determining anatomic abnormalities of the upper gastrointestinal tract, but it is a limited study for the diagnosis of GERD. Reflux may be seen during the study, but the absence of identified reflux events does not rule out the diagnosis of GERD. Conversely, some reflux events may be seen in normal individuals without disease.

Scintigraphy

Radiolabeled food materials are ingested and prolonged imaging is obtained to provide a means of determining the rate of gastric emptying and identifying reflux events. Pulmonary aspiration of a reflux event may be recorded by the presence of label within the lung fields. A negative test does not rule out the possibility of pulmonary aspiration of refluxed materials due to the episodic nature of the events. These nuclear medicine scans are not recommended for the routine evaluation of children suspected of having GERD.

Endoscopy with Biopsy

Esophagogastroduodenoscopy allows visualization of the esophageal mucosa, and permits biopsy specimens to be obtained from the proximal and distal esophagus. The stomach and duodenum are also examined. Breaks in the distal esophageal mucosa are the most reliable sign of reflux esophagitis. Mucosal erythema, pallor, and altered vascular patterns are suggestive but not specific findings of reflux. Histologic findings suggestive of gastroesophageal reflux are eosinophilia, elongation of the rete pegs, vascular hyperplasia, and dilation of intercellular spaces.

Extraesophageal reflux (reflux reaching the hypopharynx causing laryngeal irritation) is difficult to definitively diagnose. There is a poor correlation between the visual appearance of the larynx on fiberoptic examination and the results of pH probes and esophageal biopsies.[9] A reflux event that spills into the endolarynx will not be readily cleared, causing prolonged caustic irritation to the laryngeal structures. The number of extraesophageal reflux events required to cause pathologic changes within the larynx therefore will be much less than the number of events required to produce esophageal pathology.

Treatment of GERD

Medical treatment of GERD is reserved for children with excessive emesis episodes, irritability related to gastroesophageal reflux, failure to thrive, or recurrent respiratory symptoms. Antacids neutralize gastric acid. High doses of aluminum medications may reach toxic levels in children, causing neutropenia, anemia and neurotoxicity.[10] Only sporadic use of aluminum-containing antacids is recommended in children.

Prokinetic agents increase the resting tone of the LES, increasing esophageal peristalsis and accelerating gastric emptying. All these mechanisms reduce gastroesophageal reflux events. Cisapride provides the greatest prokinetic effect and is least likely to induce bronchospasm. Cases of prolonged Q-T interval and fatal arrhythmias have been associated with cisapride when used concurrently with macrolide antibiotics and antifungal medications.[11] The use of cisapride should be limited to select infants failing dietary changes and antisecretory medical therapy. Careful monitoring is required for the duration of its use, limiting the utility of this medication.

Metoclopramide facilitates gastric emptying; it is associated with lethargy, irritability, and may in rare cases cause irreversible tardive dyskinesia. Sucralfate adheres to the surface of the gastric ulcers and protects the esophageal mucosa from the corrosive effects of gastric acid. As it contains aluminum, care must be taken in children.

Histamine receptor antagonist (H$_2$ blockers), ranitidine and cimetidine, suppress gastric acid production. They reduce the symptoms of GERD and promote healing of the histologic changes associated with esophagitis.

While H$_2$ blockers are often the starting point of medical treatment for gastroesophageal reflux, proton pump inhibitors (PPIs) are the most effective acid suppressants. Lansoprazole (Prevacid) and omeprazole (Prilosec) come in formulations that are easily administered and well tolerated in children. While once daily treatment is the norm, impedance probe verified breakthrough of acid production warrants twice daily treatment. There is concern regarding the safety of prolonged PPI use. An increased risk of osteoporosis and associated bone fractures has been described with treatment durations longer than one year. Increased rates of community-acquired pneumonia, gastroenteritis, and *Candida* infections have also been associated with prolonged use of PPIs.[12]

Surgical treatment of GERD is reserved for patients with severe, medically refractory gastroesophageal reflux symptoms. Fundoplication procedures, of which the Nissen procedure is the most common, attempt to recreate a functional LES by wrapping a portion of the greater curvature of the stomach around the esophagus. The primary complication associated with this procedure is gas-bloat syndrome, retching, gagging, dumping syndrome, and recurrent reflux symptoms.

Dysphagia in Children

Swallowing is an intricate process that requires multiple cranial and cervical nerves and the precise coordination of numerous muscles of the lips, tongue, palate, pharynx, larynx, esophagus, and chest. Any condition that upsets the delicate interplay between components of the swallowing mechanism may result in dysphagia.

Changes associated with the growth and maturational development of the upper aerodigestive tract in children may create pathophysiology that differs substantially from that seen in adults with feeding and swallowing disorders. Specifically, the anatomy of the oral cavity and the anatomic relationships of the mouth, pharynx, and larynx undergo continual change over the first several years of life. Similarly, the process of food ingestion evolves from reflexive sucking to mastication and the neurologic control mechanisms that coordinate swallowing with respiratory activity undergo continual development. If the child is unable to adapt to changes in structure or if neurologic function is impaired, swallowing will be compromised, and problems may arise that could lead to chronic pulmonary disease or malnutrition.

The improved survival rates of children with a history of prematurity, low birth weight, and complex medical conditions that affect the structure and function of various components of the swallowing mechanism has resulted in an increased incidence of pediatric dysphagia.[13–16] In view of this increase, there is a high likelihood of encountering these patients in clinical practice.

Normal Swallowing Physiology

The neural control of swallowing is complex. Afferent sensory inputs are integrated in the brainstem, and efferent pattern generators direct the motor responses to produce an efficient and safe swallow. A sequential discharge of neurons is provided to the muscles in the pharynx, larynx, and esophagus. Four neural components have been well described: (1) afferent sensory fibers contained in the cranial nerves; (2) efferent motor fibers contained in the cranial nerves and the ansa cervicalis; (3) cerebral, midbrain, and cerebellar fibers that synapse in the midbrain; and (4) the paired swallowing centers located in the brainstem.[17,18]

Three Phases of Swallowing

The act of swallowing (deglutition) allows food or liquid bolus to be transported from the mouth to the pharynx and esophagus, through which it enters the stomach. Normal deglutition is a synchronized process that involves an intricate series of voluntary and involuntary neuromuscular contractions. This process is typically divided into three distinct phases: oral, pharyngeal, and esophageal. Each of these phases facilitates a specific function. Problems in one or more phases of swallowing constitute dysphagia.

Oral Phase

The oral phase is under voluntary neural control and begins with the introduction of food material into the mouth. Coordinated contractions of the tongue and muscles of mastication modulated by mechanoreceptors organize this material into a bolus. The tongue elevates as the bolus is held in the central groove of the tongue, and moves in a peristaltic fashion against the palate. The posterior propulsion of the bolus by the tongue into the pharynx triggers the onset of the involuntary swallow reflex.

This phase requires complex sensory and motor integration. The facial nerve innervates muscles of the face, and branches of the mandibular division of the trigeminal nerve innervate muscles associated with mandibular movement. The tongue requires coordinated movement of four intrinsic muscles innervated by the hypoglossal nerve, and four extrinsic muscles innervated by branches from the ansa cervicalis.[17] The vagus and glossopharyngeal nerves innervate the muscles of the palate, pharynx, and larynx. Branches from the maxillary division of the trigeminal, facial, glossopharyngeal, and vagus nerves provide sensory innervation. Neural control of the swallowing process is at the level of the brainstem in infancy—it is predominantly a reflexive act. As cortical maturation occurs and experience with food materials accumulates, increasing volitional control is acquired.

Pharyngeal Phase

The pharyngeal phase of swallowing is largely involuntary. Pharyngeal swallows are initiated in an ordered sequential pattern in response to stimulation by food or secretions in the pharynx. Tactile receptors in the pharynx provide sensory stimulation to the medullary swallowing center via the trigeminal, glossopharyngeal, and vagus nerves.[19] The medullary swallowing center initiates a swallow by stimulating the nucleus ambiguus and the dorsomedial vagal nucleus. The soft palate closes against the posterior pharyngeal wall to isolate the nasopharynx from the oropharynx as food is propelled posteriorly. The bolus is propelled through the oropharynx by the contraction of the pharyngeal muscles against the base of the tongue. Proprioceptive feedback adjusts the peristaltic activity for different food bolus sizes and consistencies.[20]

The pharynx serves as a conduit for food as well as air exchange. Precise coordination of breathing and swallowing is thus necessary during feeding. With the initiation of the swallow, respiration is concurrently inhibited and the larynx is pulled superiorly and anteriorly; this effectively moves the laryngeal inlet out of the direct path of the bolus. The true and false vocal folds close, and the epiglottis retroflexes over the laryngeal inlet with laryngeal elevation to further protect the distal airway. The upper esophageal inlet is pulled open with laryngeal elevation, and the peristaltic contractions of the pharyngeal constrictor muscles propel the bolus into the esophagus.

Food material falling into the laryngeal inlet stimulates mechanoreceptors and chemoreceptors, resulting in vocal cord closure and apnea. Apnea will be sustained until the noxious stimulus is cleared from the larynx. Hypoxia may result in the neonate due to the lack of respiratory reserve. An additional response to stimulation is the cough reflex; this may be triggered by direct laryngeal stimulation or stimulation of receptors within the trachea. It is important to note, however, that this reflex is absent in 75% of premature infants and 50% of newborns.[21] Additionally, it may be compromised in infants who are neurologically impaired.

Esophageal Phase

The esophagus is a conduit between the pharynx and the stomach, with muscular sphincters at either end in tonic contraction to keep the esophagus closed between swallows. The UES relaxes during swallowing, and is actively opened by laryngeal elevation to allow the food bolus to enter the esophagus. Peristaltic contractions propel the bolus down into the stomach. The LES relaxes to allow passage of the bolus. Tonic contraction of the LES prevents the reflux of gastric contents into the lower esophagus. Propagation of the peristaltic wave is dependent on the intrinsic myenteric plexus and vagal efferents.

Aspiration

Aspiration is the passage of solid or liquid material below the level of the vocal folds; the potential for this to occur is greatest during the pharyngeal phase of swallowing. Aspiration of small volumes of material may be cleared from the airway by normal mucociliary clearance or a cough. Large volumes of aspirated material may, however, reach the distal airway, leading to the possibility of aspiration pneumonia. Because oral secretions are laden with high concentrations of bacteria from the oral cavity, aspiration of these secretions may lead to chronic lung damage over time.[22] For children whose strength and endurance is compromised due to developmental, neurologic, or other medical conditions, fatigue during feeding can increase the risk of aspiration.[23]

Signs and Symptoms of Swallowing Disorders

The presentations of feeding and swallowing disorders are diverse, with signs and symptoms that may range from obvious problems such as projectile vomiting, coughing, or choking to more subtle silent aspiration. Affected neonates may exhibit sucking difficulty, slow sucking, or sucking that is unaccompanied by effective swallow. If left untreated, these symptoms may result in failure to thrive. Parents or clinicians may see delayed or restricted oral motor skills for intake of food or liquid, retention of food in the mouth, coughing and gagging when feeding, nasal reflux of food or liquid, failure to gain weight, or respiratory symptoms (apnea, cyanosis, retractions, tachypnea, stridor) during or shortly after feeding.

Dysphagia should be suspected in children who have repeated episodes of respiratory infections and suffer chronic bronchial congestion. Children with metabolic disease, neuromotor impairment, or craniofacial anomalies are often affected with disorders of feeding and swallowing. Dysmorphic features often indicate the presence of syndromes commonly associated with dysphagia (e.g., Cornelia de Lange syndrome, Pierre Robin syndrome, velocardiofacial syndrome, VACTERL association—vertebral defects, anal atresia, cardiac defects, tracheoesophageal fistula, renal anomalies, and limb abnormalities).[24]

Classification of Etiologies of Dysphagia in Children

The causes of pediatric dysphagia fall within five broad categories: structural abnormalities, neurologic conditions, cardiorespiratory problems, behavioral issues, and inflammatory or metabolic disorders.[25] Young children can have difficulties in swallowing that involve one or several of these issues.

Structural Abnormalities

Any anatomic abnormality from the nasal cavity to the gastrointestinal tract can potentially disrupt any phase of swallowing. Children with defects in the oral cavity or oropharynx, such as congenital craniofacial syndromes, cleft lip or palate, or macroglossia, may experience difficulty in the oral phase. Children with congenital defects of the larynx or trachea may develop feeding difficulties secondary to airway compromise during swallowing. Esophageal abnormalities may interfere with the transport of food material into the distal digestive tract. All these problems may create discomfort during feeding and may lead to feeding refusal and the development of behavioral feeding problems. In children who have undergone reconstructive procedures to correct anatomic anomalies, the behavioral issues may continue to predominate, thus perpetuating feeding problems.

Neurologic Conditions

Neurologic disorders comprise the most common etiology of pediatric feeding and swallowing disorders. Neuromotor impairment as a result of cortical dysfunction, abnormalities in the brainstem, or cervical cord injuries impacts the strength and efficiency of the oral and pharyngeal phases of swallowing, the adequacy of coordination of airway protection and swallowing, as well as overall alertness and the postural control necessary for safe and efficient feeding. In addition, these patients frequently present with esophageal issues such as impaired motility or GERD, further complicating their management.

Cardiorespiratory Problems

Cardiorespiratory compromise often affects an infant's ability to initiate or sustain a coordinated suck–swallow–breathe sequence. Feeding often results in accompanying apnea or episodes of bradycardia, thereby affecting feeding endurance and often preventing adequate food intake. Problems with respiratory compromise may result in poor coordination or inappropriate timing of airway protection during swallowing, resulting in coughing, choking, or episodes of apnea, bradycardia, chronic noisy breathing, or wheezing, as well as chronic or recurrent pneumonia, bronchitis, or atelectasis.

Behavioral Issues

Behavior-based feeding problems may stem from psychosocial factors, such as dysfunctional feeder–child interaction, poor environmental stimulation, conditioned dysphagia (a phobic response resulting from an aversive oral or pharyngeal experience or a painful feeding experience such as choking), or negative feeding behaviors. Behavioral responses exhibited by the child may include refusal to eat, rejection of certain foods or textures, and gagging or vomiting. Careful evaluation to eliminate the possibility of underlying physiologic factors before focused behavioral treatment of maladaptive feeding behaviors is essential.

Metabolic and Inflammatory Disorders

Metabolic abnormalities such as hereditary fructose intolerance or endocrine problems can interfere with swallowing. More commonly, inflammatory conditions such as GERD or eosinophilic esophagitis (EE) or food allergies can interfere with the development or maintenance of normal oral motor and feeding patterns. In young children, elimination of foods previously taken well is a hallmark of esophageal inflammation. EE is characterized by marked infiltration of the submucosa with eosinophils seen in esophageal biopsies. Gross disruption of esophageal architecture on esophagoscopy, with narrowings, furrows, or series of ring-like structures, have been described in children with EE. Treatment of EE includes the administration of swallowed aerosolized fluticasone as well as elimination of suspect foods that may be causing allergy. Allergy testing is important to identify foods that could be eliminated from the diet to reduce esophageal irritation.[26]

Diagnostic Evaluation of Dysphagia in Children

Imaging Studies

Videofluoroscopic Swallow Study

The videofluoroscopic swallow study (VFSS) is often considered the gold standard for evaluating infants and children with swallowing disorders.[27] The VFSS allows for noninvasive assessment of the oral, pharyngeal, and esophageal phases of swallowing and the interrelationship of these phases. Additionally, VFSS enables the determination of consistencies and conditions for safe swallowing and allows a trial of compensatory and therapeutic techniques to improve the safety and efficiency of swallowing. These interventions include examining the patient's response to other textures, alternating presentations of liquid and solids, and exploring the therapeutic efficacy of modifications in bolus volume, nipple, or utensil types; pace of presentation; and body posture.

The disadvantages of VFSS include use of ionizing radiation with exposure to both the child and the feeder. Assessment of compensatory strategies such as positioning alterations, oral motor strategies, or alternation of food and liquid consistencies adds to the overall exposure time. Additionally, adding barium to liquid and food sometimes decreases a child's willingness to drink or eat during the study. Moreover, because adding barium significantly increases viscosity, preparing a true thin liquid is not possible. Last, the VFSS is not feasible for patients who take extremely limited amounts of liquid or food orally, as the child needs to ingest a sufficient amount of contrast for adequate imaging.

Esophagram and Upper Gastrointestinal Radiographic Studies

The esophagram and upper gastrointestinal radiographic studies examine the anatomy and function of the esophagus, stomach, and duodenum. Dynamic images are obtained as the bolus passes through the oropharynx, into the esophagus, and into the stomach. Careful assessment for a possible tracheoesophageal fistula requires an adequate volume of contrast to distend the esophagus. In patients who cannot swallow an adequate volume of contrast, a tube is passed into the esophagus, providing a means of demonstrating the fistulous tract. Abnormalities such as esophageal strictures, webs, vascular rings, foreign bodies, or achalasia may be identified (**Figs. 12.1** and **12.2**).

Fiberoptic Endoscopic Evaluation of Swallowing

First described by Langmore et al in 1988,[28] fiberoptic endoscopic evaluation of swallowing (FEES) was initially used in the assessment of adults with feeding disorders. FEES has been used to evaluate children since the early 1990s.[29]

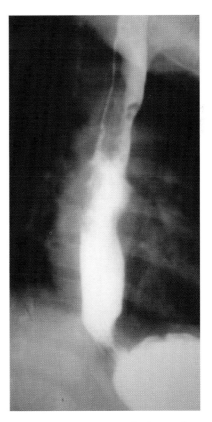

Figure 12.1 Esophagram of a 2-year-old infant with acute dysphagia to solids and mild stridor. Filling defect in mid-esophagus suggests foreign bodies.
Image courtesy: David E. Tunkel, M.D.

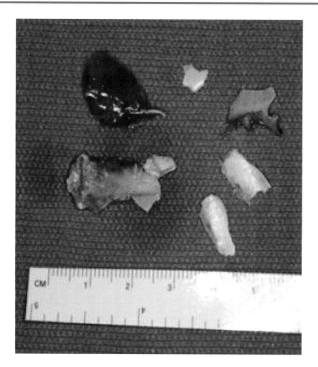

Figure 12.2 Pieces of crab shells removed at rigid esophagoscopy. *Image courtesy*: David E. Tunkel, M.D.

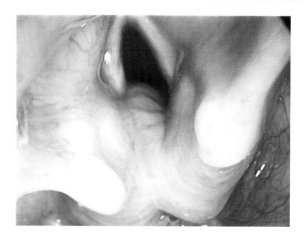

Figure 12.3 Laryngoscopic view of the larynx of a toddler with Opitz G-BBB syndrome and chronic aspiration of liquids. Wide interarytenoid distance and redundant mucosa suggested the presence of laryngeal cleft, which was confirmed by palpation.
Image courtesy: David E. Tunkel, M.D.

Indications for Pediatric FEES

The decision to use FESS for a child with feeding and/or respiratory symptoms depends on several clinical factors.[30] Children who have never been fed orally or who accept only limited oral intake are poor candidates for VFSS. Such children can have FEES to assess laryngopharyngeal structure and function as well as management of secretions, sensory awareness, and spontaneous swallowing sequences.

The FEES examination is performed with the child resting in a sitting position in the lap of a caregiver. No sedation is required for the examination. An anatomic assessment of the larynx, vocal fold mobility, and hypopharynx is performed (**Fig. 12.3**). Food materials are offered that are developmentally appropriate, often using dyed liquids as well as easy-to-visualize solids and semi-solids. The efficiency the swallow is assessed, and the ability to protect the airway from various textures and presentation styles determined.

Fiberoptic Endoscopic Evaluation of Swallowing with Sensory Testing

Performed as an adjunct to FEES, fiberoptic endoscopic evaluation of swallowing with sensory testing (FEESST) offers a tool to further investigate the neural control of swallowing and airway protection.[31] Stimulation of the supraglottic mucosa induces a sequence of neurologic events that result in vocal fold closure and a subsequent swallow. Intact laryngopharyngeal sensation is necessary to protect

the airway from aspiration, and this protection is mediated through the laryngeal adductor reflex (LAR).

FEEST was developed as a precise method of assessing laryngopharyngeal sensation. In infants and children, this is assessed by administering an air pulse calibrated for duration and intensity (ranging from 2.5 to 10 mm Hg) to the aryepiglottic fold region, and observing the induction of a swallow, a cough, or vocal fold closure. The stimulation threshold required to induce the LAR should be determined for each side of the larynx. A sensory threshold greater than 4.5 mm Hg strongly correlates with a positive history of aspiration pneumonia. There is a strong correlation in children with laryngomalacia and GERD. Feeding problems are also common in this group. Sensory thresholds within the larynx on FEEST are elevated in these children, with the thresholds normalizing and the swallowing problems resolving after treatment with antireflux medications.[32]

Nuclear Medicine Scans

Nuclear medicine scans may be used in the assessment of gastric emptying and gastroesophageal reflux. They are also used as a tool for demonstrating aspiration of oral secretions.

Technetium Scan

Technetium scans are useful in the evaluation of children with gastric motility problems. Technetium is mixed with familiar food and administered to the patient. Frequent images are then obtained by a gamma camera for 1 hour; delayed images are obtained for up to 24 hours. Reflux events can be demonstrated by identifying labeled material in the esophagus. The reflux event may deposit gastric contents into the hypopharynx, where it can be cleared through normal pharyngeal contractions or aspirated. The amount of material collecting in the airway is then quantified.

Thallium Scan

Intravenously injected thallium, which is concentrated in the functioning salivary gland tissues, is excreted into the mouth with saliva. This can be used to quantify oral secretions aspirated over time. Images of labeled secretions are obtained with a gamma camera. In normal studies, the label is found in the salivary glands and stomach, with low levels in the oral cavity, pharynx, and esophagus. In children who aspirate oral secretions, label is also seen throughout the lung fields. A thallium scan is useful in determining the need for surgical intervention to prevent chronic, life-threatening pulmonary disease.

Management Approaches

Management decisions for infants and children with feeding and swallowing problems should be made only after a detailed medical history, clinical feeding observations, and a thorough diagnostic assessment. In the setting of complex medical and developmental conditions, decisions are best made through a multidisciplinary team approach. The treating clinician must have a clear understanding of the interplay between anatomic abnormalities, medical conditions, the level of functioning, and behavioral factors.

The goal of treatment is to maximize each child's nutritional status in the context of safe and efficient feeding.[33] This frequently involves modifications in the volume, consistency, texture, or temperature of foods and liquids; the use of adaptive oral feeding utensils or equipment (e.g., bottle nipples with varying size, shape, and flow rates) to increase liquid tolerance; or repositioning the head and body to allow for better airway protection or more efficient passage of a food bolus through the oropharynx. For example, tilting the head forward widens the vallecular space, thereby diverting food away from the laryngeal inlet. When appropriate, parents or caregivers also may be provided with exercises to strengthen or improve the coordination of weak muscles of the child's face, tongue, lips, and palate. In patients with a tracheotomy there is a loss of normal subglottic pressure, which may interfere with airway protection. Capping the tracheotomy or placing a speaking valve onto the tracheotomy can normalize this pressure.

Children with psychosocial or behavioral components associated with their dysphagia are generally responsive to behavior therapy. A structured therapeutic program includes techniques such as rewarding successive approximations of targeted behaviors and offering positive reinforcement through praise, access to favorite toys or music, clapping, or any similar age-appropriate reward. Optimally, the gradual advancement of rewarded goals eventually leads to full oral feeding. Behavior therapy is also used to overcome conditioned food refusal (i.e., a learned aversion to feeding) associated with a previous anatomic abnormality that has been corrected.

For many children with neurologic or anatomic abnormalities, safe oral feeding is extremely difficult or impossible. Deciding whether to pursue efforts at oral feeding requires judicious consideration of the potential risks of aspiration and chronic lung disease versus the convenience and emotional rewards of oral feeding. Supplementing a child's nutrition by nasogastric or gastrostomy feedings may be either essential or prudent in terms of the child's overall development and well-being.

References

1. de Lorimier AA, Harrison MR. Esophageal atresia: embryogenesis and management. World J Surg 1985;9(2):250–257
2. Sutliff KS, Hutchins GM. Septation of the respiratory and digestive tracts in human embryos: crucial role of the tracheoesophageal sulcus. Anat Rec 1994;238(2):237–247
3. Kluth D, Steding G, Seidl W. The embryology of foregut malformations. J Pediatr Surg 1987;22(5):389–393
4. Holder TM, Cloud DT, Lewis JE Jr, Pilling GP IV. Esophageal atresia and tracheoesophageal fistula. A survey of its members by the Surgical Section of the American Academy of Pediatrics. Pediatrics 1964;34:542–549
5. Putnam PE, Orenstein SR, Pang D, Pollack IF, Proujansky R, Kocoshis SA. Cricopharyngeal dysfunction associated with Chiari malformations. Pediatrics 1992;89(5 Pt 1):871–876
6. Azizkhan RG, Tapper D, Eraklis A. Achalasia in childhood: a 20-year experience. J Pediatr Surg 1980;15(4):452–456
7. Euler AR, Byrne WJ. Twenty-four-hour esophageal intraluminal pH probe testing: a comparative analysis. Gastroenterology 1981;80(5 Pt 1):957–961
8. Tutuian R, Vela MF, Shay SS, Castell DO. Multichannel intraluminal impedance in esophageal function testing and gastroesophageal reflux monitoring. J Clin Gastroenterol 2003;37(3):206–215
9. McMurray JS, Gerber M, Stern Y, et al. Role of laryngoscopy, dual pH probe monitoring, and laryngeal mucosal biopsy in the diagnosis of pharyngoesophageal reflux. Ann Otol Rhinol Laryngol 2001;110(4):299–304
10. Tsou VM, Young RM, Hart MH, Vanderhoof JA. Elevated plasma aluminum levels in normal infants receiving antacids containing aluminum. Pediatrics 1991;87(2):148–151
11. Piquette RK. Torsade de pointes induced by cisapride/clarithromycin interaction. Ann Pharmacother 1999;33(1):22–26
12. Ali T, Roberts DN, Tierney WM. Long-term safety concerns with proton pump inhibitors. Am J Med 2009;122(10):896–903
13. Arvedson JC. Assessment of pediatric dysphagia and feeding disorders: clinical and instrumental approaches. Dev Disabil Res Rev 2008;14(2):118–127
14. Hawdon JM, Beauregard N, Slattery J, Kennedy G. Identification of neonates at risk of developing feeding problems in infancy. Dev Med Child Neurol 2000;42(4):235–239
15. Lefton-Greif MA. Pediatric dysphagia. Phys Med Rehabil Clin N Am 2008;19(4):837–851
16. Newman LA, Keckley C, Petersen MC, Hamner A. Swallowing function and medical diagnoses in infants suspected of Dysphagia. Pediatrics 2001;108(6):E106

17. Dodds WJ, Stewart ET, Logemann JA. Physiology and radiology of the normal oral and pharyngeal phases of swallowing. AJR Am J Roentgenol 1990;154(5):953–963

18. Miller AJ. Deglutition. Physiol Rev 1982;62(1):129–184

19. Kahrilas PJ. Pharyngeal structure and function. Dysphagia 1993;8(4):303–307

20. Miller AJ. The search for the central swallowing pathway: the quest for clarity. Dysphagia 1993;8(3):185–194

21. Loughlin GM, Lefton-Greif MA. Dysfunctional swallowing and respiratory disease in children. Adv Pediatr 1994;41:135–162

22. Boesch RP, Daines C, Willging JP, et al. Advances in the diagnosis and management of chronic pulmonary aspiration in children. Eur Respir J 2006;28(4):847–861

23. Friedman B, Frazier JB. Deep laryngeal penetration as a predictor of aspiration. Dysphagia 2000;15(3):153–158

24. Cooper-Brown L, Copeland S, Dailey S, et al. Feeding and swallowing dysfunction in genetic syndromes. Dev Disabil Res Rev 2008;14(2):147–157

25. Burklow KA, Phelps AN, Schultz JR, McConnell K, Rudolph C. Classifying complex pediatric feeding disorders. J Pediatr Gastroenterol Nutr 1998;27(2):143–147

26. Putnam PE. Eosinophilic esophagitis in children: clinical manifestations. Gastroenterol Clin North Am 2008;37(2):369–381

27. Logemann JA. Approaches to management of disordered swallowing. Baillieres Clin Gastroenterol 1991;5(2):269–280

28. Langmore SE, Schatz K, Olsen N. Fiberoptic endoscopic examination of swallowing safety: a new procedure. Dysphagia 1988;2(4):216–219

29. Willging JP, Miller CK, Link DT, Rudolph CD. Use of FEES to assess and manage pediatric patients. In: Langmore SE, ed. Endoscopic Evaluation and Treatment of Swallowing Disorders. New York: Thieme;2001:213–234.

30. Willging JP. Benefit of feeding assessment before pediatric airway reconstruction. Laryngoscope 2000;110(5 Pt 1):825–834

31. Willging JP, Thompson DM. Pediatric FEESST: fiberoptic endoscopic evaluation of swallowing with sensory testing. Curr Gastroenterol Rep 2005;7(3):240–243

32. Thompson DM, Rutter MJ, Rudolph CD, Willging JP, Cotton RT. Altered laryngeal sensation: a potential cause of apnea of infancy. Ann Otol Rhinol Laryngol 2005;114(4):258–263

33. Prasse JE, Kikano GE. An overview of pediatric dysphagia. Clin Pediatr (Phila) 2009;48(3):247–251

13 Recurrent Respiratory Papillomatosis

Rose Stavinoha and Farrel Joel Buchinsky

Recurrent respiratory papillomatosis (RRP) is an uncommon disease caused by two common viruses: human papillomavirus (HPV) 6 and HPV 11. The disease is a tremendous burden to affected children and their families because of dysphonia, airway obstruction, and the need for repeated surgery. Papillomas (warts) may be present at any point along the upper aerodigestive tract but the vocal folds are the predominant site of the lesions and hence dysphonia is typically the first symptom. Notwithstanding the fact that voice is a quintessential human characteristic, abnormalities in a young child's voice often receive little attention. If left unchecked, the papillomas can grow to obstruct the airway and lead to dyspnea and stridor. The primary goal of management is symptomatic relief by removing papillomas but even with aggressive surgical treatment, recurrence is the norm.

Clinical Course

Normal phonation is dependent on the vocal folds being able to vibrate freely in response to positive subglottic pressure. The presence of these wart-like lesions or papillomas impedes the motion of the mucosal wave that should occur on the vocal folds (**Figs. 13.1** and **13.2**). The corollary is true—papilloma may be present in the larynx or the airway, but as long as it is not located where it would interfere with voice production, the voice may be normal. The unsuspecting clinician may initially manage children with RRP as chronic cough, recurrent pneumonia, upper respiratory infections, croup, asthma, or allergies. Since RRP is rare, there is often a

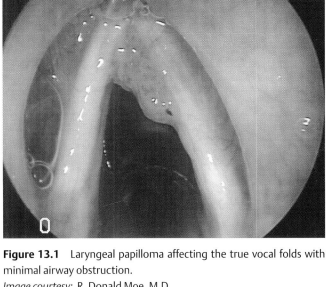

Figure 13.1 Laryngeal papilloma affecting the true vocal folds with minimal airway obstruction.
Image courtesy: R. Donald Moe, M.D.

delay of many months between the onset of symptoms and diagnosis of RRP. For children with RRP, the median age at diagnosis is 3.1 years and, on average, they undergo more than 20 surgeries for RRP during their lifetime.[1]

At any one point in time, an individual may have a disease that spans the spectrum from mild to severe. The most widely used method to document the instantaneous severity is the Derkay-Coltrera staging system. The scheme assigns a numerical score to describe the type of lesion

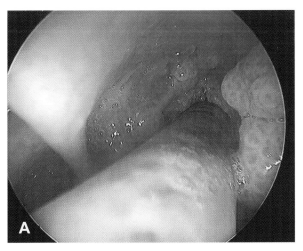

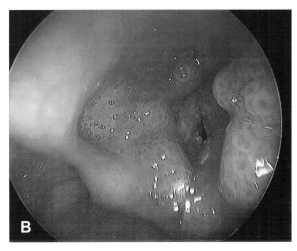

Figure 13.2A, B Laryngeal papilloma affecting the larynx with severe airway obstruction.
Image courtesy: Juan Bonilla, M.D.

(surface lesion vs. raised lesion vs. bulky lesion) according to the subsites affected with a final numerical score defining the overall current extent of disease.[2]

The natural course and duration of RRP is highly variable. In essence, RRP is a benign neoplasm but may cause significant morbidity and even death in severe cases. One patient may have an aggressive course, requiring surgical excision of papilloma every few days or weeks, and such a patient is often a candidate for adjuvant therapies. Others may require only periodic surgical interventions every several months or years. "Aggressiveness" is a label often attached to those with a greater frequency of surgeries or a greater number of lifetime surgeries or distal spread to the trachea (**Fig. 13.3**), bronchi, and pulmonary parenchyma or those who ever undergo tracheostomy for RRP. The average child with active RRP requires 5.1 procedures per year with a range from 0.4 to 22 procedures per year, according to a 2003 report from the RRP task force national registry.[1] Eventually most children with RRP go into remission. Among 165 pediatric cases followed-up for a median period of 1.7 years (range, 0.01 to 4.6), 22% went into remission.[3] By 3.6 years following diagnosis, 44% had gone into remission. Even with remission, dysphonia seldom resolves and there is always the possibility of recurrence of RRP.[4,5]

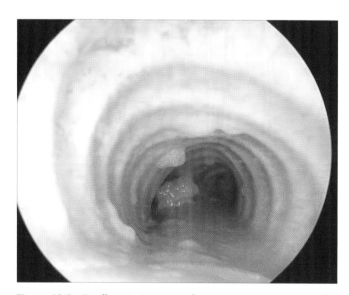

Figure 13.3 Papillomata in a case of recurrent respiratory pappillomatosis with distal spread to the trachea.
Image courtesy: David E. Tunkel, M.D.

The variable behavior of RRP is poorly understood. Epidemiological data indicate that younger patients tend to have a more aggressive disease[1,6] and decreased likelihood of remission. Remission aside, even for those still with active disease, most children require less surgery over time[7,8] (**Fig. 13.4**). In the more ominous cases, the disease may progress to include pulmonary lesions[9] (1%) or even malignant transformation. Reported malignancy rates have ranged from 2% of 244 cases[10] to 13% of 38 cases in those enrolled in an interferon trial.[11] Malignancy was almost

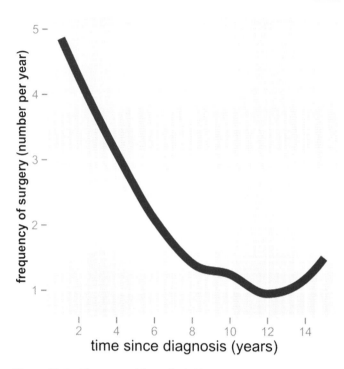

Figure 13.4 The Hospital for Sick Children in Toronto chronicled the number of surgical interventions in their cohort of patients. Adjuvant pharmacologic therapy (interferon or cidofovir) was used in less than one-fifth of cases. A locally smoothed estimate shows how, as a group, patients who still had recurrent respiratory pappillomatosis had a decelerating rate of surgeries over time.

Adapted from: Hawkes M, Campisi P, Zafar R, et al. Time course of juvenile onset recurrent respiratory papillomatosis caused by human papillomavirus. *Pediatr Infect Dis J* 2008;27(2):149–154.

always associated with HPV 11 and not with HPV 6, occurred many years after diagnosis,[12] and commonly occurred in the setting of pulmonary RRP.

Epidemiology and Virology

Two population-based systematic studies have calculated the incidence in North America at 0.2 to 1.1 per 100,000 people younger than 18 years. The prevalence of the disease is roughly four to five times the incidence.[13,14] In 2010, Campisi and colleagues created a national database in Canada for RRP affecting children younger than 14 years of age to follow incidence over time. A study published in 1995, estimated a higher incidence of 4.3 per 100,000 children in the United States.[5] This estimate relied on a survey of board-certified otolaryngologists and may be less accurate than the more recent population-based studies.

HPV is a double-stranded DNA capsid virus categorized into more than 180 identified genotypes which have different tissue preferences and clinical manifestations. HPV 6 and 11 account for the overwhelming majority of RRP cases.[15] HPV 6 and 11 confer a low risk for malignant transformation compared with HPV 16 and 18. For many years, investigators have noted an association between aggressive clinical course and HPV 11 (rather than HPV 6) and young age (rather than older children). Buchinsky et al analyzed the relevant strength of the association between HPV type, age, and course.[6] Age was more strongly associated with clinical course than was HPV type.

Epidemiological analysis has led to the presumption that RRP in children is caused by vertical transmission of HPV from the maternal genital tract to the fetus at the time of birth. The virus then remains dormant for months or years. While millions of women have genital HPV 6 and 11, relatively few children develop RRP. Even in the setting of vaginal delivery with visible condyloma acuminata the probability of subsequent RRP is low (1 in 144 being the highest risk reported).[16] Cesarean section (C-section) is associated with a lower incidence but it is not absolutely protective. C-section has been considered as a preventative strategy but has not been adopted because of the morbidity, mortality, and economic cost of C-section in the light of low RRP incidence. Further, the majority of cases of RRP occur in the absence of maternal condyloma. Exposure to HPV is necessary but is not sufficient. An underlying genetic susceptibility may explain the different clinical courses and exact mode of transmission. Further research is needed regarding factors affecting the development and clinical course of RRP.[17,18]

Management

No cure exists. Initial treatment involves surgical intervention where the aim is to improve voice, prevent airway obstruction, and avoid iatrogenic complications while awaiting remission. Many agents have been used over the years as an adjuvant to surgery but surgical removal has been the mainstay of treatment.

Surgical

Papillomas are debulked via endoscopic surgical excision or ablation with microlaryngoscopy. Ideally the surrounding normal tissue should be preserved as much as possible while debriding just the obstructing lesions. Injury to surrounding tissues causes scarring or stenosis, which may lead to permanent dysphonia and/or airway compromise. A biopsy should initially be obtained to confirm the diagnosis. During subsequent surgeries, periodic pathologic surveillance can monitor for atypia and malignant transformation.

There are several methods to debulk the papillomas. The original method involves the use of microlaryngeal instruments such as a pair of cupped biopsy forceps. If the forceps were wielded with little precision, the surrounding normal tissue could have been avulsed, which could have lead to scar formation. Seeking greater precision, surgeons have used laser ablation, using both line of sight and fiber-delivered CO_2 lasers. Laser risks include airway fire and injury from the laser beam. HPV DNA can be found in the laser plume of smoke, and in one in vivo experiment, bovine papillomavirus in the laser plume was able to establish

disease in calves.[19] Thus concern about contagion of surgical workers exists, and safety precautions are advised.

In the past 10 years, powered microdebriders with laryngeal blades have become the most commonly used device for excision of laryngotracheal papilloma. One study of microdebrider use for RRP showed reduced operative and anesthesia time, and avoidance of thermal injury to surrounding tissues when compared with the CO_2 laser.[20] An American Society of Pediatric Otolaryngology survey in 2004 documented that the microdebrider had supplanted the CO_2 laser as the most widely used device for RRP treatment.[21] It must be noted however that there have not been any randomized, controlled studies to compare treatment outcomes of CO_2 laser ablation or microdebrider excision of laryngeal papillomas. Holler and colleagues published a prospective cohort study in 2009 which compared the voice outcomes of 11 children with RRP treated with CO_2 laser or microdebrider.[22] The objective acoustic evaluations performed between each group demonstrated that microdebrider resulted in better acoustic results.

Other ablative angiolytic lasers have also been used recently, including, the 585-nm pulsed dye laser and the 532-nm pulsed potassium-titanyl-phosphate laser. Both lasers are absorbed by hemoglobin and selectively target the vascular papilloma lesions. These lasers allow for in-office treatment in older children and adults. A prospective, longitudinal study by Hartnick et al involving 23 pediatric patients found the 585-nm pulsed dye laser may allow more aggressive surgical excision of papillomas at the anterior commissure disease as epithelial damage is reduced with this device.[23]

Tracheotomy is occasionally undertaken for children with life-threatening airway obstruction from aggressive RRP. Surgeons are reluctant to place a tracheotomy as it has been suggested that the chronic irritation may activate or contribute to the spread of disease to the lower respiratory tract. If tracheotomy is performed, then early decannulation is advised when the disease can be managed by endoscopic techniques alone.

Adjuvants

Numerous adjuvant therapies have been used to treat RRP. The most widely accepted indications for use of adjuvants include surgical frequency more than four per year, rapid regrowth of papilloma with airway compromise, and distal spread of disease to multiple sites. A comprehensive review article by Gallagher and Derkay[24] describe multiple adjuvants that have been tried to treat RRP including acyclovir, ribavirin, indole-3-carbinol, cyclooxygenase-2 inhibitors, retinoids, and zinc. The two adjuvants probably most widely used and studied are interferon and cidofovir.

Interferon has been the subject of two randomized trials.[25,26] Both studies demonstrated some improvement when the drug was administered to treat aggressive disease. Unfortunately the improvement was found to be only temporary or required the ongoing administration of a drug with bothersome and toxic adverse effects such as fever, flu-like symptoms, seizures, decrease in growth rate, and leukopenia.

There has been wide adoption of cidofovir therapy for RRP most commonly as an intralesional injection or less commonly as an intravenous systemic treatment. The drug is a cytosine nucleotide analog and suppresses DNA replication through selective uptake by the viral DNA polymerase. While that mechanism holds against cytomegalovirus (the original indication for the drug), the same mechanism of action does not apply as well for HPV since HPV does not encode its own DNA polymerase. Pharmacology aside, there have been promising outcomes documented in multiple small case series but there has only been one randomized, double-blind, placebo-controlled trial. McMurray et al[27] found significant improvements, such as reduced Derkay severity score, over time in those receiving cidofovir. However, even those who received placebo improved over time. A major weakness of the study was that concerns about toxicity resulted in regulatory approval only being granted for a cidofovir intralesional injection concentration of 0.3 mg/mL—well below what most practitioners were using. Only much later were the investigators permitted to use the concentration of 5 mg/mL. Concerns over the oncogenic potential of cidofovir led the RRP task force in 2005 to recommend limiting the use of adjuvant cidofovir to severely recalcitrant RRP cases.[28,29] In contrast to these previous recommendations, a recent study of histologic specimens of RRP patients over time found no worsening of dysplastic progression and recommended additional investigation.[30]

Control of gastroesophageal reflux has been found to correlate with decreased rate of recurrence of RRP in several case reports. A small series of children with RRP studied by McKenna and Brodsky in 2005[31] found that control of extraesophageal reflux disease improved control of RRP resistant to earlier therapies. Although further study is needed, it may be worthwhile to treat patients with antireflux medication if they have aggressive disease.

Numerous adjuvants have strong support, with plausible mechanisms of action and anecdotal reports of clinical success. The small number of patients, the variable and unpredictable natural history, and the lack of controlled randomized studies make the support for most of these adjuvants quite problematic.

The most tangible hope for prevention of RRP lies in vaccination. A quadrivalent HPV vaccine has been developed which protects against HPV types 6, 11, 16, and 18. It is currently approved by the U.S. Food and Drug Administration for the prevention of cervical carcinoma, dysplasia, and genital warts. Widespread vaccination with this particular vaccine could potentially reduce newborn exposure to HPV 6 and HPV 11 by eliminating the maternal and paternal reservoir and theoretically prevent RRP. However, the reasonable expectation may be possible only if there is high penetration of the quadrivalent vaccine in the world population, a goal that may not be possible due to cost, competition, or the perception by some of unpalatable moral ramifications. Additionally, such potential benefits would take years to manifest, and affected RRP patients would not benefit.

Quality of Life and Psychosocial Considerations

RRP is frequently extremely burdensome and life altering to both patients and their families as they deal emotionally and physically with RRP and its treatment.

RRP places a large economic burden on individual patients, their families, and society. In the United States, the average lifetime cost to treat one patient with RRP has been estimated between $ 43,267 and $ 218,067.[32 see erratum] A cross-sectional study by Chadha and colleagues used validated measures of health utility (a measure of where someone feels that they are on the spectrum between death and perfect health), voice-related quality of life, and psychosocial impact to assess the burden of RRP on children and families.[13] The study found that the impact of RRP on health utility was comparable to many other chronic diseases of childhood such as cystic fibrosis. Voice disturbance is the predominant factor affecting quality of life. Interestingly, it was also found that health utility and voice-related quality of life outcomes did not correlate well with the Derkay-Coltrera severity score. In terms of family burden, the contributing factors include the need for multiple hospital visits, social stigma of the disease, and parental anxiety about the health of the affected child and unaffected siblings. The co-occurrence of RRP in siblings is rare but has been observed.[5]

Parents of children with RRP often experience shame and embarrassment as they come to terms with the fact that their child probably contracted the etiologic agent from the mother's genital tract.

There are currently two groups available to assist patients and families with the psychological and social issues surrounding RRP as well as the current research and information about the disease: the Recurrent Respiratory Papillomatosis Foundation in Lawrenceville, New Jersey, and the International RRP Information, Support and Advocacy Center based in Bellingham, Washington.

References

1. Reeves WC, Ruparelia SS, Swanson KI, Derkay CS, Marcus A, Unger ER. National registry for juvenile-onset recurrent respiratory papillomatosis. Arch Otolaryngol Head Neck Surg 2003;129(9):976–982

2. Derkay CS, Malis DJ, Zalzal G, Wiatrak BJ, Kashima HK, Coltrera MD. A staging system for assessing severity of disease and response to therapy in recurrent respiratory papillomatosis. Laryngoscope 1998;108(6):935–937

3. Ruparelia S, Unger ER, Nisenbaum R, Derkay CS, Reeves WC. Predictors of remission in juvenile-onset recurrent respiratory papillomatosis. Arch Otolaryngol Head Neck Surg 2003;129(12):1275–1278

4. Ilmarinen T, Nissilä H, Rihkanen H, et al. Clinical features, health-related quality of life, and adult voice in juvenile-onset recurrent respiratory papillomatosis. Laryngoscope 2011;121(4):846–851

5. Derkay CS. Task force on recurrent respiratory papillomas. A preliminary report. Arch Otolaryngol Head Neck Surg 1995;121(12):1386–1391

6. Buchinsky FJ, Donfack J, Derkay CS, et al. Age of child, more than HPV type, is associated with clinical course in recurrent respiratory papillomatosis. PLoS ONE 2008;3(5):e2263

7. Hawkes M, Campisi P, Zafar R, et al. Time course of juvenile onset recurrent respiratory papillomatosis caused by human papillomavirus. Pediatr Infect Dis J 2008;27(2):149–154

8. Silverberg MJ, Thorsen P, Lindeberg H, Ahdieh-Grant L, Shah KV. Clinical course of recurrent respiratory papillomatosis in Danish children. Arch Otolaryngol Head Neck Surg 2004;130(6):711–716

9. Armstrong LR, Derkay CS, Reeves WC. Initial results from the national registry for juvenile-onset recurrent respiratory papillomatosis. RRP Task Force. Arch Otolaryngol Head Neck Surg 1999;125(7):743–748

10. Dedo HH, Yu KC. CO(2) laser treatment in 244 patients with respiratory papillomas. Laryngoscope 2001;111(9):1639–1644

11. Gerein V, Rastorguev E, Gerein J, Draf W, Schirren J. Incidence, age at onset, and potential reasons of malignant transformation in recurrent respiratory papillomatosis patients: 20 years experience. Otolaryngol Head Neck Surg 2005;132(3):392–394

12. Lie ES, Engh V, Boysen M, et al. Squamous cell carcinoma of the respiratory tract following laryngeal papillomatosis. Acta Otolaryngol 1994;114(2):209–212

13. Chadha NK, Allegro J, Barton M, Hawkes M, Harlock H, Campisi P. The quality of life and health utility burden of recurrent respiratory papillomatosis in children. Otolaryngol Head Neck Surg 2010;143(5):685–690

14. Campisi P, Hawkes M, Simpson K; Canadian Juvenile Onset Recurrent Respiratory Papillomatosis Working Group. The epidemiology of juvenile onset recurrent respiratory papillomatosis derived from a population level national database. Laryngoscope 2010;120(6):1233–1245

15. Wiatrak BJ, Wiatrak DW, Broker TR, Lewis L. Recurrent respiratory papillomatosis: a longitudinal study comparing severity associated with human papilloma viral types 6 and 11 and other risk factors in a large pediatric population. Laryngoscope 2004;114(11 Pt 2, Suppl 104):1–23

16. Silverberg MJ, Thorsen P, Lindeberg H, Grant LA, Shah KV. Condyloma in pregnancy is strongly predictive of juvenile-onset recurrent respiratory papillomatosis. Obstet Gynecol 2003;101(4):645–652

17. Buchinsky FJ, Derkay CS, Leal SM, Donfack J, Ehrlich GD, Post JC. Multicenter initiative seeking critical genes in respiratory papillomatosis. Laryngoscope 2004;114(2):349–357

18. Bonagura VR, Vambutas A, DeVoti JA, et al. HLA alleles, IFN-gamma responses to HPV-11 E6, and disease severity in patients with recurrent respiratory papillomatosis. Hum Immunol 2004;65(8):773–782

19. Garden JM, O'Banion MK, Bakus AD, Olson C. Viral disease transmitted by laser-generated plume (aerosol). Arch Dermatol 2002;138(10):1303–1307

20. Patel N, Rowe M, Tunkel D. Treatment of recurrent respiratory papillomatosis in children with the microdebrider. Ann Otol Rhinol Laryngol 2003;112(1):7–10

21. Schraff S, Derkay CS, Burke B, Lawson L. American Society of Pediatric Otolaryngology members' experience with recurrent respiratory papillomatosis and the use of adjuvant therapy. Arch Otolaryngol Head Neck Surg 2004;130(9):1039–1042

22. Holler T, Allegro J, Chadha NK, et al. Voice outcomes following repeated surgical resection of laryngeal papillomata in children. Otolaryngol Head Neck Surg 2009;141(4):522–526

23. Hartnick CJ, Boseley ME, Franco RA Jr, Cunningham MJ, Pransky S. Efficacy of treating children with anterior commissure and true vocal fold respiratory papilloma with the 585-nm pulsed-dye laser. Arch Otolaryngol Head Neck Surg 2007;133(2):127–130

24. Gallagher TQ, Derkay CS. Pharmacotherapy of recurrent respiratory papillomatosis: an expert opinion. Expert Opin Pharmacother 2009;10(4):645–655

25. Leventhal BG, Kashima HK, Weck PW, et al. Randomized surgical adjuvant trial of interferon alfa-n1 in recurrent papillomatosis. Arch Otolaryngol Head Neck Surg 1988;114(10):1163–1169

26. Healy GB, Gelber RD, Trowbridge AL, Grundfast KM, Ruben RJ, Price KN. Treatment of recurrent respiratory papillomatosis with human leukocyte interferon. Results of a multicenter randomized clinical trial. N Engl J Med 1988;319(7):401–407

27. McMurray JS, Connor N, Ford CN. Cidofovir efficacy in recurrent respiratory papillomatosis: a randomized, double-blind, placebo-controlled study. Ann Otol Rhinol Laryngol 2008;117(7):477–483

28. Donne AJ, Hampson L, He XT, et al. Potential risk factors associated with the use of cidofovir to treat benign human papillomavirus-related disease. Antivir Ther 2009;14(7):939–952

29. Derkay C; Multi-Disciplinary Task Force on Recurrent Respiratory Papillomas. Cidofovir for recurrent respiratory papillomatosis (RRP): a re-assessment of risks. Int J Pediatr Otorhinolaryngol 2005;69(11):1465–1467

30. Gupta HT, Robinson RA, Murray RC, Karnell LH, Smith RJ, Hoffman HT. Degrees of dysplasia and the use of cidofovir in patients with recurrent respiratory papillomatosis. Laryngoscope 2010;120(4):698–702

31. McKenna M, Brodsky L. Extraesophageal acid reflux and recurrent respiratory papilloma in children. Int J Pediatr Otorhinolaryngol 2005;69(5):597–605

32. Bishai D, Kashima H, Shah K. The cost of juvenile-onset recurrent respiratory papillomatosis. Arch Otolaryngol Head Neck Surg 2000;126(8):935–939. Erratum in: Arch Otolaryngol Head Neck Surg 2009;135(2):208

14 Inflammatory Airway Disease
Kara K. Prickett and Steven E. Sobol

Respiratory infections are the leading cause of death among children less than 5 years of age, with significant morbidity and mortality attributed to acute inflammatory obstruction of the airway.[1] The anatomy of the pediatric airway leaves children particularly susceptible to obstructive respiratory compromise. Children have proportionately larger heads, larger tongues, and less cervical support than adults, leading to relative narrowing of the upper airway in the supine position. The pediatric airway is narrowest in the subglottis, where the outer diameter is fixed by the cricoid and loosely adherent mucosa allows for significant changes in inner diameter in the setting of inflammatory infiltrates. Turbulent flow of air through the narrowed subglottis is perceived as stridor. Children presenting with acute onset of stridor or rapidly progressing symptoms must be promptly managed to avoid complications.

Croup

The term "croup" was introduced into the medical lexicon in the late 1700s as a derivation of the Anglo-Saxon and Scottish terms for a loud or harsh cry, and was used to describe illness caused by diphtheria. Today, croup describes laryngotracheobronchitis, a virally mediated condition characterized by inflammatory obstruction of the glottic and subglottic airways.

Epidemiology

Croup has been implicated in up to 90% of cases of infectious upper airway obstruction. Children under 6 years of age are affected most commonly, with peak incidence between 6 and 36 months. Males are affected 1.5 times as often as females.[2] The incidence of croup peaks in the autumn and mid-winter, corresponding with epidemiology of common viral illnesses in children.

Pathophysiology

Most cases of croup are caused by the human parainfluenza viruses. The inflammatory response to infection, rather than direct viral damage to the epithelium, is likely responsible for most clinical symptoms. Viral titers have been found to be waning at the time of symptom onset.[1] Increased capillary permeability contributes to edema and the formation of thick secretions. Subglottic narrowing leads to the characteristic inspiratory stridor.

Host factors that may contribute to more severe infection are targets of current investigation. Defective suppression of the immunologic response to viral antigens and infection with atypical pathogens has been linked to prolonged or severe symptoms. Respiratory syncytial virus, *Mycoplasma pneumoniae*, herpes simplex virus, paramyxovirus, adenovirus, and varicella have all been reported as etiologic agents. More recently, human metapneumovirus and coronavirus have also been linked to croup.[1]

Clinical Presentation

After 1 or 2 days of viral prodrome, hoarseness, inspiratory stridor, and a seal-like, barking cough develop in most patients. Symptoms worsen at night or with agitation and gradually resolve over 3 to7 days. Less than 5% of children with croup require hospitalization, and of those admitted, only 1 to 3% require intubation.[3] Rapid onset of symptoms (<12 hours) or signs of extreme toxicity should alert the clinician to both the potential need for rapid airway management and the consideration of other possible diagnoses. The differential diagnosis of croup is shown in **Table 14.1**.

Spasmodic croup is a well-described, but poorly-understood, clinical syndrome of barking cough, stridor, and respiratory distress, which occurs almost exclusively at night. Patients lack the viral prodrome associated with classic croup. Symptoms are typically self-limited, and may resolve before arrival in the emergency department. Children with spasmodic croup are often older than the classic young child with viral laryngotracheobronchitis. Recurrence over several subsequent nights is common.[4] The etiology of spasmodic croup is unknown, but may be related to atopy.[5]

Evaluation and Initial Management

The diagnosis of croup can usually be made clinically. When the initial diagnosis is made by an experienced practitioner using clinical criteria, only 2% of cases are eventually given an alternate diagnosis. Several scoring systems have been developed to stratify patients by disease severity. The Westley Croup Scoring System is widely used in treatment trials, but has not been validated as an effective tool for clinical decision making. [5]

In the stable child, birth history, history of earlier intubations, and recent exposures should be obtained. The absence of a cough should lead the clinician to consider alternative diagnoses. Children under 6 months of age should be examined for cutaneous hemangiomas, as symptoms of subglottic hemangioma may mimic those of croup.

Radiographic findings of the characteristic "steeple sign" or dilation of the hypopharynx are 92% specific for croup

Table 14.1 Differential Diagnosis of Croup

Congenital	Laryngomalacia
	Vocal fold paralysis
	Laryngeal web
	Subglottic stenosis
	Subglottic hemangioma
	Tracheomalacia
Vascular	Innominate artery compression
	Double aortic arch
	Aberrant subclavian artery
	Pulmonary artery sling
Infectious/Inflammatory	Recurrent respiratory papillomatosis
	Epiglottitis
	Peritonsillar abscess
	Deep neck space infection
	Diphtheria
	Bacterial tracheitis
	Mycobacteria
	Laryngeal candidiasis
	Angioedema
	Wegener granulomatosis
	Sarcoidosis
	Extraesophageal reflux
Traumatic/Toxic	Acquired subglottic stenosis
	Inhalational injury
	Foreign body
Neoplastic	Benign or malignant lesions

Adapted from: Sobol SE, Zapata S. Epiglottitis and croup. *Otolaryngol Clin North Am* 2008;41(3):551–566.

(**Fig. 14.1**).[6] Because the sensitivity of neck radiographs ranges from 50 to 93%, a normal radiograph does not rule out the diagnosis.[7] Laboratory studies typically yield non-specific signs of inflammation or viral infection. Flexible fiberoptic laryngoscopy may rule out other glottic or supraglottic pathology, but provides limited examination of the subglottis.

Definitive Therapy

Systemic corticosteroids are the mainstay of treatment for croup.[8] Oral or intramuscular dosing is preferred due to ease of administration and low cost, but recent research has shown nebulized budesonide to be equally efficacious.[8,9] The most common regimens consist of single doses of prednisolone 1 mg/kg or dexamethasone 0.6 mg/kg. No data are available on the utility of multiple-dose regimens.

Helium–oxygen mixtures (heliox) can decrease work of breathing in patients with narrowed airways, as the lowered density of such inhaled mixtures can maintain or improve flow of air even with reduced airway caliber. Promising results have been obtained in several small, uncontrolled reviews, but randomized trials have thus far shown only statistically insignificant trends toward improvement in children treated with heliox.[10]

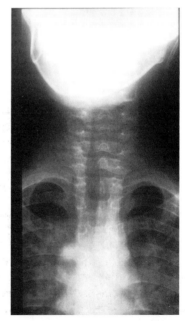

Figure 14.1 An anteroposterior radiograph typical of a patient with croup. Edema in the subglottis produces the "steeple" appearance. Dilation of the hypopharynx due to forceful inspiration against an obstructed subglottis is best appreciated on a lateral film.

The effectiveness of inhaled racemic epinephrine has been proven in several well-designed trials.[11] Alpha-adrenergic effects decrease capillary permeability, while beta-2 effects contribute to smooth muscle relaxation.[12] Overnight observation after treatment with racemic epinephrine, while once standard of practice, is no longer considered imperative. Recent studies have shown that it is safe to discharge patients after 2 to 4 hours of observation if clinical signs of croup do not return.[13]

Hospitalization is indicated for severe symptoms, failure to improve, and poor access to follow-up care.[4] Treatment is largely supportive, as there is no evidence to support the use of antibiotics, antitussives, or decongestants. Similarly, recent studies have failed to show any benefit for children treated with humidified air or mist therapy.[14] Current evidence-based recommendations for pharmacotherapy in croup are summarized in **Table 14.2**. The need for intubation has decreased markedly in the era of widely available corticosteroids, and tracheotomy is rarely performed. When intubation is necessary, the smallest effective endotracheal tube should be selected to minimize trauma to the already inflamed airway.

Otolaryngologists are often asked to evaluate patients with atypical croup. Atypical patients may present outside the classic age range, with severe or prolonged symptoms, or with multiple episodes of recurrent croup. Evaluation by an otolaryngologist is also warranted when an acquired or congenital abnormality of the larynx and/or trachea is suspected. Ideally, direct laryngoscopy and rigid bronchoscopy are performed approximately 4 weeks after resolution of the acute illness so that acute and chronic components of airway narrowing may be accurately differentiated.

Epiglottitis (Supraglottitis)

Epiglottitis, or supraglottitis, is a diffuse, bacterially mediated inflammation of the supraglottic larynx. After a dramatic decline in the incidence of epiglottitis during the mid 1990s, new-found public skepticism of childhood vaccinations has brought the discussion—and diagnosis—of epiglottitis back to the mainstream.

Epidemiology

Before widespread vaccination, incidence of acute epiglottitis ranged from 6 to 34 cases per 100,000 persons per year.[15] Reported cases dropped by more than 90% after the introduction vaccines for *Haemophilus influenzae* type b (Hib). In 2004, estimates ranged from 0.02 cases to 0.77 cases per 100,000 persons.[16] Though epiglottitis is more common during the winter months, the seasonal variability is not as pronounced as with croup. Most cases occur in children between the ages of 2 and 7 years, with males affected 1.2 to 4 times more commonly than females.[4] The average age of affected children has increased in a stepwise fashion over the past 15 years; at many children's hospitals, teenagers present with epiglottitis more commonly than do young children.[17]

Table 14.2 Evidence-Based Recommendations for Pharmacotherapy in Croup

	Drug	Severity of Croup	Quality of Evidence	Recommendation
Highly effective	Oral corticosteroids	Mild to severe	High	Consider single dose in all patients (0.15–0.6 mg/kg dexamethasone or 1 mg/kg prednisolone)
	Inhaled corticosteroids	Mild to severe	High	Consider in patients unable to tolerate PO administration (2 mg budesonide)
	Intramuscular corticosteroids	Moderate to severe	High	Consider in patients unable to tolerate PO administration (0.6 mg/kg dexamethasone)
	Inhaled racemic epinephrine	Moderate to severe	High	Consider in patients needing immediate symptomatic relief (0.5 cc of 2.25% diluted in 2.5 cc saline)
	Inhaled L-epinephrine	Moderate to severe	High	Consider in patients needing immediate symptomatic relief (5 cc of 1:1000 L-epinephrine)
Possibly effective	Heliox	Mild to severe	Moderate	Safe, not currently recommended
Ineffective	Humidified air	Mild to severe	High	Not recommended

PO: per os (by mouth).

Pathophysiology

The symptoms of acute epiglottitis are caused by inflammatory edema of the supraglottic mucosa with preservation of patency at and below the glottis. In the prevaccine era, the vast majority of cases were caused by Hib, with nearly half of patients having concomitant Hib infections of the lungs, skin, middle ear, or meninges.[18] Affected children often have a history of asthma or allergies, raising the question of whether chronic inflammation may decrease mucosal barriers to bacterial entry.

In the postvaccine era, *Streptococcus* species have emerged as the leading causes of epiglottitis in many communities, while some studies show continued frequent isolation of *Haemophilus* species.[19] *Staphylococcus aureus*, *Moraxella catarrhalis*, *Klebsiella pneumoniae*, *Pasteurella multocida*, *Pseudomonas*, and *Neisseria* species have all been identified, as have *Candida* and viral pathogens.[17,20] Vaccine failure occurs in 2 to 11% of patients and tends to be concentrated in patients receiving the polysaccharide vaccine rather than the more immunogenic protein conjugate vaccines.[20]

Clinical Presentation

Pediatric patients have rapid onset of high fever, odynophagia, drooling, and respiratory distress evolving over a period of hours. Generally, children with epiglottitis appear toxic and anxious. The adoption of a "sniffing" or "tripod" position, with the waist flexed and neck extended, is indicative of significant airway obstruction. Clinical signs and symptoms may be more varied in older children and adults, thus requiring a high index of clinical suspicion for diagnosis.

Evaluation and Initial Management

Classically, patients in whom epiglottitis was suspected were left undisturbed in quiet, dark rooms until the operating room could be readied for intubation or tracheotomy. When children present with fulminant epiglottitis, these tenets are still followed at most institutions. Protocols can help ensure the rapid coordination of services and specialists needed to care for infectious airway obstruction (**Fig. 14.2**).

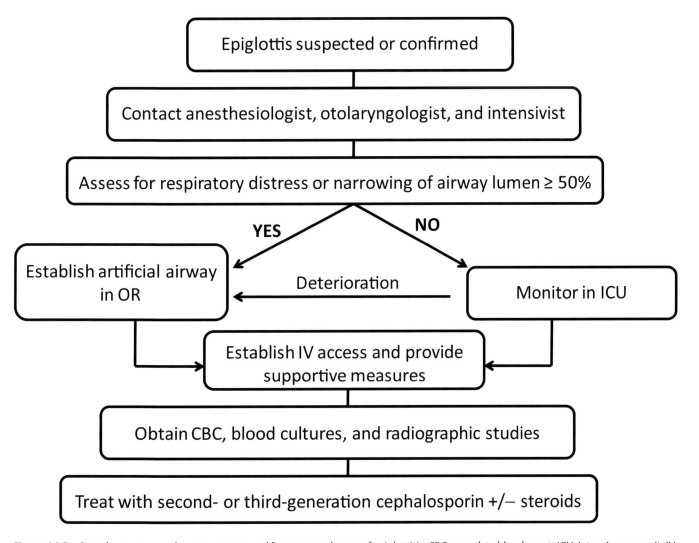

Figure 14.2   Sample emergency department protocol for suspected cases of epiglottitis. CBC, complete blood count; ICU, intensive care unit; IV, intravenous; OR, operating room.

Mask ventilation with orotracheal intubation is attempted first. The orotracheal tube may be left in place, or controlled conversion to nasotracheal intubation or even tracheostomy may be undertaken. Since the mid-1970s, the literature has supported nasotracheal intubation in children due to the morbidity associated with pediatric tracheotomy.[21]

Once the airway has been secured, further diagnostic work-up may be considered. History may help differentiate epiglottitis from inhalation injury, angioedema, or caustic ingestion. Blood cultures and cultures from the epiglottis are typically performed. Though diagnostic yield is highly variable, blood cultures tend to be more useful than direct swabs of the epiglottis.[21] Lateral neck radiographs (**Fig. 14.3**) have relatively poor sensitivity (70%) and specificity (31 to 64%), and are of limited utility.[22]

The majority of patients under 10 years of age will require airway intervention, but stable adults and older children have been increasingly managed with careful observation.[15,21] Factors associated with the need for intervention include rapid symptom onset, stridor, intolerance of secretions, and diabetes mellitus.[23]

Definitive Management

Once the airway is controlled, broad-spectrum antibiotic therapy is instituted until culture results are available. Ampicillin/sulbactam or a second-or third-generation cephalosporin is routinely used with good results.[16] Retrospective studies have not shown benefit from treatment with steroids, but they are often prescribed in an attempt to decrease airway edema.[15] Extubation may be considered in the presence of an air leak around the endotracheal tube or after direct visualization of the epiglottis confirms improvement.

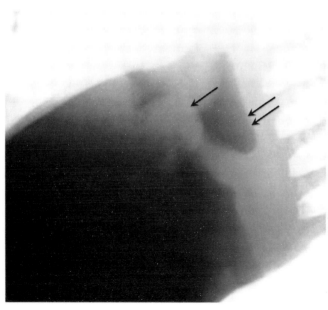

Figure 14.3   Lateral neck radiograph demonstrating epiglottis thickening (thumb sign [arrow]) and dilation of the hypopharynx [double arrow] in a patient with acute epiglottitis.

Bacterial Tracheitis

Bacterial tracheitis (BT), also known as pseudomembranous croup or bacterial laryngotracheobronchitis, was initially described by Jones et al and Han et al in 1979.[24,25] Despite advances in imaging and endoscopy, diagnosis remains difficult, and many patients are unsuccessfully treated for croup before BT is suspected. Because aggressive management of the airway may be necessary to prevent obstruction by thick secretions, prompt recognition and treatment of BT is essential.

Epidemiology

Approximately 2% of children hospitalized for croup are eventually diagnosed with bacterial tracheitis. Estimated incidence is less than 0.1 cases per 100,000 children per year with a male predominance.[26] Seasonal variation mimics that of croup. Cases of BT have been reported in children as young as 4 weeks old, but the mean age of affected children is 5.2 years.[26] The original literature reported mortality rates ranging from 6 to 40%. While deaths are rare in the era of modern antibiotics and endoscopic airway management, serious complications such as acute respiratory distress syndrome, postobstructive pulmonary edema, or multisystem organ failure may occur in up to one-third of patients.

Pathophysiology

There is considerable evidence to suggest that BT represents a superinfection of the trachea and bronchi in children already affected by viral respiratory illness.[24,26] Virally induced impairment of mucociliary clearance and disruption of mucosal barriers are thought to facilitate the entry of bacteria into the mucosal lining of the airways. Thick secretions contribute to airway obstruction and prevent inhaled medications from contacting the respiratory mucosa.[24] Methicillin-sensitive *S. aureus* (MSSA) is by far the most commonly identified pathogen. Other implicated organisms include *M. catarrhalis, H. influenzae, S. pneumoniae,* and *Branhamella catarrhalis.*[27]

Clinical Presentation

Patients with BT typically experience a prodrome of coryza, hoarseness, and a croup-like cough. After hours to days, an abrupt clinical decline is heralded by the rapid onset of high fever and stridor. Importantly, cough remains a prominent symptom. Unlike epiglottitis, BT tends not to limit the patient's ability to lie flat or tolerate his secretions. Progression of illness is rapid—87% of the patients who require mechanical ventilation are intubated within 24 hours of presentation.[26]

Evaluation and Initial Management

Any patient with severe respiratory distress should be considered for diagnostic and therapeutic rigid endoscopy and intubation in the operating room. The presence of thick, purulent secretions or pseudomembranes filling the subglottis and trachea is diagnostic of BT. The pseudomembranes of BT separate from the tracheal walls easily, without bleeding, unlike the fixed pseudomembranes seen in diphtheria. The supraglottis may show mild edema, but generally retains a normal appearance.

Radiographs of the neck are often indistinguishable from those of patients with croup, though hazy irregularities within the tracheal lumen may suggest the presence of purulent debris. Chest radiographs show coincident pneumonia in 60 to 100% of patients with BT.[24] Laboratory studies show leukocytosis with bandemia. In contrast to epiglottitis, however, blood cultures are uniformly negative.[24]

Patients with chronic tracheostomy tubes who are suspected of developing BT present a special challenge. Staphylococcal species and gram-negative organisms can be routinely cultured from the tracheal aspirates of these patients, making the differentiation of colonization and infection difficult. Previous culture data should be reviewed, and a change in the dominant organism should raise the index of suspicion for acute infection when symptoms of respiratory infection are present.

Definitive Management

Most patients with BT require formal control of the airway. Frequent suctioning is essential and repeated endoscopy may be needed to clear the trachea of sloughed tissue and debris.[27] The need for tracheotomy should be carefully considered in patients with BT. Endotracheal tubes may become obstructed with inspissated secretions, and can be difficult to replace in emergent situations.

Limited evidence suggests there may be a more subacute form of BT that can be safely managed without intubation. Patients suitable for conservative management tend to be older and tend to lack pulmonary involvement at the time of diagnosis. These patients should be closely monitored in the intensive care setting.

The decision to extubate is guided by clinical improvement, a decrease in the quantity of secretions suctioned from the trachea, and the presence of a leak around the cuff of the endotracheal tube. Extubation is often possible within 72 to 96 hours, though longer courses of 5 to 9 days of mechanical ventilation are not uncommon.[27]

Antibiotic choice should reflect the dominance of MSSA as the causative organism, but should also cover other common respiratory pathogens. Oxacillin or vancomycin is commonly combined with a third-generation cephalosporin for broad initial coverage.[2,27] Culture-directed therapy should be employed as soon as possible and continued for 10 to 14 days. The diagnosis of BT in patients with a chronic tracheostomy tube can be challenging, given that the trachea may be colonized by bacteria. In this population, BT should be suspected when the patient develops symptoms of acute infection, increased secretions, or increased ventilator settings, and should be confirmed by tracheoscopy with culture. In addition to culture-directed systemic antibiotics, aerosolized antibiotic therapy may be helpful in this population.

Rare Causes of Inflammatory Airway Obstruction in Children

Diphtheria

Laryngeal diphtheria continues to appear in epidemic fashion in areas where vaccines are not routinely used. *Corynebacterium diphtheriae* uses mucosal epithelial cells as a platform for elaboration of a potent exotoxin. The toxin causes tissue damage and local necrosis, leading to the formation of characteristic pseudomembranes. Membranes coat the mucosal surfaces of the upper respiratory tract and may cause sudden respiratory compromise if aspirated. Young children are typically affected, with disease in patients over the age of 15 relatively uncommon.[28] Treatment consists of prompt respiratory isolation, mechanical removal of the pseudomembranes, and treatment of the patient and exposed contacts with erythromycin or penicillin. Antitoxin should be obtained from the Centers for Disease Control and Prevention for treatment of confirmed cases.

Tuberculosis

Though rare in the antibiotic era, pulmonary tuberculosis may involve the major airways. Children are prone to extraluminal compression by bulky hilar nodes. Intraluminal obstruction may occur when granulomatous material infiltrates the airway walls. Frank respiratory distress and pneumothorax from erosion of a lymph node through the bronchial wall is rare, but life-threatening.[29] Surgical intervention consists of intraluminal or extraluminal enucleation of the obstructing nodes. Fibrous stenosis of affected bronchi may occur years later, requiring segmental resection of the involved airways or sequestered segments of lung.[29]

Wegener Granulomatosis

Wegener granulomatosis (WG) is characterized by the triad of necrotizing granulomatous inflammation, proliferative glomerulonephritis, and vasculitis. Primarily a disease of young adults, WG has been diagnosed in children as young as 8 years old.[30] Head and neck manifestations are seen in nearly all patients, with laryngeal and subglottic involvement occurring in 16 to 23% of cases.[31] Active patients may have circumferential edema and friable mucosa; nonspecific scar tissue may be the only finding in patients in remission. A positive serum c-anti-neutrophil cytoplasmic antibody is specific for WG, and diagnosis is confirmed with biopsy. Treatment options include glucocorticoids, immunosuppressants, laser ablation, airway reconstructive surgery, or tracheostomy. Approximately 50% of patients require surgical airway intervention.[30,31]

Sarcoidosis

Sarcoidosis is a chronic inflammatory condition that causes the formation of noncaseating granulomas. Most commonly seen in young adults, sarcoidosis may also present in young children with a triad of uveitis, arthritis, and rash. The pathophysiology is related to persistent T-cell activation and cytokine release. The lungs and lower airways are most commonly affected, but the larger airways and larynx may also be involved.[29] The supraglottic tissues are classically thickened, irregular, and edematous. Diagnosis is confirmed with biopsy. Treatment options include systemic or intral-

esional steroids, cytotoxic agents, and surgical debulking, with tracheostomy reserved for only the most serious cases.

Summary

Historically, inflammatory obstruction of the pediatric airway had devastating consequences. Medical advances that include vaccines, antibiotics, and steroids have led to a dramatic decline in morbidity and mortality attributed to inflammatory airway disease. However, prompt evaluation and management with a low threshold for endoscopy to achieve definitive diagnosis and control of the airway remains essential. Protocols for management of impending airway obstruction are often helpful to ensure the rapid coordination of available of trained personnel, equipment, and services for these patients.

References

1. Loughlin GM, Moscona A. The cell biology of acute childhood respiratory disease: therapeutic implications. Pediatr Clin North Am 2006;53(5):929–959, ix–x
2. Cherry JD. Clinical practice. Croup. N Engl J Med 2008;358(4):384–391
3. To T, Dick P, Young W, Hernandez R. Hospitalization rates of children with croup in Ontario. Paediatr Child Health (Oxford) 1996;1:103–108
4. Sobol SE, Zapata S. Epiglottitis and croup. Otolaryngol Clin North Am 2008;41(3):551–566, ix
5. Westley CR, Cotton EK, Brooks JG. Nebulized racemic epinephrine by IPPB for the treatment of croup: a double-blind study. Am J Dis Child 1978;132(5):484–487
6. Mills JL, Spackman TJ, Borns P, Mandell GA, Schwartz MW. The usefulness of lateral neck roentgenograms in laryngotracheobronchitis. Am J Dis Child 1979;133(11):1140–1142
7. Wright RB, Pomerantz WJ, Luria JW. New approaches to respiratory infections in children. Bronchiolitis and croup. Emerg Med Clin North Am 2002;20(1):93–114
8. Klassen TP, Craig WR, Moher D, et al. Nebulized budesonide and oral dexamethasone for treatment of croup: a randomized controlled trial. JAMA 1998;279(20):1629–1632
9. Fifoot AA, Ting JY. Comparison between single-dose oral prednisolone and oral dexamethasone in the treatment of croup: a randomized, double-blinded clinical trial. Emerg Med Australas 2007;19(1):51–58
10. Weber JE, Chudnofsky CR, Younger JG, et al. A randomized comparison of helium-oxygen mixture (Heliox) and racemic epinephrine for the treatment of moderate to severe croup. Pediatrics 2001;107(6):E96
11. Kristjánsson S, Berg-Kelly K, Winsö E. Inhalation of racemic adrenaline in the treatment of mild and moderately severe croup. Clinical symptom score and oxygen saturation measurements for evaluation of treatment effects. Acta Paediatr 1994;83(11):1156–1160
12. Kelley PB, Simon JE. Racemic epinephrine use in croup and disposition. Am J Emerg Med 1992;10(3):181–183
13. Prendergast M, Jones JS, Hartman D. Racemic epinephrine in the treatment of laryngotracheitis: can we identify children for outpatient therapy? Am J Emerg Med 1994;12(6):613–616
14. Moore M, Little P. Humidified air inhalation for treating croup. Cochrane Database Syst Rev 2006;3:CD002870
15. Guldfred LA, Lyhne D, Becker BC. Acute epiglottitis: epidemiology, clinical presentation, management and outcome. J Laryngol Otol 2008;122(8):818–823
16. Shah RK, Roberson DW, Jones DT. Epiglottitis in the *Hemophilus influenzae* type B vaccine era: changing trends. Laryngoscope 2004;114(3):557–560
17. Smith PJ, Singleton JA. Vaccination coverage estimates for selected counties: achievement of Healthy People 2010 goals and association with indices of access to care, economic conditions, and demographic composition. Public Health Rep 2008;123(2):155–172
18. Rabe EF. Infectious croup; *Hemophilus influenzae* type B croup. Pediatrics 1948;2(5):559–566
19. Torkkeli T, Ruoppi P, Nuutinen J, Kari A. Changed clinical course and current treatment of acute epiglottitis in adults a 12-year experience. Laryngoscope 1994;104(12):1503–1506
20. Tanner K, Fitzsimmons G, Carrol ED, Flood TJ, Clark JE. *Haemophilus influenzae* type b epiglottitis as a cause of acute upper airways obstruction in children. BMJ 2002;325(7372):1099–1100
21. Mayo-Smith MF, Spinale JW, Donskey CJ, Yukawa M, Li RH, Schiffman FJ. Acute epiglottitis. An 18-year experience in Rhode Island. Chest 1995;108(6):1640–1647
22. Stankiewicz JA, Bowes AK. Croup and epiglottitis: a radiologic study. Laryngoscope 1985;95(10):1159–1160
23. Katori H, Tsukuda M. Acute epiglottitis: analysis of factors associated with airway intervention. J Laryngol Otol 2005;119(12):967–972
24. Jones R, Santos JI, Overall JC Jr. Bacterial tracheitis. JAMA 1979;242(8):721–726
25. Han BK, Dunbar JS, Striker TW. Membranous laryngotracheobronchitis (membranous croup). AJR Am J Roentgenol 1979;133:53-8
26. Tebruegge M, Pantazidou A, Thorburn K, et al. Bacterial tracheitis: a multi-centre perspective. Scand J Infect Dis 2009;41(8):548–557
27. Kasian GF, Bingham WT, Steinberg J, et al. Bacterial tracheitis in children. CMAJ 1989;140(1):46–50

28. Galazka AM, Robertson SE. Diphtheria: changing patterns in the developing world and the industrialized world. Eur J Epidemiol 1995;11(1):107–117

29. Papagiannopoulos KA, Linegar AG, Harris DG, Rossouw GJ. Surgical management of airway obstruction in primary tuberculosis in children. Ann Thorac Surg 1999;68(4):1182–1186

30. Gubbels SP, Barkhuizen A, Hwang PH. Head and neck manifestations of Wegener's granulomatosis. Otolaryngol Clin North Am 2003;36(4):685–705

31. Gluth MB, Shinners PA, Kasperbauer JL. Subglottic stenosis associated with Wegener's granulomatosis. Laryngoscope 2003;113(8):1304–1307

15 Evaluation and Management of Upper Airway Obstruction in Children

Nicholas Smith, Aliza P. Cohen, and Michael J. Rutter

Causes of airway obstruction in children encompass a wide spectrum of anomalies that may involve not only the larynx and trachea, but also other anatomic sites from the nasal vestibule to the subsegmental bronchi. This chapter presents an overview of the diagnosis and management of these anomalies, focusing on those that are commonly encountered and those that are significant, though infrequently encountered. Causes of airway obstruction will be discussed below from proximal to distal fashion anatomically.

Supralaryngeal

Congenital Nasal Pyriform Aperture Stenosis

Congenital nasal pyriform aperture stenosis (CNPAS) is a relatively uncommon developmental anomaly characterized by bony overgrowth of the medial aspect of the nasal process of the maxilla. Because the pyriform aperture is the narrowest section of the bony nasal skeleton, even minor anatomic abnormalities in the cross-sectional area of the aperture substantially affect airflow by increasing nasal airway resistance. CNPAS typically presents during the first few months of life, when infants are obligate nasal breathers. Although it sometimes occurs as an isolated anomaly, it is generally associated with a single central upper incisor.

Neonates present with a spectrum of symptoms resulting from nasal obstruction, including cyanosis, apnea, feeding difficulties, and labored breathing. These symptoms may mimic the symptoms observed in patients with bilateral choanal atresia (described further); as such, evaluation for suspected choanal atresia is sometimes performed, yielding negative results. Clinicians may thus be falsely reassured that there is no substantial nasal obstruction.

The diagnosis of CNPAS is established by anterior rhinoscopy, which reveals an anterior bony obstruction of the nasal vestibule. This is confirmed by computed tomography (CT), which may also confirm the presence of a single central upper incisor and other midline anomalies of the central nervous system.

Management depends on the severity of symptoms. In patients with mild symptoms, expectant management may be all that is required until growth results in increased nasal airway size. In more severely affected patients, surgical enlargement is indicated. This is best performed through a sublabial approach, exposing the pyriform aperture, and using a diamond burr to remove the excessive bone of the nasal process of the maxillary crest. Temporary nasal stents are generally placed for 2 to 4 weeks postoperatively.

Choanal Atresia

Although several theories of the embryogenesis of choanal atresia have been proposed, this anomaly is believed to result from the persistence of the nasal buccal membrane. The nasal obstruction may be membranous, bony, or a combination of both; however, the latter is most commonly seen. The atresia may be unilateral or bilateral, with a likely ratio of 1:1. Both unilateral and bilateral disease may be associated with other congenital anomalies; the most widely recognized association is with CHARGE syndrome (*c*oloboma, *h*eart defects, *a*tresia, *r*etardation of growth and development, *g*enitourinary disorders, and *e*ar abnormalities).[1]

Given that neonates are obligate nasal breathers during the first 6 weeks of life, apnea in children with bilateral disease may occur during quiet respiration irrespective of the underlying disease process causing the nasal obstruction. Apnea is not observed when neonates are agitated, as they breathe by mouth when crying. Once the crying subsides, they are again at risk for apnea. Complete obstruction of the posterior nasal passage by choanal atresia prevents normal drainage of nasal secretions into the nasopharynx. These secretions must therefore drain anteriorly and are characteristically copious and tenacious.

We recommend evaluating nasal passages with a thin (1.9 mm) flexible nasal endoscope. Airway management of a patient with bilateral disease is placement of an oral airway or intubation. This approach stabilizes the child until CT can be performed and, if appropriate, until genetic assessments can be performed. We advise radiologic evaluation with bone/window high-resolution, thin-section CT imaging. The quality of the image is greatly enhanced by removing all nasal sections with a soft suction catheter immediately before the scan. A thin atretic plate at the posterior choana is usually seen; this plate is often both bony and membranous. Frequently, an associated prominence of the bony margins of the choana is revealed, with bony overgrowth of the vomer in the midline or medialization of the lateral nasal walls.

Unless there are contraindications for surgery (e.g., extreme prematurity or multiple congenital anomalies), patients should undergo early surgical repair.[2] Although surgical approaches may be either transpalatal or transnasal, the latter is preferable in most children. This approach involves endoscopically guided removal of the atretic plate using urethral dilators, backbiting forceps, drills, powered microdebrider cutters, or a combination of these instruments. For cases in which there is prominence of the bony margins of the choana, the posterior aspect of the vomer may be removed to form a common cavity at the level of the atretic plate. Whereas transnasal stents were formerly placed for several weeks postoperatively, the current trend is toward either shorter periods of stenting or no stenting at all. Because both options carry the risk of the patient developing secondary choanal stenosis, adjuvant therapy such as topical application of steroid nasal drops may be used.

Patients with unilateral choanal atresia are generally not diagnosed until later in childhood, when they present with unilateral rhinorrhea and nasal obstruction that necessitate a CT evaluation. Transnasal repair of the atresia is generally performed after 2 years of age. Nasal obstruction at birth in the subset of patients with choanal atresia associated with CHARGE syndrome is more severe than in other patients. Because the level of obstruction in these children is not restricted to the choana and may include pharyngomalacia, hypopharyngeal collapse, and laryngomalacia, repair of the choanal atresia may not preclude the need for tracheostomy placement. If other levels of obstruction are recognized initially, placement of a tracheostomy tube and late repair of the choanal atresia may be the most appropriate management strategy. Regardless of whether the atresia is unilateral or bilateral or whether surgical repair is undertaken early or late, outcomes are less successful in these patients.

Nasolacrimal Duct Cysts

Nasolacrimal duct cysts result from the failure of the nasolacrimal duct to recanalize during embryogenesis. This anomaly may arise either unilaterally or bilaterally. Patients typically present with nasal obstruction caused by a large cyst under the inferior turbinate, occluding the anterior nasal airway. Swelling of the nasolacrimal sac in the medial canthal area may also be observed. Epiphora is evident, as tears cannot drain. If the cyst is infected, as is frequently the case, there may be abscess formation in the nasolacrimal sac region, and the neonate may be septic. The diagnosis is established with anterior rhinoscopy and CT imaging of the nasal passages. Patients are managed by transnasal endoscopic removal or marsupialization of the cyst, with placement of nasolacrimal duct catheters if required.

Retrognathia/Glossoptosis

Retrognathia is a descriptive term for mandibular hypoplasia. A consequence of the hypoplasia is crowding of the tongue posteriorly and superiorly, which may cause airway obstruction and a cleft of the secondary palate, as the palate anlagen are unable to close around the cephalically displaced tongue. Retrognathia is associated with several abnormalities, including Pierre Robin sequence (short mandible, cleft palate), Treacher Collins syndrome (mandibulo-facial dysostosis), and Stickler syndrome. The severity of retrognathia is not always a reliable indicator of the severity of obstruction or of problems that may occur with intubation. Obstructing retrognathia generally becomes evident during the neonatal period; however, problems may develop later in life. Such problems are often triggered by incidental surgical procedures or with the insidious onset of severe sleep apnea caused by glossoptosis or adenotonsillar hypertrophy.

The management of neonates involves prone positioning and the use of high-flow nasal cannula; occasionally, a nasal trumpet is useful. Continuous positive airway pressure (CPAP) is often unsuccessful, as the mask tends to exacerbate the retrognathia. Because infants have difficulty feeding, placement of a nasogastric tube placement is often required. For children with persistent airway compromise, intubation is desirable though challenging.

In infants who suffer with significant obstructive symptoms or feeding difficulties, the standard of care is placement of a tracheotomy. In most nonsyndromic children, catch-up growth of the mandible will permit decannulation within 1 to 2 years. If catch-up is not apparent at 1 year of age, mandibular distraction should be considered.[3] Although this procedure is controversial, in select cases it may be an effective alternative to tracheotomy placement. Distraction may be performed without placement of a tracheotomy tube; however, in some instances it is prudent to perform distraction while the airway is secured with a tracheotomy tube.

Because of the association between retrognathia and tracheobronchomalacia, some children continue to have symptoms of obstruction after tracheotomy placement. In this setting, performing flexible bronchoscopy through the tracheotomy tube is diagnostic, and management with CPAP, bi-level positive airway pressure, or ventilation is sometimes necessary. In infants with isolated tracheomalacia, replacing the tracheotomy tube with a longer tube that lies close to carina may be all that is required. A surgical alternative for the management of severe intrathoracic tracheomalacia is aortopexy.

Supraglottic

Laryngomalacia

Laryngomalacia is the most common cause of stridor in infants. Although stridor is generally mild, it is exacerbated by crying, excitement, feeding, or lying in a supine position. In about 10% of cases, symptoms worsen during sleep. Approximately 50% of children with laryngomalacia experience an exacerbation of symptoms during the first 6 months of life; however, virtually all children have spontaneous resolution of symptoms by 1 year of age. For children with severe laryngomalacia (5 to 10%), surgical intervention is required. Symptoms in these children may include apneic spells, cyanosis, severe retractions, and failure to thrive. In very severe cases, cor pulmonale is seen.

The diagnosis is generally confirmed by transnasal flexible

laryngoscopy. Bronchoscopic evaluation is not indicated unless symptoms are severe enough to warrant intervention or the observed degree of laryngomalacia is disproportionate to the severity of the symptoms. Characteristic findings on flexible laryngoscopy include short aryepiglottic folds, with prolapse of the cuneiform cartilages (50%). In addition, a tightly curled omega-shaped (Ω) epiglottis is sometimes (15 to 20%) observed. Flexible laryngoscopy may also show cricoid irritation and edema. Gastroesophageal reflux disease is frequently associated with laryngomalacia. This condition is usually managed with either an H_2 antagonist or a proton-pump inhibitor.

For the subset of children who require surgical intervention, supraglottoplasty with division of the short aryepiglottic folds, and if indicated, removal of the cuneiform cartilages (if these are excessively mobile) is remarkably effective.[4] If there is any risk of edema, overnight intubation is warranted. For children in whom supraglottoplasty is ineffective, consideration should be given to whether there is any underlying neurologic component. Although neurologic problems may be quite subtle initially, they may become more evident with age. This particular group of children is far more likely to require tracheotomy placement.

Cysts

Supralaryngeal cysts encompass several diverse pathologic entities, including lingual thyroglossal duct cysts, vallecular cysts, laryngoceles, and saccular cysts. These cysts typically become evident during the neonatal period and are associated with a muffled cry and apneic spells that may be life threatening.

Lingual thyroglossal duct cysts usually occur in tongue base near the epiglottis; they tend to be midline and deep to the mucosa. Although these cysts are frequently asymptomatic in older children, they may be life threatening in neonates. Affected infants require surgical intervention. A transoral cyst excision is a straightforward and effective technique for managing the disease. Special care should be taken on the induction of general anesthesia in neonates, as the airway is susceptible to complete obstruction during induction.

In contrast to thyroglossal duct cysts, vallecular cysts are thin-walled cysts near the glottic surface of the epiglottis. These cysts can easily be marsupialized.

Laryngoceles and saccular cysts occur when the laryngeal ventricle is obstructed. Although endoscopic marsupialization may be attempted, recurrence is frequent and placement of a tracheotomy is often required. An open surgical approach with dissection of the cyst through the thyrohyoid ligament enables complete cyst removal and is thus curative.

For all of these cysts, transnasal flexible laryngoscopy suggests the diagnosis and formal bronchoscopic evaluation of the airway confirms it. A CT scan with contrast enhancement is useful in ensuring that a lingual thyroid is not mistaken for a lingual thyroglossal duct cyst and delineates the extent of disease.

Supraglottic Infection

Effective pediatric immunization programs have virtually eliminated supraglottic infections such as diphtheria (a century ago) and epiglottitis (2 decades ago). The *Haemophilus influenzae* type B vaccination has virtually eliminated epiglottitis. Although it still occurs, it is more frequently a disease of older age groups with less acute airway obstruction or is due to less virulent organisms. While intubation of patients with these disorders may be challenging in the acute phase of disease, it is nevertheless the preferred method of securing the airway. In the event that the airway cannot be secured, the surgeon should be prepared to proceed directly to an emergent tracheotomy if required.

Glottic

Laryngeal Webs

Laryngeal webs may be either congenital or acquired. Congenital webs are a consequence of embryologic failure of laryngeal recanalization of the glottic airway in the early weeks of embryogenesis. Acquired webs are generally posttraumatic in origin, either iatrogenic in nature or the result of direct trauma or inhalational injuries. Although congenital laryngeal webs have been described in the supraglottic, glottic, and subglottic regions and may occur anteriorly or posteriorly, anterior glottic webs comprise more than 95% of cases. Associated congenital anomalies are seen in up to 60% of patients, and there is a strong association between anterior glottic webs and velocardiofacial syndrome.[5] The web may be the only early manifestation of this disorder.

Congenital anterior glottic webs manifest with varying degrees of glottic airway compromise. The severity of symptoms correlates with the size and position of the web. Although some anterior glottic webs are gossamer thin, most are thick and are associated with a subglottic "sail" that compromises the subglottic lumen. Thin webs may elude detection, as neonatal intubation for airway distress may lyse the web, which is curative. In infants with moderate to severe webs, biphasic stridor and retractions become increasingly evident as the infant grows and are particularly evident when the infant is feeding or upset.

In children with minor webs, early intervention is unwarranted, though it is desirable to intervene before school age to improve voice. In children with thick webs, open reconstruction with either reconstruction of the anterior commissure or placement of a laryngeal keel is indicated.[6] Intervention with the carbon dioxide (CO_2) laser usually leads to recalcitrant web re-formation. The presence of thick membranous webs may require temporary placement of a tracheotomy to allow growth before elective laryngeal repair is performed. Repair is usually performed before the child reaches school age.

Vocal Cord Paralysis

Vocal cord paralysis may be congenital or acquired and unilateral or bilateral. In most cases, bilateral vocal cord paralysis is congenital. Unilateral paralysis is generally an acquired problem caused by damage to the recurrent laryngeal nerve. In view of the length and course of the left recurrent nerve, this nerve is far more likely to be damaged than the right recurrent laryngeal nerve. Risk factors for acquired paralysis are patent ductus arteriosus ligation (particularly in neonates weighing less than 1500 g), cardiac surgery, and esophageal surgery (especially tracheoesophageal fistula repair). In older children, thyroid surgery is an additional risk factor. Children with unilateral vocal cord paralysis generally have an acceptable airway, but have a breathy voice and are at a slightly higher risk of aspiration. For the most part, these children ultimately become asymptomatic with compensation of the functional vocal cord and do not require surgical intervention.

Congenital cord paralysis is usually idiopathic, but may also be associated with central nervous system pathology such as hydrocephalus and Chiari malformation of the brainstem. When the underlying cause is corrected, the paralysis may be reversible. Most children with bilateral vocal cord paralysis present with significant airway compromise, but have an excellent voice and usually do not aspirate unless there are associated central nervous system abnormalities.

In an infant with stridor and retractions caused by bilateral vocal cord paralysis, placing a tracheotomy is indicated. Stabilization can be achieved with intubation, with CPAP, or high-flow nasal cannula as an alternative temporizing measure. Up to 50% of children with congenital idiopathic bilateral vocal cord paralysis have spontaneous resolution of their paralysis by 1 year of age.[7] Surgical intervention to achieve decannulation is thus usually delayed until after 1 year. Similarly, children with acquired bilateral vocal cord paralysis may have spontaneous recovery several months after recurrent laryngeal nerve injury if the nerve is stretched or crushed but otherwise intact.

Because no particular surgical approach for managing bilateral paralysis yields a universally acceptable outcome, several surgical options have been used.[8] The aim of surgery is twofold: (1) to achieve an adequate decannulated airway while maintaining voice and (2) to prevent aspiration. Surgical options include laser cordotomy, partial or complete arytenoidectomy (endoscopic or open), vocal process lateralization (open or endoscopically guided), and posterior cricoid cartilage grafting. In a child with a tracheotomy, it is often desirable to maintain the tracheotomy to ensure an adequate airway before decannulation. In a child without a tracheotomy, a single-stage procedure can be performed.

Acquired bilateral vocal cord paralysis is usually more recalcitrant to treatment than idiopathic cord paralysis, and more than one procedure may be required to achieve decannulation. In patients who have undergone any such procedures, postextubation stridor may respond to CPAP or high-flow nasal cannula. A child's postoperative risk of aspiration should be assessed by a video swallow study before resuming a normal diet. During the initial weeks following surgery, there is sometimes an increased aspiration risk with certain food textures, particularly thin fluids.

Posterior Glottic Stenosis

Although posterior glottic stenosis (PGS) is usually a consequence of prolonged intubation, other contributing synergistic factors include endotracheal tube size, patient agitation, laryngeal inflammation, and oral tube placement. Because these are also risk factors for the development of subglottic stenosis (SGS), both conditions frequently coexist. Cricoarytenoid fixation may also coexist and may mimic PGS. Furthermore, PGS may mimic bilateral vocal cord paralysis. The diagnosis is best made by performing rigid bronchoscopy, with an attempt to splay the vocal cords. Flexible bronchoscopy is not a reliable diagnostic tool in this condition.

Although several schemas for classifying the severity of PGS have been proposed, the system put forth by Bogdasarian and Olson[9] is the most widely used. These authors divide PGS into four types and advocate a graded surgical approach based on the extent of the pathology. PGS is best treated through an open approach, with the division of the posterior plate of the cricoid and placement of a cartilage graft to distract the scar tissue while remucosalization and healing occur. If associated SGS is present, an anterior graft may also be placed if required. In selected cases of isolated PGS, the posterior cartilage graft may be placed endoscopically.[10]

Clinical outcomes in children with PGS are not as impressive as those achieved in children with SGS; patients with PGS have been found to have a restenosis rate of at least 15%.[11] Success rates are markedly improved for children with interarytenoid adhesions (Bogdasarian and Olson type I), as the interarytenoid scar band responds well to endoscopic excision.

Papillomatosis

Recurrent respiratory papillomatosis (RRP), also referred to as juvenile laryngeal papillomatosis, is the most common infective lesion of the larynx in children. The etiology of RRP is infection of the upper airway with human papillomavirus (HPV) types 6 and 11, and less commonly, types 16 and 18. RRP is frequently associated with transplacental transmission of maternal HPV; however, contact with active cervical HPV during delivery is also considered a causal factor. Although genital papillomas are extremely common, RRP is extremely rare and the relative risk of acquiring RRP is low.

Nearly 75% of children with RRP are diagnosed by age 5. Although the condition typically presents with hoarseness, stridor caused by airway obstruction is also common and often precipitates otolaryngologic referral. Initial evaluation is performed with flexible transnasal laryngoscopy, which may reveal a laryngeal mass; however, microlaryngoscopy and bronchoscopy with biopsy of the papillomas are required for a definitive diagnosis and for serotyping lesions for prognostic purposes. Serotypes 16 and 18 are associated with more aggressive disease and a higher risk of malignant transformation.

Although the course of the disease is both variable and unpredictable, RRP tends to recur locally and, in severe cases, spreads throughout the respiratory tract. Surgical intervention should be based on debulking gross disease without attempting complete removal of the affected tissue, so as to avoid laryngeal scarring or stenosis. The most widely used surgical procedure is suspension laryngoscopy with tumor removal using the CO_2 laser, microforceps, or the microdebrider. In patients with extensive disease, surgery should be aimed at reducing the tumor burden, decreasing the spread of disease, creating a patent airway, improving voice quality, and lengthening the intervals between surgical interventions. In children with severe RRP, tracheotomy placement may be required; however, this is often at the cost of disseminating disease beyond the glottis.

Cidofovir and bevacizumab are currently the most enthusiastically embraced adjunctive treatment modalities. However, innoculation with polyvalent HPV vaccine is the brightest hope for the future.

Subglottic

Subglottic Cysts

Subglottic cysts are most commonly a consequence of the prolonged intubation of a premature infant. These cysts are often multiple, and may be superficial and thin walled or may lie deep in the submucosal layer. Although the pathogenesis of subglottic cysts is unlike that of SGS, both problems may coexist. Management includes deroofing the cyst using microlaryngeal instrumentation, powered instrumentation, CO_2 laser, or Bugbee electrocautery. As subglottic cysts tend to recur, follow-up bronchoscopy is essential. Removal may need to be performed on several occasions before complete resolution is attained.

Subglottic Hemangioma

Subglottic hemangiomas are the most common neoplasm affecting the airway in children. These lesions follow the same natural history as their cutaneous counterparts, having a phase of proliferation followed by a phase of spontaneous involution; however, subglottic lesions expand and involute more rapidly. They typically proliferate during the first 12 months of life and spontaneously regress over an additional 12 months or more. Most patients present in the first few weeks or months of life, and the earlier the presentation, the more severe the problem and the higher the likelihood that intervention will be required. Although 50% of children with a subglottic hemangioma also have a cutaneous hemangioma, the risk of having a subglottic hemangioma if a cutaneous hemangioma is present is generally very low. An exception to this is hemangiomas that arise in a beard distribution; 65% of patients with these lesions have associated airway involvement.[12]

The classic symptoms of subglottic hemangioma include progressive stridor and retractions, often exacerbated by upper respiratory tract infections. Worsening respiratory difficulty in an infant demands a transnasal flexible laryngoscopy with the patient awake. The most common laryngeal pathologies (laryngomalacia, vocal cord paralysis, laryngeal cysts) are clearly visible. If, however, there is not a clear cause for the stridor, airway films and a rigid bronchoscopy are indicated. Airway films show a subglottic narrowing, which is frequently asymmetric. On bronchoscopy, the hemangioma always looks more impressively obstructive than the child's clinical presentation suggests. The hemangioma is compressible, may have vascular markings, and more commonly arises to the left of the midline. It is important to perform the bronchoscopy with the patient under spontaneous ventilation, while avoiding intubation, as this may compress the lesion, making diagnosis more challenging. Biopsy is not indicated. A deeply seated subglottic hemangioma may be confused with a subglottic cyst.

Airway compromise frequently occurs before involution, thus necessitating intervention. Over the past decade, the management of subglottic hemangioma has evolved significantly, and a wide range of interventions and treatment approaches have been reported. Currently, first-line management involves a trial of propranolol, with surgery (tracheotomy or open excision) being reserved for patients who are unresponsive to treatment.[13]

SGS

SGS can be either congenital or acquired. Congenital SGS is comparatively rare and is thought to result from failure of the laryngeal lumen to recanalize; it is one of a continuum of embryologic failures that include laryngeal atresia, stenosis, and webs. In the neonate, SGS is defined as a lumen 4 mm in diameter or less at the level of the cricoid. Acquired SGS is more common and is generally a sequela of prolonged intubation of the neonate. A useful and practical guide is that the outer diameter of a 3.0 endotracheal tube is 4.3 mm, and if air leaks around the tube at less than 20 cm of subglottic pressure of water, the subglottis is not stenotic.

Levels of disease severity are graded according to the Myer-Cotton grading system (grades I to IV), with grade I ranging from no obstruction to 50% obstruction and grade IV being no detectable lumen.[14] Mild SGS may manifest in recurrent upper respiratory infections (often diagnosed as croup) in which minimal subglottic swelling precipitates airway obstruction. More severe cases may present with acute airway compromise at delivery. If endotracheal intubation is successful, the patient may require intervention before extubation. When intubation cannot be achieved, tracheotomy placement at the time of delivery may be lifesaving. It is important to note that infants typically have few symptoms, and because growth of the child exceeds growth of the airway, even those with grade III stenosis may not be symptomatic for weeks or months.

Congenital SGS is often associated with other congenital head and neck lesions and syndromes (e.g., a small larynx in a patient with Down syndrome). After initial management of SGS, the larynx will grow with the patient and may not require further surgical intervention; however, if initial management requires intubation, there is considerable risk of developing an acquired SGS in addition to the underlying congenital SGS.

Radiologic evaluation of an airway that is not intubated may give the clinician clues about the site and length of the stenosis. The single most important investigation is a high-kilovoltage airway film. This is taken not only to identify the classic "steepling" observed in patients with SGS, but also to identify possible tracheal stenosis.

Evaluation of SGS, whether it is congenital, acquired, or a combination of both, requires endoscopic assessment; ideally, this is done with a Hopkins rod rigid telescope. Precise evaluation of the endolarynx should be performed, including grading of the SGS. Stenosis caused by scarring, granulation tissue, submucosal thickening, or a congenitally abnormal cricoid can be differentiated from SGS with a normal cricoid, but endoscopic measurement with endotracheal tubes or bronchoscopes is required for an accurate evaluation.

The greatest risk factor for developing acquired SGS is prolonged intubation with an inappropriately large endotracheal tube. The appropriate endotracheal tube size is not the largest that will fit, but rather the smallest that allows for adequate ventilation. Ideally, the tube should leak air around it, with subglottic pressures below 25 to 30 cm of water. Other cofactors for the development of acquired SGS include gastroesophageal reflux and eosinophilic esophagitis.

Children with mild acquired SGS may be asymptomatic or minimally symptomatic. Observation rather than intervention may thus be appropriate. This is often the case for children with grades I or II disease. Those with more severe disease are symptomatic, with either tracheal dependency or stridor and exercise intolerance. Unlike congenital SGS, acquired stenosis is unlikely to resolve spontaneously and thus requires intervention. In children with mild symptoms and a minor degree of SGS, endoscopic intervention may be effective, with scar division and balloon dilation being the most effective approach.

More severe forms of disease are better managed with open airway reconstruction. Laryngotracheal reconstruction using costal cartilage grafts placed through the split lamina of the cricoid cartilage is reliable and has withstood the test of time.[15,16] Costal cartilage grafts may be placed through the anterior lamina of the cricoid cartilage, the posterior lamina of the cricoid cartilage, or both. This is usually performed as a two-stage procedure, maintaining the tracheal tube and temporarily placing a suprastomal laryngeal stent above the tracheal tube. Alternatively, in selective cases, a single-stage procedure may be performed, with removal of the tracheal tube on the day of surgery and with the child requiring intubation for a 1- to 14-day period. For the management of severe SGS, better results may be achieved with cricotracheal resection (CTR) than with laryngotracheal reconstruction; however, CTR is a technically demanding procedure that carries a significant risk of complications.[17]

Patients should be optimized before undergoing surgery. Preoperative evaluation includes assessment and management of gastroesophageal reflux, eosinophilic esophagitis, and low-grade tracheal infection, particularly methicillin-resistant *Staphylococcus aureus* and *Pseudomonas*.

Tracheal

Complete Tracheal Rings

Complete tracheal rings are a rare but life-threatening anomaly. They present with insidious worsening of respiratory function over the first few months of life and with stridor, retractions, and marked exacerbation of symptoms during intercurrent upper respiratory tract infections. Children with distal tracheal stenosis usually have a characteristic biphasic wet-sounding breathing pattern that transiently clears with coughing. The risk of respiratory failure increases with age. Over 80% of children with complete tracheal rings have other congenital anomalies that are usually cardiovascular in origin.

Although the diagnosis is established with rigid bronchoscopy, an initial high-kilovolt airway radiograph may reveal tracheal narrowing. Bronchoscopy should be performed with great caution, using the smallest possible telescopes, as any airway edema in the region of the stenosis may turn a narrow airway into an extremely critical airway. The location, extent, and degree of stenosis are all relevant; however, if the airway is exceptionally narrow, it may be more prudent just to establish the diagnosis rather than risk-causing posttraumatic edema by forcing a telescope through a stenosis. As 50% of children have a tracheal inner diameter of about 2 mm at the time of diagnosis, the standard interventions for managing a compromised airway are not applicable. More specifically, the smallest endotracheal tube has an outer diameter of 2.9 mm and the smallest tracheotomy tube has an outer diameter of 3.9 mm; as such, the stenotic segment cannot be intubated. Extracorporeal membrane oxygenation may thus be left as the only viable alternative for stabilizing the child. This situation is best avoided by performing bronchoscopy with the highest level of care. In view of frequent cardiovascular anomalies, investigation should include a high-resolution, contrast-enhanced CT scan of the chest and an echocardiogram.

Most children with complete tracheal rings require tracheal reconstruction.[18] The recommended surgical technique is the slide tracheoplasty.[19] This approach yields significantly better results than any other form of tracheal reconstruction and is applicable to all anatomic variants of complete tracheal rings.

Tracheomalacia

Tracheomalacia is the most common congenital tracheal anomaly. Most children are either asymptomatic or minimally symptomatic, and most cases involve posterior malacia of the trachea, with associated broad tracheal rings. Commonly associated abnormalities include laryngeal clefts, tracheoesophageal fistulae, and bronchomalacia. Presenting symptoms include a honking cough, wheezing, dying spells, and respiratory distress when agitated.

The diagnosis is established with rigid or flexible bronchoscopy, while maintaining spontaneous respiration. The key elements of diagnosis include: (1) ascertaining the severity of the malacia; (2) ascertaining the location of the malacia, particularly the possible presence of associated bronchomalacia; and (3) determining whether positive pressure support improves the malacia. Mild tracheomalacia improves with time and is therefore managed expectantly; however, more severe cases warrant intervention.[20] Tracheotomy placement, with the tip of the tracheotomy tube

bypassing the malacic segment, remains the most common intervention. Positive pressure support delivered down the tracheotomy tube assists with associated bronchomalacia. An alternative surgical procedure for isolated tracheomalacia is aortopexy, with thymectomy and anterior suspension of the ascending arch of the aorta to the posterior periosteum of the sternum. Although the placement of intratracheal stents is alluring, it is presently discouraged.

Conclusion

Obstruction of the pediatric airway is often best considered anatomically in a proximal to distal fashion. Obstruction at or above the vocal folds may be rapidly and safely evaluated with transnasal flexible laryngoscopy at the bedside in an awake child. If no pathology is found, then by implication the pathology is more distal and rigid bronchoscopy in an anesthetized child is indicated. Given that most causes of pediatric airway obstruction are proximal, operative evaluation is required only in a minority of cases.

References

1. Keller JL, Kacker A. Choanal atresia, CHARGE association, and congenital nasal stenosis. Otolaryngol Clin North Am 2000;33(6): 1343–1351, viii

2. Samadi DS, Shah UK, Handler SD. Choanal atresia: a twenty-year review of medical comorbidities and surgical outcomes. Laryngoscope 2003;113(2):254–258

3. Mandell DL, Yellon RF, Bradley JP, Izadi K, Gordon CB. Mandibular distraction for micrognathia and severe upper airway obstruction. Arch Otolaryngol Head Neck Surg 2004;130(3):344–348

4. Denoyelle FM, Mondain M, Gresillon N, Roger G, Chaudre F, Garabedian EN. Failures and complications of supraglottoplasty in children. Arch Otolaryngol Head Neck Surg 2003;129(10):1077–1080, discussion 1080

5. Miyamoto RC, Cotton RT, Rope AF, et al. Association of anterior glottic webs with velocardiofacial syndrome (chromosome 22q11.2 deletion). Otolaryngol Head Neck Surg 2004;130(4): 415–417

6. Wyatt ME, Hartley BE. Laryngotracheal reconstruction in congenital laryngeal webs and atresias. Otolaryngol Head Neck Surg 2005;132(2):232–238

7. Miyamoto RC, Parikh SR, Gellad W, Licameli GR. Bilateral congenital vocal cord paralysis: a 16-year institutional review. Otolaryngol Head Neck Surg 2005;133(2):241–245

8. Hartnick CJ, Brigger MT, Willging JP, Cotton RT, Myer CM III. Surgery for pediatric vocal cord paralysis: a retrospective review. Ann Otol Rhinol Laryngol 2003;112(1):1–6

9. Bogdasarian RS, Olson NR. Posterior glottic laryngeal stenosis. Otolaryngol Head Neck Surg 1980;88(6):765–772

10. Inglis AF Jr, Perkins JA, Manning SC, Mouzakes J. Endoscopic posterior cricoid split and rib grafting in 10 children. Laryngoscope 2003;113(11):2004–2009

11. Rutter MJ, Cotton RT. The use of posterior cricoid grafting in managing isolated posterior glottic stenosis in children. Arch Otolaryngol Head Neck Surg 2004;130(6):737–739

12. Orlow SJ, Isakoff MS, Blei F. Increased risk of symptomatic hemangiomas of the airway in association with cutaneous hemangiomas in a "beard" distribution. J Pediatr 1997;131(4):643–646

13. Javia LR, Zur KB, Jacobs IN. Evolving treatments in the management of laryngotracheal hemangiomas: will propranolol supplant steroids and surgery? Int J Pediatr Otorhinolaryngol 2011;75(11):1450–1454

14. Myer CM III, O'Connor DM, Cotton RT. Proposed grading system for subglottic stenosis based on endotracheal tube sizes. Ann Otol Rhinol Laryngol 1994;103(4 Pt 1):319–323

15. Cotton RT, Gray SD, Miller RP. Update of the Cincinnati experience in pediatric laryngotracheal reconstruction. Laryngoscope 1989;99(11):1111–1116

16. Cotton RT. The problem of pediatric laryngotracheal stenosis: a clinical and experimental study on the efficacy of autogenous cartilaginous grafts placed between the vertically divided lamina of the cricoid cartilage. Laryngoscope 1991;101(12 Pt 2 Suppl 56):1–34

17. White DR, Cotton RT, Bean JA, Rutter MJ. Pediatric cricotracheal resection: surgical outcomes and risk factor analysis. Arch Otolaryngol Head Neck Surg 2005;131(10):896–899

18. Rutter MJ, Cotton RT. Tracheal stenosis and reconstruction. In: Mattei P, ed. Surgical Directives: Pediatric Surgery. Philadelphia, PA; Lippincott, Williams & Wilkins;2003:151-156

19. Rutter MJ, Cotton RT, Azizkhan RG, Manning PB. Slide tracheoplasty for the management of complete tracheal rings. J Pediatr Surg 2003;38(6):928–934

20. McNamara VM, Crabbe DC. Tracheomalacia. Paediatr Respir Rev 2004;5(2):147–154

16 Laryngotracheal Reconstruction

David L. Mandell and Deepak Mehta

For those clinicians who have dedicated themselves to the field of pediatric upper airway obstruction, subglottic stenosis is a well-known disorder, representing the most common laryngotracheal anomaly requiring tracheostomy in infants.[1] The unique knowledge, skills, and procedures required to comprehensively manage this clinical entity have been a significant factor in the emergence of pediatric otolaryngology as a distinct subspecialty unto itself. Despite the broadening experience with airway anomalies, its treatment remains challenging and ever-evolving, necessitating constant development of new techniques and surveillance of changing trends.

Etiology

The subglottis is the narrowest portion of the pediatric laryngotracheal airway, with a diameter of 4.5 to 5.5 mm in full-term newborns, and of just 3.5 mm in preterm newborns.[1] The subglottis is also notoriously unforgiving when instrumented by an endotracheal tube, given that it is the only site within the upper airway which is completely encircled by a ring of cartilage (the cricoid). It is estimated that the majority of cases of pediatric subglottic stenosis are acquired, as a result of injury from an indwelling endotracheal tube. Conversely, it has been estimated that as few as 5% of all cases of subglottic stenosis are congenital.[2] Of course, the true prevalence of congenital cases are unknown, since any subglottic stenosis that is found after endotracheal intubation is by definition deemed to be acquired, and it is not possible to know if a preexisting congenital stenosis might have been present.

The mechanism by which an endotracheal tube may precipitate the development of subglottic stenosis is believed to be related to pressure necrosis from the tube. Subglottic mucosal ulceration occurs, followed by eventual cricoid cartilage exposure, chondritis, and necrosis. Granulation tissue appears as a result of this cascade of events and the injured tissue can subsequently mature into a fibrotic scar.[3] Other factors that might potentiate the development of subglottic stenosis in this setting include excessive tube movement and/or repeated extubations/intubations. Elements that have been traditionally associated with laryngeal inflammation and poor wound healing, such as bacterial infection, laryngopharyngeal reflux, and poor nutritional status, are also likely involved in this pathological process.

History

Acquired subglottic stenosis became an increasingly encountered entity as a direct consequence of the introduction and subsequent popularity of long-term endotracheal intubation as a viable option for maintaining life support for premature newborns in the 1960s.[4] As these patients eventually graduated from the intensive care unit (ICU) and their pulmonary status improved with time, subglottic stenosis was often the only remaining reason for the ongoing need for a tracheostomy tube. The desire to achieve tracheostomy decannulation in this population of patients gave rise to rapid developments in the field of laryngotracheal reconstruction in the 1970s.[5]

Fearon and Cotton are credited with performing the first reliably successful open pediatric airway reconstructions by expanding the lumen of the cricoid cartilage and placing costal cartilage grafts to maintain airway patency.[6,7] Results were dramatic, and over the course of time it was found that there were no long-term adverse effects on laryngeal growth.[7] However, decannulation is not possible in all patients, and the success of the operation was less robust for the most severe, high-grade stenoses. In 1993, Monnier et al described the cricotracheal resection operation, in which the stenotic segment was resected entirely, followed by an end-to-end tracheal-to-laryngeal anastomosis, with high decannulation rates.[8] When examining the outcomes of all of these open surgical reconstructive techniques as a whole, the overall pediatric decannulation rate is estimated to be 91%.[5] These reconstructive approaches have withstood the test of time and remain the core surgical procedures used to this day for most cases of mature, acquired subglottic stenosis.

Current improvements in endotracheal tube design and management (including using an appropriately sized tube that allows a leak at 20 cm water pressure),[3] have resulted in the incidence of subglottic stenosis falling to less than 1%.[9] However, prolonged endotracheal intubation is still considered the primary cause of acquired subglottic stenosis in pediatric patients today.

Clinical Evaluation and Diagnosis

Most patients with acquired subglottic stenosis will present either as infants in the ICU who have failed repeated endotracheal extubation attempts, or as children already with tracheostomy tubes who present in the outpatient setting with families interested in pursuing tracheostomy decannulation. Children with congenital subglottic stenosis, which is generally less severe than acquired stenosis, may present with recurrent croup.

Direct microlaryngoscopy with rigid bronchoscopy is the standard mechanism for assessing subglottic stenosis. The length, severity, consistency (soft vs. hard), and degree of inflammation and granulation tissue (or lack thereof) of the stenosis should be noted, as these findings have therapeutic implications.[3] The severity of a mature subglottic stenosis can be "graded" using the Myer–Cotton grading chart, in which the largest endotracheal tube that can be placed with an air leak between 10 and 25 cm water pressure is chosen and compared with the expected normal-sized tube for the patient's age.[10] Based on this system, Grade I = 0 to 50% obstruction, Grade II = 51 to 70% obstruction, Grade III = 71 to 99% obstruction, and Grade IV = no detectable lumen (**Fig. 16.1**).[10]

With regards to congenital subglottic stenosis, it is believed that the most common endoscopic finding is an elliptical cricoid, in which the transverse diameter is less than the anteroposterior diameter.[1] Another recognized pattern of congenital subglottic stenosis involves the first tracheal ring being trapped within the cricoid cartilage.[1] Other anomalies, such as laryngeal cleft, may coexist with congenital subglottic stenosis and should be ruled out.[1]

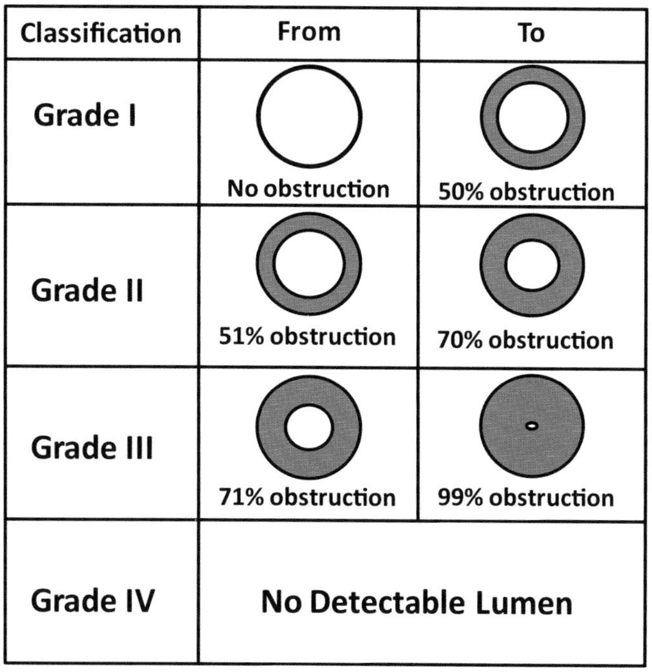

Classification	From	To
Grade I	No obstruction	50% obstruction
Grade II	51% obstruction	70% obstruction
Grade III	71% obstruction	99% obstruction
Grade IV	**No Detectable Lumen**	

Figure 16.1 Myer–Cotton grading system of laryngeal stenosis.[10]

Reprinted with permission from: Myer CM III, O'Connor DM, Cotton RT. Proposed grading system for subglottic stenosis based on endotracheal tube sizes. *Ann Otol Rhinol Laryngol* 1994;103(4 Pt 1):319–323.

During endoscopy, the cricoarytenoid joints should be palpated to test for passive mobility. If the arytenoid cartilages do not move freely along the cricoarytenoid joints, posterior glottic stenosis is likely present, resulting from interarytenoid and/or cricoarytenoid joint scarring. Failure to recognize posterior glottic stenosis preoperatively can lead to failure of laryngotracheal reconstruction.

Dynamic airway assessment is also required to assess vocal fold mobility, laryngomalacia, and tracheomalacia.[3] Dynamic assessment can be performed with flexible laryngoscopy with the patient wide awake (including in the office setting and/or rigid bronchoscopy with spontaneous respiration in the operating room (or ICU) setting.[11]

Preoperative Management

When assessing a potential candidate for laryngotracheal reconstruction, the effect of the airway stenosis on the child's overall quality of life should be determined. The amount of respiratory compromise and pulmonary reserve of a potential laryngotracheal reconstruction candidate should be assessed. Pediatric pulmonologists are often asked to provide preoperative clearance and approval for a reconstruction procedure, helping to ensure that the patient's lungs are healthy enough to allow for the rigors of the reconstruction and the expected permanent removal of the tracheostomy tube.

Laryngopharyngeal reflux of gastric contents is felt by many to have the ability to compromise laryngotracheal wound healing after surgery. As such, it is considered routine practice to attempt to diagnose and treat such reflux before surgery. Diagnostic techniques can include 24-hour dual-probe pH studies, esophagoscopy with biopsy, contrast esophagram and/or impedance probe testing (which can identify nonacid reflux).[11] Eosinophilic esophagitis, if present and untreated, is also felt to be a likely contributing factor to laryngeal inflammation and failure of reconstructive pediatric airway surgery, and thus its possible presence should be investigated with preoperative esophageal biopsy.[11,12] Laryngopharyngeal reflux can be treated with H_2 blockers and proton-pump inhibitors, and if unresponsive, may require Nissen fundoplication.[1]

The swallowing status of the patient should be determined preoperatively, and assessment for potential aspiration should be undertaken, either with modified barium swallow study, and/or a functional endoscopic evaluation of swallowing. Aspiration is not necessarily a contraindication to reconstructive surgery, but identifying aspiration may allow for more appropriate postoperative expectations, and feeding therapies geared toward managing and minimizing aspiration can be instituted.

Correctable upper airway obstruction (e.g., adenotonsillectomy for adenotonsillar hypertrophy, maxillofacial surgery for midface or mandibular hypoplasia, or supraglottoplasty for severe laryngomalacia) can be performed before laryngotracheal reconstruction if needed.

Open Surgical Techniques

Mild cases of subglottic stenosis (Grade I) often do not require open surgical reconstruction, as they frequently do not cause significant upper airway obstruction.[1] Mature, fibrotic subglottic stenoses that are causing markedly symptomatic airway obstruction and/or are associated with tracheostomy dependence can be well-managed with either augmentation (laryngotracheal reconstruction) or resection (cricotracheal resection) techniques.

Laryngotracheal reconstruction, in which the cricoid cartilage is divided anteriorly and/or posteriorly to allow for cartilage graft augmentation, is generally accepted as the standard of care in most cases of mature pediatric laryngotracheal stenosis that require intervention.[3] Costal cartilage is the most commonly utilized grafting material, although cartilage grafts from many other sites can be used. Thyroid alar cartilage grafts have risen in popularity recently, primarily due to their ease of harvest.[3] However, thyroid alar grafts are limited by the size and thickness of the graft and therefore are useful in only selected cases.

Lower grade stenoses (such as Grade II and mild Grade III) may be managed by dividing the anterior cricoid and placing a single anterior cartilage graft. However, if such stenoses are also associated with posterior glottic stenosis (with impaired mobility of the true vocal folds bilaterally), the cricoid should also be split posteriorly, with a posterior cartilage graft placed in addition to the anterior one.

If an augmentation procedure is performed for a Grade IV or a high Grade III stenosis, combined anterior and posterior cartilage grafting is the preferred technique. However, some authors feel that this more severe category of stenosis is more amenable to cricotracheal resection, in which diseased subglottic tissue that might not support cartilage grafting can be completely resected.[11] However, if the stenotic segment is too long, or if it is too close to the inferior surface of the true vocal folds (within 1 to 2 mm), anterior and posterior cartilage graft augmentation may still be the procedure of choice.[11] If a high-grade subglottic stenosis coexists with posterior glottic stenosis, a cricotracheal resection with a posterior cricoid split and posterior cartilage graft can be performed.[11]

Anterior Cricoid Split

Cricoid split (anterior laryngotracheal decompression) can be used in newborns with subglottic stenosis.[13] Infants must have an isolated subglottic stenosis that is the cause of repeated failed extubation attempts, and must have adequate cardiopulmonary reserve. Typically, the anterior cricoid split operation is performed in a single stage, with endotracheal intubation for 4 or 5 days afterwards.[1] Some authors prefer to use a thyroid ala cartilage graft during cricoid split procedures, turning the procedure into a laryngotracheal reconstruction.[1] Recently, endoscopic anterior cricoid split has been described with good success.[14]

Single-Stage Laryngotracheal Reconstruction

A single-stage procedure is one in which, after the reconstruction, the patient leaves the operating room without a tracheostomy tube. The airway is stented with an endotracheal tube, and when the tube is removed (usually 1 week later), the reconstruction is presumably complete and well-healed.[3] Depending on surgeon's preference, microlaryngoscopy and bronchoscopy may be performed just before extubation, and if the reconstruction is felt to be healing well, the endotracheal tube can either be removed at that time, or replaced with a smaller diameter tube which can be removed later in the ICU setting whenever the patient is ready and fully weaned off of the ventilator.

Single-stage procedures can be considered when only an anterior graft is used, with or without a posterior cricoid split.[3] However, with better intensive care this has been successfully used for posterior grafts as well. A single-stage reconstruction is less likely to be successful in patients with other synchronous airway lesions, particularly tracheomalacia. Single-stage procedures should also be avoided in patients whose anatomy makes reintubation technically difficult should an emergency arise.

One of the major drawbacks of performing laryngotracheal reconstruction in a single stage is the need for very labor-intensive and demanding postoperative care. Most require significant doses of sedatives and analgesics, which can be associated with complications such as weakened respiratory drive and medication withdrawal. The surgeon should be aware of complications such as atelectasis and pneumonia, tube blockage with secretions, and tube dislodgement. Also, the possibility exists that a new tracheotomy may need to be performed if the patient is not able to remain extubated.

Multistage Laryngotracheal Reconstruction

When laryngotracheal reconstruction is performed in multiple stages, the initial reconstruction is supported by an indwelling stent while the tracheostomy site remains patent and cannulated.[15] A T-tube can be used for this purpose; such a tube serves the dual purpose of stenting opening the airway while simultaneously allowing for respiration via the stoma. T-tubes can become occluded if too small in diameter, and thus are generally not used under the age of 4 years. Alternatively, a short stent can be used; this type of stent is considered "short" because it ends just proximal to the tracheostomy stoma. Such a stent is typically sutured into place above the stoma, allowing uninhibited ongoing use of traditional tracheostomy tubes. Whichever type of stent is used, it can remain in place as long as is necessary, can be removed at a later date while maintaining the tracheostomy site intact, and tracheostomy decannulation can then proceed in a relatively leisurely fashion whenever the patient is deemed ready.

Staging the reconstruction is a wise choice in the following situations: (1) Grade IV and high Grade III subglottic stenosis, in which the reconstruction is more complex and likely to take longer to heal; (2) patients with poor respiratory reserve who may not be easy to wean off of the ventilator after prolonged intubation; (3) patients with multiple synchronous airway lesions; and (4) patients with compromised wound healing, in which case long-term stenting is desirable.[3]

Cricotracheal Resection

In the cricotracheal resection procedure, the anterior and lateral portions of the cricoid cartilage are excised, whereas the posterior cricoid plate is preserved.[8] The trachea inferior to the resection is then anastomosed to the remaining cricothyroid segment. A pedicled tracheal mucosal graft can be used to line the posterior cricoid plate. The risk of dehiscence can be minimized by employing maneuvers to reduce anastomotic tension, such as suprahyoid release, tracheal mobilization, and chin-to-chest sutures. The addition of cricotracheal resection to the armamentarium of procedures for subglottic stenosis has further improved the success rate of decannulation, especially for the highest grade stenoses.[5]

Postoperative Care

Routine postoperative care after open airway reconstruction typically involves prophylaxis with broad-spectrum antibiotics, with particular attention to prophylaxis against bacteria that may be associated with failure of airway surgery such as *Pseudomonas aeruginosa* and *Staphylococcus aureus*).[11] Antireflux medication (typically proton-pump inhibitors) is routinely given as well. Sedation and analgesia are titrated to achieve the goals of maintaining patient comfort and minimizing undesired patient movement, while simultaneously trying to prevent cardiopulmonary depression and decrease the likelihood of sedative withdrawal, which can complicate the process of weaning young patients off mechanical ventilation.[16]

During the early postoperative period after any open airway reconstruction, most authors recommend routine endoscopic surveillance of the airway under anesthesia, so that wound healing can be assessed and steps can be taken to address potential problems (such as granulation tissue formation or early restenosis that may be amenable to dilatation) before mature restenosis occurs.[11]

Endoscopic Management

With the rousing success of the laryngotracheal reconstruction procedures introduced in the 1970s, older techniques such as laryngotracheal dilatation with bougienage, which had been attempted sporadically in the first half of the 20th century, fell by the wayside.[5] However, endoscopic techniques, and in particular laryngotracheal dilatation

procedures, have been making a comeback. This recent trend in pediatric airway management has been spurred on by the modern progression toward minimally invasive surgery, the desire to avoid prolonged postoperative ICU stays and their related complications, and the ever-increasing skill level and advanced instrumentation acquired by pediatric airway surgeons.

Currently, it appears that endoscopic management of subglottic stenosis is a reasonable option in the following scenarios: (1) to prevent endotracheal tube-related subglottic injury from progressing to a mature stenosis when active subglottic inflammation and granulation tissue are identified; (2) to attempt to maintain airway patency and promote appropriate wound healing when a reconstructed subglottis is showing signs of inflammation and restenosis in the early postoperative period; (3) to temporarily improve a relatively mature stenotic subglottic airway (with dilatation), thus potentially allowing more time to pass for an infant to grow and become medically stabilized before an open reconstruction is performed; and (4) to possibly avoid tracheotomy altogether, especially with balloon dilatation in the very young infant, or in cases of a soft subglottic stenosis.

The current thinking is that endoscopic techniques for laryngotracheal stenosis are best suited for less severe and less mature stenoses.[17] Although endoscopic posterior cricoid split with costal cartilage grafting has been described,[18] most endoscopic techniques do not involve cartilage grafting.

Balloon Dilatation

Any technique to dilate the stenotic pediatric subglottis may yield similar initial results, but the theoretical benefit of balloon dilatation over bougienage or rigid bronchoscopic dilatation is that the balloon applies dilating forces radially, thus avoiding mucosal shearing which could promote poor wound healing and restenosis. Balloon dilatation can be attempted with angioplasty balloons and Fogarty catheters, but with the recent surge in interest in this technique, pediatric airway-specific balloons are starting to be manufactured (most notably with a lumen that allows ventilation to continue even while the balloon is being deployed). A 70% success rate has been reported with balloon dilatation for acquired Grade II or Grade III Cotton subglottic stenosis in infants in the ICU.[19] After dilation, adjuvant therapies such as topical steroid or mitomycin C application are often employed.

Laser Endoscopy

Over the past quarter century, lasers have been used for a variety of purposes in the pediatric airway, including removal of laryngeal and suprastomal granulation tissue and glottic webs. For low-grade (e.g., Grade I or II) subglottic stenosis, the stenotic segment can be lasered in a staged fashion, one quadrant at a time with several weeks of healing in between treatments, or the stenosis can be lysed with radial laser incisions followed by immediate balloon dilatation.[17] Traditionally, it has been felt that management of pediatric subglottic stenosis with a laser is most appropriate for noncircumferential stenoses and for lesions that are no longer than 1 cm in length.[17]

Powered Microdebrider

The microdebrider is a thin, hollow metal tube that houses a spinning blade with simultaneous suction, allowing for precise and rapid removal of airway lesions (especially granulation tissue and cysts) with the ability to avoid damage to surrounding normal tissue. This instrument removes blood and debris while collecting tissue for histopathology and avoids the thermal injury and airway fires that can be associated with lasers. Given its larger size, however, it cannot be used through a ventilating bronchoscope, and thus its applications are generally limited to the endolarynx and subglottis. A laryngeal radiofrequency ablation (coblation) wand has also recently been introduced and may have similar applications to the microdebrider in the pediatric airway.

Adjuvant Endoscopic Therapies

The unpredictability of wound healing is a constant thorn in the side of pediatric airway surgeons; poor wound healing can undermine an initially successful procedure for laryngotracheal stenosis. Modulation of airway wound healing in a favorable fashion can be attempted with topical pharmacotherapy.

Mitomycin C is an antibiotic derived from the *Streptomyces caespitosus* bacteria. This pharmacological agent interferes with postsurgical scar formation at the molecular level.[17] It is usually applied topically at a concentration of 0.4 mg/mL for a few minutes after airway surgery has been performed. It appears to be a useful adjunct after endoscopic cold, laser, or balloon procedures, with a good safety profile, although its clinical utility is not universally agreed upon. Topical application of corticosteroids can be used in a similar fashion to minimize edema and granulation tissue formation. Topical or nebulized antibiotics can be used, in combination with systemic antibiotics, to mitigate any potential adverse effect on wound healing caused by bacterial infection.

Summary and Future Directions

The specialty of pediatric airway surgery has now reached a point where nearly all cases of laryngotracheal stenosis can be repaired by various techniques and most patients can achieve decannulation. Looking toward the future, clinicians are increasingly devoting more attention to other outcomes of laryngotracheal surgery besides decannulation, including voice and swallowing function. A normal or near-normal voice is achieved in only about 50% of children after laryngotracheal reconstruction[20]; this is an important component of these patients' quality of life which has traditionally been overlooked.

The recent rise in popularity of balloon dilatation is part of a larger trend toward performing fewer major open reconstructions with prolonged ICU stays, thus promoting faster recoveries and possible avoidance of postoperative stenting and endotracheal intubation. Endoscopic techniques are now being used more regularly to prevent mature stenoses from developing in infants who are found to have early endotracheal tube damage in the ICU setting. The future holds promise for new techniques, such as robotic pediatric laryngeal surgery, which may have the added benefits of steady, precise movements in small spaces, elimination of line-of-sight limitations by using angled endoscopes and flexible robotic instruments, and allowance of 3D-vision capabilities.[21] In place of cartilage grafting for open procedures, research is ongoing to find stable porous biomaterials that might maintain airway structure while enhancing wound healing by promoting well-vascularized mucosal growth within the reconstructed airway lumen.[22]

A variety of techniques are required, sometimes in the same patient, and constant assessment and reassessment of the stenosis has to be performed.[5] The old adage, "decision making is at least as important as the actual surgery," rings particularly true in the field of pediatric airway surgery.[3]

References

1. Schroeder JW Jr, Holinger LD. Congenital laryngeal stenosis. Otolaryngol Clin North Am 2008;41(5):865–875, viii

2. Werkhaven JA, Beste D. Diagnosis and management of pediatric laryngeal stenosis. Otolaryngol Clin North Am 1995;28(4):797–808

3. Boardman SJ, Albert DM. Single-stage and multistage pediatric laryngotracheal reconstruction. Otolaryngol Clin North Am 2008;41(5):947–958, ix

4. McDonald IH, Stocks JG. Prolonged nasotracheal intubation. A review of its development in a pediatric hospital. Br J Anaesth 1965;37:161–173

5. Santos D, Mitchell R. The history of pediatric airway reconstruction. Laryngoscope 2010;120(4):815–820

6. Fearon B, Cotton R. Surgical correction of subglottic stenosis of the larynx: preliminary report of an experimental surgical technique. Ann Otol Rhinol Laryngol 1972;81:508–513

7. Cotton R. Management of subglottic stenosis in infancy and children: review of a consecutive series of cases managed by surgical reconstruction. Ann Otol 1978;87:649–657

8. Monnier P, Savary M, Chapuis G. Partial cricoid resection and with primary tracheal anastomosis in infants and children. Laryngoscope 1993;103:1273–1283

9. Walner DL, Loewen MS, Kimura RE. Neonatal subglottic stenosis—incidence and trends. Laryngoscope 2001;111(1):48–51

10. Myer CM III, O'Connor DM, Cotton RT. Proposed grading system for subglottic stenosis based on endotracheal tube sizes. Ann Otol Rhinol Laryngol 1994;103(4 Pt 1):319–323

11. de Alarcon A, Rutter MJ. Revision pediatric laryngotracheal reconstruction. Otolaryngol Clin North Am 2008;41(5):959–980, x

12. Dauer EH, Ponikau JU, Smyrk TC, Murray JA, Thompson DM. Airway manifestations of pediatric eosinophilic esophagitis: a clinical and histopathologic report of an emerging association. Ann Otol Rhinol Laryngol 2006;115(7):507–517

13. Rethi A. An operation for cicatricial stenosis of the larynx. J Laryngol Otol 1956;70(5):283–293

14. Horn DL, Maguire RC, Simons JP, Mehta D. Endoscopic anterior cricoid split with balloon dilation in infants with failed extubation. Laryngoscope 2012;122(1):216–219

15. Wootten CT, Rutter MJ, Dickson JM, Samuels PJ. Anesthetic management of patients with tracheal T-tubes. Paediatr Anaesth 2009;19(4):349–357

16. Hammer GB. Sedation and analgesia in the pediatric intensive care unit following laryngotracheal reconstruction. Paediatr Anaesth 2009;19(Suppl 1):166–179

17. Lando T, April MM, Ward RF. Minimally invasive techniques in laryngotracheal reconstruction. Otolaryngol Clin North Am 2008;41(5):935–946, ix

18. Inglis AF Jr, Perkins JA, Manning SC, Mouzakes J. Endoscopic posterior cricoid split and rib grafting in 10 children. Laryngoscope 2003;113(11):2004–2009

19. Durden F, Sobol SE. Balloon laryngoplasty as a primary treatment for subglottic stenosis. Arch Otolaryngol Head Neck Surg 2007;133(8):772–775

20. Bailey CM, Clary RA, Pengilly A, Albert DM. Voice quality following laryngotracheal reconstruction. Int J Pediatr Otorhinolaryngol 1995;32(Suppl):S93–S95

21. Faust RA, Rahbar R. Robotic surgical technique for pediatric laryngotracheal reconstruction. Otolaryngol Clin North Am 2008;41(5):1045–1051, xi

22. Janssen LM, van Osch GJVM, Li JP, et al. Tracheal reconstruction: mucosal survival on porous titanium. Arch Otolaryngol Head Neck Surg 2009;135(5):472–478

17 Pediatric Voice

Roger C. Nuss

A child's voice changes throughout childhood, both due to normal physiologic development as well as from various pathologic conditions that may affect the vocal folds. Though many of these conditions are benign, it is important for the clinician to recognize if a child's voice is significantly deviated from the norm, and pursue an appropriate evaluation and treatment plan. A voice disturbance that persists for more than 3 months, has no clear underlying etiology, or impairs a child's intelligibility, needs to be investigated. This chapter will discuss the clinical evaluation of children with voice disorders, describe several common laryngeal pathologies that affect children, and review treatment options including voice therapy, medical management, and surgical intervention.

Vocal folds grow in length and mature structurally from infancy through adolescence. These changes do not occur in a linear manner, and are accompanied by changes in a child's fundamental frequency as well as their vocal range and control. There is a period of more rapid growth from birth through 3 years of age, then slower growth, until another period of rapid growth during adolescence and puberty. Before puberty, the larynx is similar in size for boys and girls and there is not a great deal of voice difference based on gender.[1] During puberty, the laryngeal and vocal fold growth rate is greater for boys with a corresponding greater change in fundamental frequency.[2]

The definition of what constitutes a "pediatric voice disorder" is not generally uniform, though may be understood as a perceptual deviation of at least one standard deviation from normal of the qualities of overall severity, roughness, breathiness, strain, pitch, or loudness. Voice disorders in children are felt to be fairly common, with a reported incidence ranging from 6 to 25% of children.[3-5] The most common cause of hoarseness in children—vocal fold nodules—is more common in boys than girls by an almost 2:1 ratio in school-age children. However, in the teenage population, there is a strong female preponderance.[6-8] There has been a surging interest in pediatric voice disorders over the past decade, partly due to the realization that there are therapeutic interventions which can have a positive impact on a child's voice quality and intelligibility, and partly due to technological advances in our diagnostic equipment.

Clinical Evaluation

Perceptual Measures

A clinician's ability to judge a child's voice quality may be based on observations in the office setting during conversational speech as well as parental report as to whether such speech sample is typical for their child. Beyond an informal perceptual assessment, it is also helpful to use a validated scale that may describe a child's voice quality. The Consensus Auditory-Perceptual Evaluation of Voice scale has been developed and adopted by the American Speech-Language-Hearing Association Special Interest Division 3 (Voice and Voice Disorders) as the recommended standard protocol for the perceptual assessment of disordered voices.[9] Perceptual qualities including overall severity, roughness, breathiness, strain, pitch, and loudness are rated on a visual analog scale (**Appendix I**).

Acoustic Measures

Computer-based programs to analyze voice are widely available and are a useful adjunct in creating an objective description of audible characteristics of voice. These tools may be used in children as young as 4 years of age, and sometimes even in younger children. Routine acoustic measurements include fundamental frequency, intensity, frequency and intensity perturbations (jitter and shimmer), and signal-to-noise ratio. In singers, phonation range is also measured. Variations from normative values based on age and gender may reflect on the size, tension, irregularity, biomechanics, and state of hydration of the vocal folds.

Aerodynamic Measures and Electroglottography

Aerodynamic tests allow the clinician to measure air pressure, flow rate, and resistance during voice production. Subglottic and supraglottic air pressure as well as glottic impedance and volume flow rate are recorded while a child phonates into a facemask. An inefficient glottal valve, due to a nodule or polyp, may result in higher glottal airflow and the perceptual quality of breathiness. Electroglottography is a noninvasive means of measuring vocal fold vibratory behavior. Electrodes placed on opposite side of the neck overlying the larynx allow for measurement of variation in electrical resistance (impedance) through the larynx. This measure of vocal fold contact, however, does not examine noncontact vibratory events. Both these measures are still relatively new to the pediatric population, and their value will be determined over time.

Laryngeal Examination

The laryngeal examination is typically performed after perceptual and acoustic measures have been recorded, and allows for the consolidation of all clinical information and the confirmation of a diagnosis. There are several options for obtaining an excellent view of a child's larynx. In general, most preschool and school-age children, and young teens are best examined with a flexible nasolaryngoscope passed transnasally. Either a traditional fiberoptic nasolaryngoscope or one of the newer distal-chip flexible scopes may be used, with attention to the diameter of the scope chosen appropriate to the age of the child. A mixture of 4% lidocaine solution and 0.25% oxymetazoline solution is sprayed into one of the nasal passages. The scope may be advanced through the inferior meatus or middle meatus, depending on the child's individual anatomy. A complete laryngeal examination includes visualization of the supraglottic larynx, false and true vocal folds, arytenoids, and possibly also the subglottis. Gross vocal fold speed and range of movement are noted. The patient is asked to phonate "/eeee/" at various pitches, to assess for lesions that may only be apparent at higher frequencies when the vocal folds are elongated and thinned. The use of stroboscopy may be especially helpful in assessing epithelial and subepithelial lesions, scarring, and disruptions of the mucosal wave. Supraglottic compression may reflect underlying vocal hyperfunction or compensation for vocal fold immobility or scarring. A laryngeal examination summary sheet is helpful in reporting and documenting the noted abnormalities (**Appendix II**).

Rigid laryngeal telescopes have historically provided the most optically clear, bright, and undistorted images of the larynx. These telescopes are now available in diameters as small as 6 mm, and may be tolerated in some older school-age children as well as teenagers. The use of an intraoral topical anesthetic spray may help reduce gag sensation and improve cooperation.

Vocal Fold Pathology in Children

The underlying etiology of a child's voice disorder may be related to issues that may be missed if attention is directed only to the vocal folds themselves. The patency of a child's lower airway as well as his pulmonary status should be considered for any abnormalities that may affect breath support. The presence of tracheal stenosis, tracheomalacia, or subglottic stenosis may limit airflow through the larynx and impair voice production. Lower airway reactivity with associated exercise or cold-air–induced asthma may result in increased coughing and throat clearing as well as decreased subglottic air pressure. The presence of neck muscle tension may give an important clue for underlying laryngeal strain and vocal hyperfunction.

Glottic lesions are the most common cause of a child's voice disturbance. Vocal fold nodules and polyps are epithelial lesions located in the anterior membranous vocal fold. Large vocal fold nodules may affect glottal closure, and be accompanied both by breathiness as well vocal strain/ hyperfunction (**Fig. 17.1**). Vocal fold nodule size may be graded by the examining clinician, based on a validated

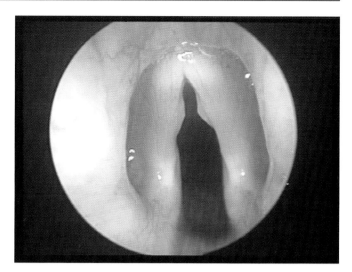

Figure 17.1 Vocal fold nodules.

scale.[10] There is a significant relationship between vocal fold nodule size and overall severity of a child's voice disturbance.[11] Subepithelial lesions, such as keratin or mucus-filled cysts, will affect vocal fold vibratory behavior, with resulting reduced range and amplitude of vocal fold mucosal wave as well as incomplete glottic closure (**Fig. 17.2**). These lesions may cause a reactive nodule on the contralateral vocal fold. Dilated and tortuous blood vessels, known as vocal fold varices, may hemorrhage within the vocal fold and result in areas of stiffness. The epithelial covering of the vocal fold may scar down to the underlying vocal ligament (sulcus vocalis)—a finding that may be congenital in nature or result from rupture of a subepithelial cyst. Iatrogenic injury to the vocal folds, as may occur from prior surgical removal of a lesion or from airway reconstructive surgery, may cause scarring of the vocal folds with loss of the normal vibratory characteristics of the mucosal wave (**Fig. 17.3**). Areas of scarred and adynamic mucosal wave may result in alterations of pitch, vocal breaks, diplophonia, loss of upper vocal range, and vocal fatigue.

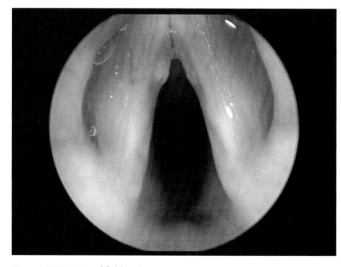

Figure 17.2 Vocal fold cyst.

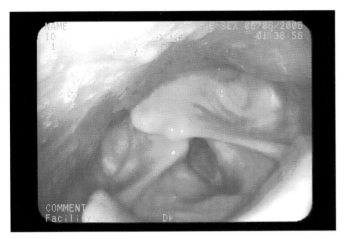

Figure 17.3 Iatrogenic scarring of vocal folds.

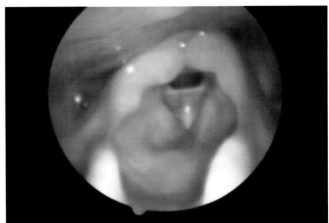

Figure 17.5 Anterior glottic web.

Vocal fold immobility may be idiopathic or congenital in nature, may have a central nervous system or brainstem etiology, or may be due to recurrent laryngeal nerve injury. The underlying cause may be mass effect causing pressure or traction on the recurrent laryngeal nerve, or direct injury to the nerve during cardiothoracic surgical procedures. In addition, prolonged endotracheal tube intubation as well as laryngeal reconstructive surgery may result in cricoarytenoid joint fixation with reduced or absent arytenoid movement. A child with unilateral vocal fold immobility will have a resulting weak and breathy voice quality, which may be associated with increased strain and decreased loudness (**Fig. 17.4**). Bilateral vocal fold immobility may allow a child to phonate with a fairly strong clear voice, though with associated stridor and dyspnea with exertion.

Congenital lesions may underlie a child's long-standing voice disorder. An anterior glottic web may result in a strained, high-pitched vocal quality, and possibly may interfere with a child's airway with resulting stridor (**Fig. 17.5**).

Infectious causes of voice disorders include self-limited viral inflammation of the larynx and vocal folds, due to rhinoviruses, parainfluenza viruses, respiratory syncytial virus, and others. A diagnosis of acute laryngitis based on a viral etiology can be managed with conservative measures. Recurrent respiratory papillomatosis caused by human papilloma virus (HPV) may result in long-term laryngeal involvement requiring multiple procedures over a patient's lifetime (**Fig. 17.6**). Various surgical instruments and techniques have evolved to treat this condition, including cold steel laryngeal instruments, carbon dioxide lasers, laryngeal microdebrider, and additional lasers with varying wavelengths and tissue effects. The underlying surgical premise is to preserve the airway, avoid any damage to the superficial lamina propria of the vocal fold, while trying to minimize the number of procedures in a given child. Ultimately, however, the greatest promise may be in the vaccination of all children, both girls and boys, before they become sexually active. Current recommendations are that all boys and girls receive the quadrivalent HPV vaccine at age 11 to 12 years.[12] With the expected decreased incidence of HPV in general, there will also be an expected decreased incidence of laryngeal papillomatosis.

Functional voice disorders may be present in the pediatric patient with a structurally normal larynx. These are more

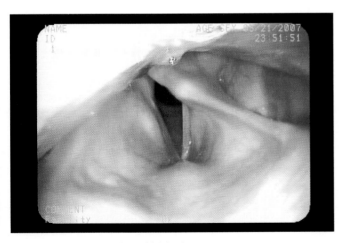

Figure 17.4 Unilateral vocal fold palsy.

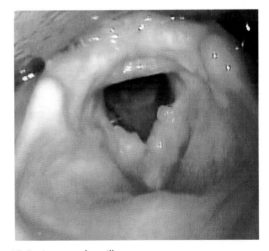

Figure 17.6 Laryngeal papilloma.

common in the adolescent years, and may manifest in near total aphonia or a severe dysphonia. The term "muscle tension dysphonia" may be used to describe this condition, with increased tension within the intrinsic laryngeal muscles and resulting inefficient and ineffective vocal production. Boys may maintain a persistently high pitch voice or hoarseness at puberty and beyond, and not be able to transition to the expected lower pitch as their larynx grows. This is referred to as a mutational voice disorder or "puberphonia." These functional voice disorders are best managed through voice therapy with an experienced speech–language pathologist.

Measurement of Impact

Quality-of-life scales may be useful to better understand the impact of a person's voice disorder on their lifestyle. The Voice Handicap Index (VHI) and the Voice-Related Quality of Life index are designed to address self-perception of emotional, physical, and functional impact in relation to voice.[13,14] A quality-of-life scale oriented toward the pediatric patient is the Pediatric Voice-Related Quality of Life scale, intended for administration with the parent(s) of a child with a voice disorder.[15]

Therapy

The ideal treatment plan for a child with a voice disorder is multifaceted. This includes education to the child and his/her parents, vocal hygiene, direct voice therapy, as well as medical and/or surgical intervention. Education requires explaining the diagnosis and nature of the voice problem in a manner appropriate to a child's age and cognitive level, with additional details provided to the parents. Visual images, review of stroboscopy recordings, and line drawings are all helpful. Improved comprehension by the patient and his/her parents will improve compliance as well as help them develop realistic expectations from treatment.

Vocal hygiene includes maintenance of good hydration, moderation of amount of voice use and volume of voice, dietary precautions to minimize laryngopharyngeal reflux, and reduction/elimination of vocal abuse. Basic vocal hygiene is reviewed with the entire family, with an emphasis on creating an atmosphere of positive reinforcement for achieving the targeted behavior. Behavioral approaches to voice hygiene are generally appropriate in the preschool and school-age group of children.

Direct voice therapy helps a child improve the manner of voice production and work toward achieving his/her best possible voice quality. Considerations involve breathing techniques to ensure proper breath support, reduction of increased neck and laryngeal muscle tension, coordination of respiration and phonation, and improvement in glottal closure. Various therapy techniques may be useful, depending on the age, developmental level, and motivation of the child.

Medical Management

Medical conditions associated with voice disorders should be recognized, appropriately evaluated, and treated in conjunction with management of the voice disorder. A diagnosis of pediatric laryngopharyngeal reflux (LPR) should be based on relevant history and symptoms, physical findings, and judicious use of testing. Findings during laryngoscopy may include posterior laryngeal mucosal hyperplasia, erythema, and pachydermia. Generalized vocal fold edema and erythema, thick mucus secretions, and lymphoid follicular hyperplasia ("cobblestoning") of the hypopharyngeal mucosa are subjective observations that may reflect inflammation and irritation of the laryngeal mucosa from LPR. Objective measures of reflux include the use of pH probe studies, impedance manometry, and esophageal endoscopy and biopsy. Of note, the pediatric gastroenterologist evaluating for gastroesophageal reflux may have a different impression of the severity of findings as compared with the pediatric otolaryngologist evaluating for LPR.[16–18] A child with a significant degree of dysphonia and notable laryngeal findings that are suggestive of LPR may warrant a trial of reflux management. This should be part of the overall management strategy, including patient and family education, improved hydration, vocal hygiene, dietary management of reflux, and direct vocal therapy. A 3-month trial of a proton pump inhibitor is reasonable, with follow-up assessment of the effects of the medication and the overall treatment plan. The strategy of prescribing a medication (proton pump inhibitor) without an overall treatment approach is not likely to be successful.

Asthma may be an important contributing factor in a child's voice disturbance. Coughing and throat clearing may traumatize the vocal folds with the subsequent development of vocal fold edema, nodules, polyps, and varices. Asthma medications, including the use of inhaled steroids and bronchodilators, may result in dehydration of the vocal folds and even some degree of vocal fold epithelial atrophy. Environmental allergies may cause vocal fold edema, increased upper airway secretions, coughing, throat clearing, and sneezing. Environmental controls at home are the first line of treatment. Antihistamines have a role as well; although they can lead to drying of the vocal folds and thicker secretions. Other medications, including nasal steroid sprays and leukotriene inhibitors, may be a part of allergy management. Sinusitis may contribute to voice disorders, due to upper aerodigestive tract inflammation, postnasal drip, and laryngeal irritation. Appropriate evaluation and treatment is an important part of improving the health of the larynx.

Surgery

Surgery is rarely indicated as a first line of treatment for the majority of pediatric voice disorders. Patient and family education, vocal hygiene, improvement of state of hydration, management of associated medical conditions, and patience are the best approach in general. There are times, however, when surgical management is called for. Vocal fold nodules that significantly impact a child's voice quality and intelligibility and persist despite an appropriate period of therapy and monitoring may be considered for surgical excision. Risks include scarring of the vocal fold as well as recurrence of the nodules. Excellent microlaryngeal surgical techniques are required, and a 1-week period of voice rest after surgery is recommended. Vocal fold cysts may mimic vocal fold nodules but can be distinguished with the use of stroboscopy. These lesions are not likely to resolve spontaneously, and may be excised with microlaryngeal surgical techniques. The goal in this instance is to avoid complications related to chronic dysphonia with compensatory hyperfunction as well as risk of cyst rupture and scarring of the vocal fold epithelium.

Unilateral vocal fold palsy is associated with a weak, breathy, and strained voice quality. Neonates and infants with this condition may also exhibit dysphagia, with a higher risk of aspiration of thin liquids. Though a period of "watchful waiting" may allow some children to compensate and achieve a safe swallow, it is appropriate even in infants and young children to consider an injection medialization of the paralyzed vocal fold. This may be accomplished safely without airway compromise, and allow for an improvement in glottal closure and airway protection. Helping a child achieve a more "normal" voice quality at this younger age might be beneficial, during which time a higher degree of neural plasticity allows for better long-term voice results.

The school-age child with newly diagnosed vocal fold immobility may make some gains in voice quality with vocal therapy. Treatment goals include decreasing breathiness, improving loudness, and improving intelligibility. If treatment goals are not met with therapy alone, there may then be consideration of a medialization procedure. Injection medialization is an appropriate technique for younger children, whereas older school-age children and adolescents may be treated more effectively with laryngeal framework surgery.

When considering injection medialization, the surgeon may choose from several options that have different periods of effectiveness. Short-lived materials include Gelfoam (Pfizer, New York, United States) and Radiesse Voice Gel (BioForm Medical, San Mateo, California, United States), which may last for a few months before they are resorbed. Longer lasting materials include abdominal fat prepared appropriately for injection or commercially available substances made of a hydroxyapatite/water-based gel that may last for several years. Laryngeal framework surgery, including vocal fold medialization, has become an accepted technique for use in older children. There are commercially available vocal fold medialization implant systems. Of these, the Montgomery Thyroplasty Implant System (Boston Medical Products, Westborough, Massachusetts, United States) offers various sizes of male and female implants, with the ability to upsize the implants as a child's larynx grows.

Additionally, the use of nerve transfers from the ansa cervicalis nerve to the affected recurrent laryngeal nerve may help improve vocal fold tone with associated improvement in adduction and voice quality. This technique may be performed in conjunction with a vocal fold medialization procedure.

Vocal fold scarring is a difficult surgical problem to resolve. The superficial lamina propria is the layer of loose connective tissue beneath the vocal fold epithelium, and is necessary to achieve the desired vocal fold vibratory characteristics. This layer does not regenerate if damaged, and loss of the superficial lamina propria results in scarring and an adynamic area of the vocal fold. This is an area of active research, including the development of synthetic materials that may be injected into the vocal fold to re-create the characteristics of this important structure and hence to improve vocal fold mucosal wave and voice quality.

Summary

Pediatric voice disorders are common, and should be evaluated and treated in the context of the severity of the problem as well the impact on the child's life. A "total body" approach encourages the clinician to consider the child, his/her family, as well as home and school environmental influences in the causes and management of a child's voice disorder. Dysphonia in children may be a congenital problem, acquired though overuse and hyperfunction, or due to an infectious/inflammatory condition. Iatrogenic injury from prolonged intubation, laryngeal surgery, or cardiothoracic surgery are possible causes of a child's voice disturbance. Neoplasms causing hoarseness need to be diagnosed and treated appropriately. Related medical conditions may cause poor breath support, airway insufficiency, or chronic irritation of the larynx and vocal folds.

A coordinated team diagnostic approach, considering the entire child, the impact of any concurrent medical conditions, and the status of the larynx and vocal folds, will allow the voice clinicians to develop an age and developmentally appropriate treatment plan. There may be roles for simple monitoring, vocal therapy, medical management, and surgical interventions. It is the role of the voice care team to make an accurate diagnosis and also to individualize the treatment plan best suited for the child with a voice disorder.

References

1. Maddern BR, Campbell TF, Stool S. Pediatric voice disorders. Otolaryngol Clin North Am 1991;24(5):1125–1140

2. Gray SD, Smith ME, Schneider H. Voice disorders in children. Pediatr Clin North Am 1996;43(6):1357–1384

3. Baynes RA. An incidence study of chronic hoarseness among children. J Speech Hear Disord 1966;31(2):171–176

4. Silverman EM, Zimmer CH. Incidence of chronic hoarseness among school-age children. J Speech Hear Disord 1975;40(2):211–215

5. Fuchs M. [Diagnostics and therapy of dysphonia suitable for the ages and developmental stages of children and adolescents (part 2)]. Laryngorhinootologie 2008;87(2):86–91

6. De Bodt MS, Ketelslagers K, Peeters T, et al. Evolution of vocal fold nodules from childhood to adolescence. J Voice 2007;21(2):151–156

7. Akif Kiliç M, Okur E, Yildirim I, Güzelsoy S. The prevalence of vocal fold nodules in school age children. Int J Pediatr Otorhinolaryngol 2004;68(4):409–412

8. Connelly A, Clement WA, Kubba H. Management of dysphonia in children. J Laryngol Otol 2009;123(6):642–647

9. Kempster GB, Gerratt BR, Verdolini Abbott K, Barkmeier-Kraemer J, Hillman RE. Consensus auditory-perceptual evaluation of voice: development of a standardized clinical protocol. Am J Speech Lang Pathol 2009;18(2):124–132

10. Shah RK, Feldman HA, Nuss RC. A grading scale for pediatric vocal fold nodules. Otolaryngol Head Neck Surg 2007;136(2):193–197

11. Nuss RC, Ward J, Huang L, Volk M, Woodnorth GH. Correlation of vocal fold nodule size in children and perceptual assessment of voice quality. Ann Otol Rhinol Laryngol 2010;119(10):651–655

12. CDC Online Newsroom – Press Briefing. "ACIP recommends all 11-12 year-old males get vaccinated against HPV". Transcript October 25, 2011. Available at: http://www.cdc.gov/media/releases/2011/t1025_hpv_12yroldvaccine.html

13. Jacobson BH, Johnson A, Grywalski C, et al. The Voice Handicap Index (VHI): development and validation. Am J Speech Lang Pathol 1997;6:66–70

14. Hogikyan ND, Sethuraman G. Validation of an instrument to measure voice-related quality of life (V-RQOL). J Voice 1999;13(4):557–569

15. Boseley ME, Cunningham MJ, Volk MS, Hartnick CJ. Validation of the Pediatric Voice-Related Quality-of-Life survey. Arch Otolaryngol Head Neck Surg 2006;132(7):717–720

16. Ali Mel-S. Laryngopharyngeal reflux: diagnosis and treatment of a controversial disease. Curr Opin Allergy Clin Immunol 2008;8(1):28–33

17. Karkos PD, Leong SC, Apostolidou MT, Apostolidis T. Laryngeal manifestations and pediatric laryngopharyngeal reflux. Am J Otolaryngol 2006;27(3):200–203

18. Gupta R, Sataloff RT. Laryngopharyngeal reflux: current concepts and questions. Curr Opin Otolaryngol Head Neck Surg 2009;17(3):143–148

Consensus Auditory-Perceptual Evaluation of Voice (CAPE-V)

Name:_____   **Date:**_____

The following parameters of voice quality will be rated upon completion of the following tasks:
1. Sustained vowels, /a/ and /i/ for 3-5 seconds duration each.
2. Sentence production:
   a.   The blue spot is on the key again.
   b.   How hard did he hit him?
   c.   We were away a year ago.
   d.   We eat eggs every Easter.
   e.   My mama makes lemon muffins.
   f.   Peter will keep at the peak.
3. Spontaneous speech in response to: "Tell me about your voice problem." or "Tell me how your voice is functioning."

> **Legend:** C = Consistent   I = Intermittent
> MI = Mildly Deviant
> MO =Moderately Deviant
> SE = Severely Deviant

SCORE

Overall Severity _____ C   I   ____/100
MI   MO   SE

Roughness _____ C   I   ____/100
MI   MO   SE

Breathiness _____ C   I   ____/100
MI   MO   SE

Strain _____ C   I   ____/100
MI   MO   SE

Pitch   (Indicate the nature of the abnormality): _____
_____ C   I   ____/100
MI   MO   SE

Loudness   (Indicate the nature of the abnormality): _____
_____ C   I   ____/100
MI   MO   SE

_____   _____ C   I   ____/100
MI   MO   SE

_____   _____ C   I   ____/100
MI   MO   SE

COMMENTS ABOUT RESONANCE: NORMAL   OTHER (Provide description):_____

ADDITIONAL FEATURES (for example, diplophonia, fry, falsetto, asthenia, aphonia, pitch instability, tremor, wet/gurgly, or other relevant terms):

Clinician:_____

Appendix I   Consensus Auditory-Perceptual Evaluation of Voice scale.
Source: Reprinted with permission from Consensus Auditory-Perceptual Evaluation of Voice: Development of a Standardized Clinical Protocol by G. B. Kempster, B. R. Gerratt, K. V. Abbott, J. Barkemeier-Kraemer, and R. E. Hillman. *American Journal of Speech-Language Pathology*, 18, 124–132. Copyright 2009 by American Speech-Language-Hearing Association. All rights reserved.

Endoscopic Evaluation of Larynx

Date of Exam:

Endoscope Used: Rigid   Flexible 2.4 mm scope

                              Distal chip scope 3.7 mm   Flexible 3.4 mm scope

Route: Transoral   Right Nasal   Left Nasal

Light source: Halogen   Xenon Stroboscopy

Topical Anesthesia: 1:1 mix (0.05 % oxymetazoline HCl : 4 % lidocaine)

                          Cetacaine

Patient Cooperation: Excellent   Very Good   Good   Fair   Poor

Exam Findings:

    Nasopharynx

    Palate Closure

    Supraglottis

    Arytenoid Movement   Right   Left
- Range
- Speed

    Vocal Fold Edge   Right   Left
- Anterior third
- Middle third
- Posterior third

    Glottal Closure   Anterior chink   Posterior chink   Hourglass closure

    Vocal Fold Movement*   Right   Left   * Stroboscopy Exams only
- Amplitude Vibration
- Mucosal Wave

    Phase Symmetry of Vocal Fold Vibration*

                Regular   Horizontal phase asymmetry   Vertical phase asymmetry

    Supraglottic Compression   None   Mild   Moderate   Severe
- Ventricular fold
- A-P Dimension

    Other Findings   None   Mild   Moderate   Severe
- Posterior mucosal hyperplasia / erythema
- Pachydermia
- Vocal fold edema
- Varices
-

Summary Diagnosis

Appendix II Laryngeal examination record.

SECTION IV: Neck Disease

18 Neck Infections
Gi Soo Lee

Pediatric neck infections are unique due to their variety of etiologies as well as the potential for severe complications. Aggressive management of the airway is often the most urgent aspect of care, and the diagnosis must be made expeditiously to prevent delay in either antibiotic or surgical management. A careful history and examination, along with judicious use of various diagnostic imaging and laboratory tests can aid the physician in determining the potential etiology. This chapter discusses the more common and uncommon causes of neck infections in the neonate to adolescent age group.

Streptococcal Pharyngotonsillitis

Bacterial pharyngitis and tonsillitis in the pediatric population can be distinguished from its viral counterpart by the absence of coryza symptoms of cough, rhinorrhea, and malaise and the greater-than-expected severity of sore throat, fever, and lymphadenopathy.[1] Bacterial pharyngotonsillitis is most commonly caused by Group A beta-hemolytic *Streptococcus pyogenes* (GABHS). In fact, while *Hemophilus influenzae* was the most commonly identified organism in the core of tonsils removed for obstructive symptoms, Group A *Streptococcus* was the predominant organism identified in those excised for chronic tonsillitis.[2] *S. pyogenes* are gram-positive cocci with multiple strains characterized by their antigenic differences in the configuration of cell wall polysaccharides. These differences are classified into groups (A, B, G, etc). GABHS is characterized by the presence of a zone of complete hemolysis when grown on agar plates, sensitivity to bacitracin, and production of specific enzymes.

Streptococcal pharyngotonsillitis presents with marked oropharyngeal erythema and pain, odynophagia, indurated palate and uvula, palatal petechiae, referred otalgia, and tender cervical lymphadenopathy. In all cases of suspected infection, obtaining a throat culture is considered the standard criterion for diagnosis. Rapid antigen detection tests (rapid strep test) have a high specificity but lower sensitivity (96 to 98% vs. 70 to 95%),[3–5] and are often used while culture results are pending to institute antibiotic therapy.

For medical therapy, penicillin is the first-line antibiotic treatment of choice. Till date, no penicillin-resistant *S. pyogenes* has been isolated in the clinical setting.[6,7] Those patients allergic to penicillins are treated with macrolides such as erythromycin or azithromycin.

Tonsillectomy is recommended after seven or more episodes of culture-proven streptococcal pharyngitis in 1 year, five episodes per year for two consecutive years, or three episodes per year for 3 years.[8] Surgical management of the asymptomatic streptococcal carrier, however, remains controversial. An estimated 15 to 20% of all schoolchildren are carriers of *Streptococcus* in their saliva or nasal secretions, depending on their location and the season, even after adequate antibiotic therapy.[9,10] These carriers may harbor infection that may then be spread to other family or school members. In some children, it may be difficult to determine whether the carrier state or an active infection exists. For this reason, it still may be reasonable to recommend a tonsillectomy even in cases in which the carrier has minimal clinical morbidity.

Streptococcal pharyngotonsillitis can result in localized and disseminated suppurative complications. Peritonsillar cellulitis can progress to peritonsillar abscess (classically referred to as a *quinsy tonsillitis* in the older literature), characterized by drooling, trismus, a "hot potato" voice, and tender cervical lymphadenopathy. Peritonsillar infection can subsequently spread medially into the retropharyngeal space or laterally into the parapharyngeal space. Either of these deep-space infections may track inferiorly into the mediastinum. Septic thrombi may also produce metastatic spread resulting in osteomyelitis, meningitis, or brain abscess. All these conditions require intravenous antibiotic therapy and deep-space infections require surgical drainage. If a peritonsillar abscess is recurrent or associated with a history of chronic tonsillar infection, tonsillectomy may be indicated.[11]

Streptococcal infections can also cause other systemic complications. *Scarlet fever* presents as a generalized, non-pruritic, erythematous, macular skin rash that is worse on the extremities. The associated "strawberry tongue" is bright red and tender due to superficial desquamation of the papillae. Typically, the rash lasts for 4 to 7 days and is accompanied by fever and arthralgias. *Rheumatic fever* is rare today with only sporadic outbreaks[12]; however, in the 1940s and 1950s, it was a complication that was seen in 3% of streptococcal pharyngitis infections.[13] Bacterial vegetations affect the mitral and tricuspid heart valves leading to murmurs, persisting relapsing fevers, and valvular stenosis or incompetence. *Septic arthritis* with painful, hot, joint effusions is a known complication of streptococcal pharyngitis. The bacteria can be isolated by needle aspiration of the effusion. Treatment with parenteral antibiotics for at least 6 weeks is necessary to avoid osteitis, arthrodesis, and long-term morbidity from restricted range of movement. *Acute post-streptococcal glomerulonephritis* can result in 10 to 15% of those streptococcal pharyngeal infections caused by certain nephritogenic strains of the bacteria. Generalized edema, hypertension, bradycardia or tachycardia, and gross hematuria/proteinuria are common signs. Treatment includes various supportive measures in addition to antihypertensives, diuretics, and strict diet and fluid management usually results in full recovery.

Non-Group A *Streptococcus* Pharyngotonsillitis

Pharyngotonsillitis can be caused by a multitude of organisms, including various anaerobic bacteria that reside in the oral cavity as normal flora. Beta-lactamase producing *Bacteroides* species, *Fusobacterium* spp., and *Haemophilus influenzae* have been isolated from tonsil cores of 73 to 80% of children with a history of GABHS tonsillitis, and from 40% of tonsils from those with non-GABHS infections.[14] Additionally, other organisms such as *Prevotella, Porphyromonas* spp., and Actinomycetes have been isolated from peritonsillar and retropharyngeal abscesses.[15] *Bacteroides*, the most common anaerobic organism isolated from tonsil tissue, has been implicated in the development of tonsillitis that may progress to frank peritonsillar abscess formation following penicillin therapy.[16–18] In this scenario, surgical incision and drainage is performed with antibiotic coverage either with clindamycin or amoxicillin/clavulanate.

Retropharyngeal Abscess

Retropharyngeal abscesses (RPAs) are uncommon but serious complications of upper respiratory tract infections that extend into the retropharyngeal lymph nodes. Suppuration of these nodes leads to abscess formation. This is nearly exclusively a pediatric diagnosis, with most incidents occurring in children in the age group of 6 months to 6 years (mean age: 3 to 5 years).[19–21] This is in contrast to parapharyngeal and peritonsillar abscesses that occur more frequently in older children and adolescents. Primary infections include pharyngotonsillitis, adenoiditis, otitis, sinusitis, and dental infections. In some instances, osteomyelitis of the spine can develop from extension of infection from the prevertebral space. Additionally, penetrating trauma can also result in retropharyngeal space infections, including foreign body impalement in the oral cavity, impacted fish bones in the oropharynx/hypopharynx, and instrumentation during surgery.

Group A *Streptococcus* is the most common bacterial cause, though other *Streptococcus* species, *Staphylococcus, Neisseria*, and *Haemophilus* species have also been cultured.[22,23] *Bacteroides* species are the most common anaerobic organisms.

Children with an RPA present with a constellation of symptoms and signs including fever, chills, decreased appetite, sore throat, odynophagia, trismus, decreased neck range of motion, torticollis, altered voice, and globus sensation. Fever and neck pain are the most common symptoms.[24] Cervical lymphadenopathy, neck swelling, oropharyngeal fullness

(usually asymmetric), stridor, and drooling are also noted.

When an RPA is suspected, a lateral neck X-ray plain film is often first performed. This is taken during inspiration with normal neck extension. However, there are some limitations to making the diagnosis with this imaging modality, therefore computed tomography (CT) is recommended in any patient with a high index of suspicion.[25] A CT scan provides much more information than a plain film, with sensitivity of 90%.[24] Positive predictive value has been estimated at 82%, and the negative predictive value has been estimated to be 100%.[26]

Determining airway stability is critical when managing a patient with retropharyngeal abscess. Patients must remain in a position of comfort, usually supine with the neck extended, as neck flexion or forcing a child to sit up can occlude the airway. Once the diagnosis is made, broad-spectrum antibiotic coverage is initiated. Clindamycin is often a first-line treatment, but due to the increasing frequency of resistant bacteria, treatment may include a combination with cefoxitin or a beta-lactamase–resistant penicillin, such as ticarcillin/clavulanate, piperacillin/tazobactam, or ampicillin/sulbactam. Close cardiopulmonary monitoring is also important. If airway compromise is impending, the examination should be done in the operating room. A needle aspiration can often decompress the lesion, followed by transoral surgical drainage. If there is extension laterally into the parapharyngeal space, the collection may need to be drained via a transcervical approach. Notably, the preferred treatment for RPAs has been controversial. Recently, some have advocated antibiosis as the primary mode of treatment, with surgery reserved for those who do not respond.[27,28]

Lemierre Syndrome

Lemierre syndrome is an anaerobic, bacteria-mediated, suppurative thrombophlebitis of the internal jugular vein that occurs as a complication of head and neck infections. Oropharyngeal processes including pharyngotonsillitis comprise 85% of the primary sites. There is mucosal invasion and spread of the infection into the lateral pharyngeal space with subsequent infiltration of the internal jugular vein either by direct extension or via lymphatic or hematogenous spread. Other primary sources of infection including parotitis, mastoiditis, otitis, and dental infections have been reported.[29,30] Lemierre syndrome usually affects healthy young adults and adolescents. The most common causative organism (in 84% of cases) is *Fusobacterium necrophorum*, a gram-negative obligate anaerobe,[29] but others, including *Bacteroides, Streptococcus*, and *Lactobacillus* species, have also been identified.

Patients will report a history of fever and acute pharyngitis or other head and neck infection, followed by neck swelling and tenderness. Septic emboli can result in empyema, lung cavitation, and hypoxia. Other complications such as septic arthritis, hepatic abscesses, and osteomyelitis have also been reported. Imaging of the neck by ultrasound or CT will demonstrate internal jugular vein thrombosis and blood cultures will confirm septicemia. Treatment involves surgical drainage of abscesses with possible ligation or excision of the affected portion of the vein, and prolonged antibiotic therapy directed at anaerobes.

Atypical Mycobacterial Infection

Nontuberculous mycobacteria (NTM) are a group of acid-fast bacilli that have been recognized as a cause of cervicofacial lymphadenitis in healthy children since 1956,[31] though they were previously identified in human secretions in 1885.[32] These organisms, collectively referred to as "atypical mycobacteria," include, among others, *Mycobacterium avium-intracellulare, M. scrofulaceum, M. kansasii, and M. bohemicum.* Endemic in the Midwest and southwest United States, they are ubiquitous in soil, water, vegetation, dairy products, and animals. Human-to-human transmission has not been documented. Affected patients are generally immunocompetent and healthy children between ages 1 to 5 years.[33,34] Incidence has been reported as 1.21 per 100,000 children per year.[35]

Infections caused by NTM generally present as chronic, nontender cervical lymphadenitis that develop over weeks to months. A single lymph node, or collection of unilateral nodes, gradually enlarges in the upper cervical or submandibular area—the "beard distribution." Occasionally it presents in the preauricular, intraparotid, or posterior neck regions. Initially, they are firm and well-circumscribed; as the disease progresses, the nodes become more superficial, and overlying skin becomes thin and violaceous. Eventually, the suppuration breaks through the skin and causes a chronic drainage. The dolor and calor usually associated with other suppurative lymphadenopathy are absent, as are generalized systemic signs of infection.

The diagnosis of NTM infection is primarily clinical, since culturing the organism is difficult and time-consuming. Purified protein derivative (PPD) tuberculin skin testing is only positive in approximately 50% of patients.[36]

Optimal treatment for cervicofacial NTM has not been established. Left untreated, the frank suppuration results in a chronically draining sinus tract that may persist for months before spontaneously resolving. This leads to significant epidermolysis and scarring. Total surgical excision of the affected lymph nodes is still considered the gold standard and the primary management strategy for infections in children. Cure rates vary from 80 to 95%.[35,37–39] For lesions not amenable to total excision (extensive draining fistulae or involvement of facial nerve), alternatives include needle aspiration, incision and drainage, and curettage. Some authors advocate these methods as primary treatment modalities and have exhibited good results.[40,41] While atypical mycobacteria are unresponsive to many common antibiotics, reports have demonstrated reasonable efficacy with the clarithromycin-based therapies.[42–45] Currently, no standardized antibiotic regimens exist, but clarithromycin alone or with a second drug such as ethambutol, rifampin, or rifabutin are most commonly utilized. The treatment is often prolonged (up to months), and may be more beneficial in early infections without suppuration.

Cat Scratch Disease

This worldwide anthropozoonosis is caused by *Bartonella henselae,* a gram-negative proteobacterium. The bacterium is present in 30 to 60% of healthy domestic and wild cats; while feline-to-feline transmission occurs via fleas, human are inoculated by direct contact (scratches or bites).[46] The incidence of this disease in United States is 1.8 to 9.3 per 100,000 persons.[47,48]

A self-limited, unilateral, and tender cervical lymphadenopathy results after exposure. This may occur up to several weeks after contact, and a 1- to 10-mm nontender papule sometimes presents at the inoculation site. Systemic signs of mild fever and malaise occur in approximately 50% of cases.[49] Serologic testing is widely available, and the organisms can be identified with Warthin-Starry stain.

The infection spontaneously resolves over months, and treatment typically is supportive. Suppuration occurs in more than 80% of patients, but only 10% of abscesses are significant enough to requires surgical intervention.[50] Complications, including Parinaud oculoglandular syndrome (preauricular lymphadenopathy and conjunctivitis), encephalitis, and hepatitis, may form in 5 to 13% of cases, especially if immunocompromised.[51] Antibiotic use is controversial, and there is no standardized regimen. Macrolides, fluoroquinolones, and sulfa-based medications can be helpful, but are often used only when complications arise.[52]

Tularemia

Tularemia is caused by *Francisella tularensis,* an aerobic gram-negative, facultative intracellular, pleomorphic coccobacillus. It is one of the most infectious bacteria known, causing illness in humans with exposure to as few as 10 to 50 organisms. *F. tularensis* is considered a category A biowarfare agent due to its high infectivity, ease of dissemination, and ability to cause substantial illness and death.[53] Natural hosts include rabbits and rodents. Biting flies and ticks are the most common vectors in the United States. There is a bimodal age prevalence: one peak at 5 to 9 years and the second at 75 years.[54]

The ulceroglandular form of tularemia is the most common in both adults and children. A primary skin ulcer forms at the site of inoculation 2 to 5 days after exposure; the painful lesion necroses and forms a black eschar—this is associated with tender lymphadenopathy. Greater than 20% of cases will suppurate if left untreated or if treatment is delayed over 2 weeks.[55] Oropharyngeal tularemia, the second most common form in children, presents with an exudative pharyngitis and tonsillitis, mucosal ulcers, stomatitis, ipsilateral adenitis, gastrointestinal symptoms, headaches, and fevers. A less common glandular form presents with lymphadenopathy only without epidermal or mucosa involvement.

The diagnosis is made clinically, with a history of animal exposure and a tick bite. Serologic testing is available, but cross-reactivity with other organisms including *Yersinia*, *Brucella*, and *Pseudomonas* makes it unreliable. Additionally, while *F. tularensis* can be cultured, its highly contagious nature makes it a danger to laboratory personnel. Streptomycin is the treatment of choice, but within 24 hours of exposure, prophylaxis with ciprofloxacin or doxycycline is recommended.

Actinomycosis

Actinomyces israelii is the cause of this chronic granulomatous infection. It is a gram-positive microaerophilic bacterium commonly found in the oropharynx; one study found a 28% incidence of *A. israelii* in tonsil tissue specimens.[56] Cervicofacial actinomycosis, which comprises 55% of all cases and makes it the most common form,[57] is thought to be due to injury to oral mucosa, secondary to maxillofacial trauma, dental infections, or surgery. The infection spreads via lymphatic or hematogenous means into adjacent tissues. Sinus tracts form followed by the emergence of firm, nontender erythematous or violaceous masses. These masses eventually suppurate and drain. True lymphadenopathy is rare. Any tissue in the head and neck region can be affected, including major salivary glands, tongue, palate, sinuses, nasopharynx, larynx, ear, and thyroid.[58–64]

Histological examination of the draining fluid will often reveal "sulfur granules"; yellow-hued flecks representing clumps of bacteria. The organism is difficult to culture and treatment includes antibiotic therapy for months to years. The bacteria are susceptible to penicillin, clindamycin, macrolides, and tetracycline. Draining masses are surgically excised.

Histoplasmosis

Histoplasmosis is an opportunistic infection caused by dimorphic fungus *Histoplasma capsulatum*. It is the most common fungal infection in humans, and is contracted by inhaling particles from bat guano or poultry droppings containing *H. capsulatum* spores. Though found worldwide, it is endemic to central and northeast United States. In these locations, 75 to 80% of the population are asymptomatic carriers.[65,66] Progressive disseminated histoplasmosis occurs in 4 to 27% of infected children, those immunocompromised, or in the elderly,[67] and may present with head and neck findings.

Most patients with acute pulmonary histoplasmosis present with a flu-like infection; symptoms include malaise, fevers, cough, mylagias, and chills. Onset is 3 to 14 days after exposure.[68] Those who develop a chronic, progressive disseminated infection often present with wart-like lesions that evolve to painful, ulcerated lesions on the aerodigestive mucosa and mimic neoplasms or granulomatous diseases. These lesions are found on the tongue, palate, buccal mucosa, and larynx.[69–71]

Diagnosis is made with sputum or blood cultures, and antigen/antibody testing. Sputum cultures are positive in 15% of acute pulmonary and 60 to 85% of chronic pulmonary histoplasmosis cases, and blood cultures are positive in 50 to 70% of progressive disseminated histoplasmosis cases.[72] No treatment is required for asymptomatic or mildly symptomatic patients. Prolonged or more severe cases are treated with itraconazole or amphotericin B.

Infectious Mononucleosis

Acute infectious mononucleosis is the most common manifestation of primary infection with Epstein–Barr virus (EBV), also known as the human herpesvirus-4. This ubiquitous gammaherpesvirus infects approximately 95% of the world's population. In the United States, 50% of children acquire the virus by the age of 5.[73] Infectious mononucleosis primarily affects adolescents and young adults. Infection in infants and younger children are often asymptomatic or mild[74]; nonetheless, children can present with the acute infection. Oral manifestations include sore throat—the most common symptom, exudative pharyngitis—the most common clinical finding, tonsillar hypertrophy with associated dysphagia or airway obstruction, and petechiae at the hard and soft palate junction (present in 25 to 60% of patients).

The enlarged and erythematous tonsils exhibit a gray, exudative membrane. This can be easily scraped off without bleeding. In younger children, respiratory distress due to obstruction may require treatment with high-dose steroids or, rarely, placement of a nasal airway or endotracheal tube. The tonsils can remain grossly hypertrophied following the resolution of infectious mononucleosis, and necessitate a future tonsillectomy.[75] However, this procedure may be associated with an increased risk of post-tonsillectomy hemorrhage.[76]

The diagnosis of infectious mononucleosis is made by a positive heterophile antibody agglutination test with confirmation by positive blood titers to the virus. Clinically, generalized cervical lymphadenopathy and hepatosplenomegaly often suggests the diagnosis. The blood smear typically displays many atypical lymphocytes. Infection with cytomegalovirus may mimic that caused by EBV but is usually less severe clinically. Low-grade fever, fatigue, and malaise may continue for months. Treatment is supportive, with rest, good oral hygiene, hydration, and use of corticosteroids for severe cases. Secondary bacterial infections or oral ulcerations can occur in the tonsils, and antibiotic therapy may be necessary.[77] The use of ampicillin, however, is associated with a greater incidence of a cutaneous papular rash.

References

1. Douglas RM, Miles H, Hansman D, Fadejevs A, Moore B, Bollen MD. Acute tonsillitis in children: microbial pathogens in relation to age. Pathology 1984;16(1):79–82

2. Brodsky L, Moore L, Stanievich J. The role of *Haemophilus influenzae* in the pathogenesis of tonsillar hypertrophy in children. Laryngoscope 1988;98(10):1055–1060

3. Schlager TA, Hayden GA, Woods WA, Dudley SM, Hendley JO. Optical immunoassay for rapid detection of group A beta-hemolytic streptococci. Should culture be replaced? Arch Pediatr Adolesc Med 1996;150(3):245–248

4. Wegner DL, Witte DL, Schrantz RD. Insensitivity of rapid antigen detection methods and single blood agar plate culture for diagnosing streptococcal pharyngitis. JAMA 1992;267(5):695–697

5. Sheeler RD, Houston MS, Radke S, Dale JC, Adamson SC. Accuracy of rapid strep testing in patients who have had recent streptococcal pharyngitis. J Am Board Fam Pract 2002;15(4):261–265

6. Gerber MA, Baltimore RS, Eaton CB, et al. Prevention of rheumatic fever and diagnosis and treatment of acute Streptococcal pharyngitis: a scientific statement from the American Heart Association Rheumatic Fever, Endocarditis, and Kawasaki Disease Committee of the Council on Cardiovascular Disease in the Young, the Interdisciplinary Council on Functional Genomics and Translational Biology, and the Interdisciplinary Council on Quality of Care and Outcomes Research: endorsed by the American Academy of Pediatrics. Circulation 2009;119(11):1541–1551

7. Markowitz M, Gerber MA, Kaplan EL. Treatment of streptococcal pharyngotonsillitis: reports of penicillin's demise are premature. J Pediatr 1993;123(5):679–685

8. Baugh RF, Archer SM, Mitchell RB, et al; American Academy of Otolaryngology-Head and Neck Surgery Foundation. Clinical practice guideline: tonsillectomy in children. Otolaryngol Head Neck Surg 2011;144(1, Suppl):S1–S30

9. Martin JM, Green M, Barbadora KA, Wald ER. Group A streptococci among school-aged children: clinical characteristics and the carrier state. Pediatrics 2004;114(5):1212–1219

10. Tanz RR, Shulman ST. Chronic pharyngeal carriage of group A streptococci. Pediatr Infect Dis J 2007;26(2):175–176

11. Wolf M, Kronenberg J, Kessler A, Modan M, Leventon G. Peritonsillar abscess in children and its indication for tonsillectomy. Int J Pediatr Otorhinolaryngol 1988;16(2):113–117

12. Veasy LG, Wiedmeier SE, Orsmond GS, et al. Resurgence of acute rheumatic fever in the intermountain area of the United States. N Engl J Med 1987;316(8):421–427

13. Denny FW, Wannamaker IW, Brink WR, et al. Prevention of rheumatic fever: Treatment of preceding streptococcal infection. JAMA 1950;143:151–153

14. Brook I, Yocum P. Comparison of the microbiology of group A and non-group A streptococcal tonsillitis. Ann Otol Rhinol Laryngol 1988;97(3 Pt 1):243–246

15. Brook I. The role of anaerobic bacteria in tonsillitis. Int J Pediatr Otorhinolaryngol 2005;69(1):9–19

16. Tunér K, Nord CE. Emergence of beta-lactamase producing anaerobic bacteria in the tonsils during penicillin treatment. Eur J Clin Microbiol 1986;5(4):399–404

17. Nord CE. The role of anaerobic bacteria in recurrent episodes of sinusitis and tonsillitis. Clin Infect Dis 1995;20(6):1512–1524

18. Reilly S, Timmis P, Beeden AG, Willis AT. Possible role of the anaerobe in tonsillitis. J Clin Pathol 1981;34(5):542–547

19. Lander L, Lu S, Shah RK. Pediatric retropharyngeal abscesses: a national perspective. Int J Pediatr Otorhinolaryngol 2008; 72(12):1837–1843

20. Schweinfurth JM. Demographics of pediatric head and neck infections in a tertiary care hospital. Laryngoscope 2006;116(6):887–889

21. Grisaru-Soen G, Komisar O, Aizenstein O, Soudack M, Schwartz D, Paret G. Retropharyngeal and parapharyngeal abscess in children—epidemiology, clinical features and treatment. Int J Pediatr Otorhinolaryngol 2010;74(9):1016–1020

22. Page NC, Bauer EM, Lieu JE. Clinical features and treatment of retropharyngeal abscess in children. Otolaryngol Head Neck Surg 2008;138(3):300–306

23. Brook I. Microbiology and management of peritonsillar, retropharyngeal, and parapharyngeal abscesses. J Oral Maxillofac Surg 2004;62(12):1545–1550

24. Grisaru-Soen G, Komisar O, Aizenstein O, Soudack M, Schwartz D, Paret G. Retropharyngeal and parapharyngeal abscess in children—epidemiology, clinical features and treatment. Int J Pediatr Otorhinolaryngol 2010;74(9):1016–1020

25. Uzomefuna V, Glynn F, Mackle T, Russell J. Atypical locations of retropharyngeal abscess: beware of the normal lateral soft tissue neck X-ray. Int J Pediatr Otorhinolaryngol 2010;74(12):1445–1448

26. Freling N, Roele E, Schaefer-Prokop C, Fokkens W. Prediction of deep neck abscesses by contrast-enhanced computerized tomography in 76 clinically suspect consecutive patients. Laryngoscope 2009;119(9):1745–1752

27. Craig FW, Schunk JE. Retropharyngeal abscess in children: clinical presentation, utility of imaging, and current management. Pediatrics 2003;111(6 Pt 1):1394–1398

28. Johnston D, Schmidt R, Barth P. Parapharyngeal and retropharyngeal infections in children: argument for a trial of medical therapy and intraoral drainage for medical treatment failures. Int J Pediatr Otorhinolaryngol 2009;73(5):761–765

29. Chirinos JA, Lichtstein DM, Garcia J, Tamariz LJ. The evolution of Lemierre syndrome: report of 2 cases and review of the literature. Medicine (Baltimore) 2002;81(6):458–465

30. Sinave CP, Hardy GJ, Fardy PW. The Lemierre syndrome: suppurative thrombophlebitis of the internal jugular vein secondary to oropharyngeal infection. Medicine (Baltimore) 1989;68(2):85–94

31. Masson AM, Prissick FH. Cervical lymphadenitis in children caused by chromogenic *Mycobacteria*. Can Med Assoc J 1956;75(10):798–803

32. Wolinsky E. Nontuberculous mycobacteria and associated diseases. Am Rev Respir Dis 1979;119(1):107–159

33. Tunkel DE, Romaneschi KB. Surgical treatment of cervicofacial nontuberculous mycobacterial adenitis in children. Laryngoscope 1995;105(10):1024–1028

34. Hazra R, Robson CD, Perez-Atayde AR, Husson RN. Lymphadenitis due to nontuberculous mycobacteria in children: presentation and response to therapy. Clin Infect Dis 1999;28(1):123–129

35. Sigalet D, Lees G, Fanning A. Atypical tuberculosis in the pediatric patient: implications for the pediatric surgeon. J Pediatr Surg 1992;27(11):1381–1384

36. Twist CJ, Link MP. Assessment of lymphadenopathy in children. Pediatr Clin North Am 2002;49(5):1009–1025

37. Suskind DL, Handler SD, Tom LW, Potsic WP, Wetmore RF.

Nontuberculous mycobacterial cervical adenitis. Clin Pediatr (Phila) 1997;36(7):403–409

38. Rahal A, Abela A, Arcand PH, Quintal MC, Lebel MH, Tapiero BF. Nontuberculous mycobacterial adenitis of the head and neck in children: experience from a tertiary care pediatric center. Laryngoscope 2001;111(10):1791–1796

39. Schaad UB, Votteler TP, McCracken GH Jr, Nelson JD. Management of atypical mycobacterial lymphadenitis in childhood: a review based on 380 cases. J Pediatr 1979;95(3):356–360

40. Alessi DP, Dudley JP. Atypical mycobacteria-induced cervical adenitis. Treatment by needle aspiration. Arch Otolaryngol Head Neck Surg 1988;114(6):664–666

41. Kennedy TL. Curettage of nontuberculous mycobacterial cervical lymphadenitis. Arch Otolaryngol Head Neck Surg 1992;118(7):759–762

42. Tessier MH, Amoric JC, Méchinaud F, Dubesset D, Litoux P, Stalder JF. Clarithromycin for atypical mycobacterial lymphadenitis in non-immunocompromised children. Lancet 1994;344(8939-8940):1778

43. Berger C, Pfyffer GE, Nadal D. Treatment of nontuberculous mycobacterial lymphadenitis with clarithromycin plus rifabutin. J Pediatr 1996;128(3):383–386

44. Luong A, McClay JE, Jafri HS, Brown O. Antibiotic therapy for nontuberculous mycobacterial cervicofacial lymphadenitis. Laryngoscope 2005;115(10):1746–1751

45. Lindeboom JA, Kuijper EJ, Bruijnesteijn van Coppenraet ES, Lindeboom R, Prins JM. Surgical excision versus antibiotic treatment for nontuberculous mycobacterial cervicofacial lymphadenitis in children: a multicenter, randomized, controlled trial. Clin Infect Dis 2007;44(8):1057–1064

46. Chomel BB, Kasten RW, Floyd-Hawkins K, et al. Experimental transmission of *Bartonella henselae* by the cat flea. J Clin Microbiol 1996;34(8):1952–1956

47. Zangwill KM, Hamilton DH, Perkins BA, et al. Cat scratch disease in Connecticut. Epidemiology, risk factors, and evaluation of a new diagnostic test. N Engl J Med 1993;329(1):8–13

48. Jackson LA, Perkins BA, Wenger JD. Cat scratch disease in the United States: an analysis of three national databases. Am J Public Health 1993;83(12):1707–1711

49. Peters TR, Edwards KM. Cervical lymphadenopathy and adenitis. Pediatr Rev 2000;21(12):399–405

50. Margileth AM. Antibiotic therapy for cat-scratch disease: clinical study of therapeutic outcome in 268 patients and a review of the literature. Pediatr Infect Dis J 1992;11(6):474–478

51. Rombaux P, M'Bilo T, Badr-el-Din A, Theate I, Bigaignon G, Hamoir M. Cervical lymphadenitis and cat scratch disease (CSD): an overlooked disease? Acta Otorhinolaryngol Belg 2000;54(4):491–496

52. Windsor JJ. Cat-scratch disease: epidemiology, aetiology and treatment. Br J Biomed Sci 2001;58(2):101–110

53. Dennis DT, Inglesby TV, Henderson DA, et al; Working Group on Civilian Biodefense. Tularemia as a biological weapon: medical and public health management. JAMA 2001;285(21):2763–2773

54. Centers for Disease Control and Prevention (CDC). Tularemia—United States, 1990-2000. MMWR Morb Mortal Wkly Rep 2002;51(9):181–184

55. Evans ME, Gregory DW, Schaffner W, McGee ZA. Tularemia: a 30-year experience with 88 cases. Medicine (Baltimore) 1985;64(4):251–269

56. Bhargava D, Bhusnurmath B, Sundaram KR, et al. Tonsillar actinomycosis: a clinicopathological study. Acta Trop 2001;80(2):163–168

57. Russo TA. Agent of actinomycosis. In: Mandell GLBJ, Dolin R, eds. Principles and Practice of Infectious Disease. 5th ed. Philadelphia: Churchill Livingstone; 2000:2645–2654

58. Lester FT, Juhasz E. Actinomycosis of the ear. Ethiop Med J 1990;28(1):41–44

59. Lahoz Zamarro MT, Laguía Pérez M, Muniesa Soriano JA, Martínez Sanz G. [Base tongue actinomycosis]. Acta Otorrinolaringol Esp 2005;56(5):222–225

60. Osborne JE, Blair RL, Christmas HE, McKenzie H. Actinomycosis of the nasopharynx: a complication of nasal surgery. J Laryngol Otol 1988;102(7):639–640

61. Thomas R, Kameswaran M, Ahmed S, Khurana P, Morad N. Actinomycosis of the vallecula: report of a case and review of the literature. J Laryngol Otol 1995;109(2):154–156

62. Altundal H, Gursoy B, Salih I, Olgaç V. Pediatric cervicofacial actinomycosis: a case report. J Dent Child 2004;71(1):87–90

63. Oysu C, Uslu C, Guclu O, Oysu A. Actinomycotic abscess of the thyroid gland in an infant. Int J Pediatr Otorhinolaryngol 2005;69(5):701–703

64. Sari M, Yazici M, Bağlam T, Inanli S, Eren F. Actinomycosis of the larynx. Acta Otolaryngol 2007;127(5):550–552

65. Odio CM, Navarrete M, Carrillo JM, Mora L, Carranza A. Disseminated histoplasmosis in infants. Pediatr Infect Dis J 1999;18(12):1065–1068

66. Lowell JR. Diagnosis of histoplasmosis. Ann Intern Med 1983;98(2):260

67. Kauffman CA. Histoplasmosis: a clinical and laboratory update. Clin Microbiol Rev 2007;20(1):115–132

68. Hage CA, Wheat LJ, Loyd J, Allen SD, Blue D, Knox KS. Pulmonary histoplasmosis. Semin Respir Crit Care Med 2008;29(2):151–165

69. Coiffier T, Roger G, Beust L, et al. Pharyngo-laryngeal histoplasmosis: one case in an immunocompetent child. Int J Pediatr Otorhinolaryngol 1998;45(2):177–181

70. Gerber ME, Rosdeutscher JD, Seiden AM, Tami TA. Histoplasmosis: the otolaryngologist's perspective. Laryngoscope 1995;105(9 Pt 1):919–923

71. Boutros HH, Van Winckle RB, Evans GA, Wasan SM. Oral histoplasmosis masquerading as an invasive carcinoma. J Oral Maxillofac Surg 1995;53(9):1110–1114

72. Wheat LJ. Improvements in diagnosis of histoplasmosis. Expert Opin Biol Ther 2006;6(11):1207–1221

73. Luzuriaga K, Sullivan JL. Infectious mononucleosis. N Engl J Med 2010;362(21):1993–2000

74. Grose C. The many faces of infectious mononucleosis: the spectrum of Epstein-Barr virus infection in children. Pediatr Rev 1985;7:35–44

75. Goode RL, Coursey DL. Tonsillectomy and infectious mononucleosis—a possible relationship. Laryngoscope 1976;86(7):992–995

76. Windfuhr JP, Chen YS, Remmert S. Hemorrhage following tonsillectomy and adenoidectomy in 15,218 patients. Otolaryngol Head Neck Surg 2005;132(2):281–286

77. Snyderman NL. Otorhinolaryngologic presentations of infectious mononucleosis. Pediatr Clin North Am 1981;28(4):1011–1016

19 Congenital Neck Masses

Tali Lando and Ian N. Jacobs

Congenital neck masses are a common problem in children. This chapter will discuss etiology as well as diagnosis and treatment of congenital neck masses. The etiology of these lesions can often be determined by characteristics on examination such as size, consistency, and location. Midline lesions include thyroglossal duct cysts (TGDC), ectopic thyroid, dermoid cysts, and thymic rests. Lateral and posterior triangle lesions include branchial anomalies (BAs) and lymphatic malformations (LMs). Upper cervical and submandibular lesions include hemangiomas and venous and lymphatic malformations.

BAs

Between the 4th and 6th week of fetal development, 6 paired branchial arches appear. Each arch is layered externally by ectoderm and internally by endoderm, with a core of mesoderm. The arches are separated by ectodermal clefts externally and endodermal pouches internally. Each arch, pouch, and cleft will form specific structures in the head and neck (**Table 19.1**). As a general rule, BAs and their associated tract lie inferior (superficial) to all embryonic derivatives of their associated arch and superior (superficial) to all derivatives of the next arch.

Imaging

Imaging can aid in diagnosis, identify anatomic relationships to neurovascular structures, and also determine the extent of the BAs. Ultrasound can differentiate cysts from lymphadenopathy, but BAs do not have a classic ultrasound appearance. Magnetic resonance imaging (MRI) is most helpful in assessing soft-tissue borders. For first BAs, high-resolution computed tomography (CT) scan can define the relationship of the sinus tract with the external auditory canal and the middle ear. Preoperative fistulography (with thin barium) has been used to study third and fourth branchial sinuses (pyriform fistulae) (**Fig. 19.1**), but inflammation and scarring can yield false-negative results.[1] A barium swallow can clarify postsurgical anatomy in recurrent lesions.

First BAs

Embryology and Anatomy

First BAs develop as a result of incomplete obliteration of the cleft between the mandibular process of the first arch (Meckel cartilage) and the second arch (Reichert cartilage). They represent between 7 and 10% of all BAs.[2,3] First BAs

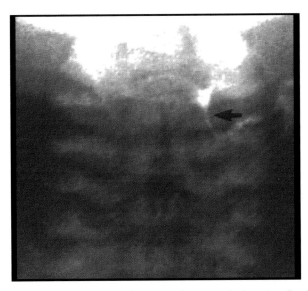

Figure 19.1 A pharyngoesophagram with contrast leakage into fistula.

course close to the parotid gland and the superficial parotid lobe may overlie a component of the lesion. The relationship between first BAs and the facial nerve is variable, but identification of the facial nerve should be a component of most, if not all surgical plans for these lesions. The tracts are more likely to be superficial or deep to the facial nerve, but may also intercalate split between nerve branches.[3,4]

Clinical Presentation and Diagnosis

First BAs appear in front of, below, or behind the pinna. They can be confused with dermoid cysts or preauricular pits and cysts, which are developmentally distinct entities formed from failure of fusion of the auricular hillocks. As a result, they are often not diagnosed or completely treated for years.[3] Clinical presentation is variable: parotid symptoms include a mass or cystic swelling which increases with inflammation; auricular symptoms involve fullness in the ear canal (with or without chronic discharge) in the presence of a normal tympanic membrane; and cervical symptoms consist of swelling or drainage in the neck, just posterior to the mandible. Misdiagnosed intraparotid cysts or parotid tumors may be embryonic remnants of the first branchial cleft.

Fistulae and sinuses from the first branchial cleft are rare and account for less than 8% of all BAs.[4] Tract openings can occur anywhere in the external ear canal (EAC), middle ear cleft, postauricular region or neck over the angle of the mandible, below the hyoid and anterior

Table 19.1 Embryonic Derivatives of the Branchial Apparatus

First arch

Cartilage (Meckel): Sphenomandibular ligament, anterior malleolar ligament, malleus, and the incus (excluding the manubrium of the malleus and the long process of the incus). Bony derivatives contribute to the formation of the ramus of the mandible and the maxilla.

Mesenchymal component: Muscles of mastication—temporalis, masseter, and the medial and lateral pterygoid muscles. Tensor tympani, tensor veli palatine, anterior belly of the digastric, and mylohyoid muscles.

Blood supply: Facial artery.

Innervation: Mandibular portion of the trigeminal nerve (V3).

First cleft[a]

Dorsal portion: External auditory meatus.

Middle portion: Concha cavum.

Ventral portion: Obliterates. Pinna develops around dorsal end of the first branchial cleft from the six tubercles or hillocks of His. Membrane at the bottom of the groove becomes outer squamous layer of tympanic membrane. First cleft separates the mandibular process from the second branchial arch.

First pouch

Ventral portion: Eustachian tube. Dorsal portion of the first and second pharyngeal pouches; contributes to formation of the middle ear, tubotympanic recess, and mastoid antrum.

Second arch

Cartilage (Reichert): Stylohyoid ligament, styloid process, manubrium of the malleus, long process of the incus and stapes suprastructure. (Stapes footplate is mostly derived from the otic capsule.) Part of the body and both of the lesser cornu of the hyoid bone.

Mesenchymal component: Muscles of facial expression, posterior belly of digastric, stylohyoid, and stapedius muscle.

Blood supply: Stapedial artery (should degenerate before birth).

Innervation: Facial nerve (CNVII).

Second cleft

Obliterated.

Second pouch

Endodermal layer: Epithelial lining of the palatine tonsil. Mesodermal layer: palatine tonsil itself.

Third arch

Cartilage: Remaining parts of the body and the greater cornu of the hyoid.

Mesenchymal component: Stylopharyngeus muscles.

Blood supply: Common carotid and proximal portions of the internal and external carotid artery.

Innervation: Glossopharyngeal nerve (CN IX).

Third cleft

Obliterated.

Third pouch

Inferior parathyroids and thymus. Opens into the pharynx at the level of pyriform fossa anterior to fold formed by the internal laryngeal nerve.

Fourth–sixth arch

Cartilage: Laryngeal framework including the thyroid, cricoid, arytenoid, corniculate, and cuneiform cartilages.

Mesenchymal component: Fourth arch—cricothyroid and inferior constrictor muscles and superior part of the esophagus, composed of striated muscle. Sixth arch—remaining extrinsic and intrinsic muscles of the larynx.

Blood supply: Fourth arch—right subclavian and aortic arch. Sixth arch—pulmonary artery and ductus arteriosus.

Innervation: Fourth arch—superior laryngeal nerve. (The superior laryngeal nerve gives sensation to the larynx and motor innervation to the cricothyroid. Pharyngeal constrictors are innervated by the pharyngeal branch of the vagus and upper esophagus by the recurrent laryngeal branch.) Sixth arch—recurrent laryngeal nerve.

Fourth–sixth clefts

Obliterated.

Fourth pouch

Superior parathyroid glands and ultimobranchial body (opens in the region of the pyriform sinus posterior to the internal branch of the superior laryngeal nerve or upper esophagus). Sixth pouch—obliterated.

[a]The first branchial cleft is unique because it is the only cleft that is not completely obliterated by the 8th week of gestation.

to the sternocleidomastoid muscle (SCM). A membranous attachment between the tract and the tympanic membrane is present in 10% of patients.[3]

Work classified first BAs based on clinical and histological features.[5] Type I lesions are duplications of the cartilaginous EAC containing squamous epithelium only. Typically, a cystic mass in the postauricular area extends anteromedially, paralleling the EAC, and passing lateral to the facial nerve to end at the bony meatus. Type II lesions are more common. Classically, a sinus tract from an external opening high in the neck along the anterior border of the SCM passes superficial or deep to the facial nerve, in close relation to the parotid gland. The tract ends blindly near the floor of the cartilaginous EAC or opens into the canal to form a complete fistula. Although the Work classification system is time-honored, the value of such classification for clinical treatment has been questioned.

Second BAs

Embryology and Anatomy

Second arch anomalies, the most common BAs, represent between 69 and 93% of all BAs.[1,2] Tracts pass from an external opening in the mid to lower neck, anterior to the border of the SCM, deep to the platysma, and along the carotid sheath. They course between the internal and external carotid arteries after passing superficial to the glossopharyngeal and hypoglossal nerves. In the case of true fistulae, the tract then dives below the stylohyoid ligament and opens internally in the oropharynx at the level of the tonsillar fossa. The second, third, and fourth BAs have a similar exit point in the neck because embryologically they all share a common external opening—the cervical sinus of His.

Clinical Presentation and Diagnosis

Second cleft fistulae are generally diagnosed early in infancy or childhood. Patients complain of recurrent neck drainage that often increases with upper respiratory tract infections (URIs). This is due to the respiratory epithelium lining the tract that increases secretion production in the presence of inflammation or infection. In contrast, cysts may be diagnosed later in adulthood as nontender neck masses that may enlarge during an URI. These sinuses are usually right-sided and occur more often in girls.[1] Between 2 and 13% occur bilaterally.[6] Bilateral lesions with concomitant preauricular sinuses may suggest a syndromic diagnosis such as branchio-oto-renal syndrome.

Third and Fourth BAs

Embryology and Anatomy

Third arch anomalies are uncommon. Persistent fistulae of the third branchial cleft and pouch course along the anterior border of the SCM (between the middle and the lower third) and pass deep to the internal carotid artery. The tract courses the between the glossopharyngeal nerve and hypoglossal

nerve below or loops around the hypoglossal nerve. If there is an internal opening, it pierces the thyrohyoid membrane and enters the pharynx in the region of the pyriform sinus. Third BAs originate from the base (cranial end) of the pyriform sinus and pass above the superior laryngeal nerve, whereas the tract of fourth BAs originates from the apex (caudal end) of the pyriform sinus and passes through the cricothyroid membrane beneath the superior laryngeal nerve.[7]

Fourth branchial malformations are rare (**Fig. 19.1**). The course of the anomalous tract depends on its sidedness. Left-sided lesions descend into the mediastinum and loop around the aortic arch, medial to the ligamentum arteriosus; the tract then ascends into the neck and enters the pharynx at the level of the pyriform sinus or cervical esophagus. Right-sided lesions loop around the subclavian artery and pass deep to the internal carotid artery, then ascending to the level of the hypoglossal nerve. The tract then descends and enters the pharynx.

Clinical Presentation and Diagnosis

The second, third, and fourth BAs have a similar external cervical presentation because embryologically they all share a common external opening—the cervical sinus of His. Neck masses originating from the third and fourth branchial apparatus often present lower in the neck, and are most often on the left side.

Third and fourth BAs can be grouped together as "pyriform sinus tracts." Pyriform sinus tracts should be considered in any child with recurrent left neck abscesses or suppurative thyroiditis.[8] Direct laryngoscopy with identification of a fistulous opening confirms the diagnosis (**Fig. 19.2**).

Management/Treatment

With all these lesions, surgical intervention may be delayed in young infants with uncomplicated courses until at least 2 or 3 years of age. Whenever possible, excision should be postponed until any acute infection has been well treated.

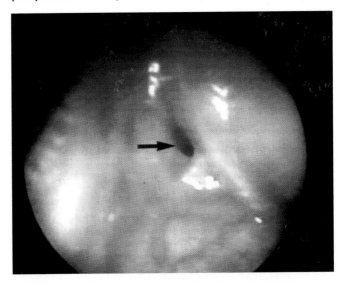

Figure 19.2 Endoscopic localization of a pyriform sinus tract.

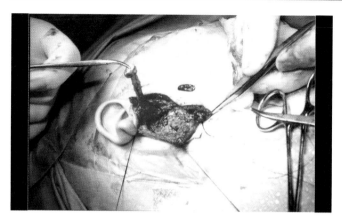

Figure 19.3 Complete excision of first branchial cleft anomalies including facial nerve dissection.

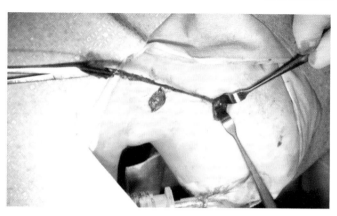

Figure 19.4 Stepladder incision to excise second branchial cleft tract.

In some refractory cases, long-term oral or parenteral antibiotic therapy may be required until the time of excision to prevent reinfection.

First BAs

Surgical excision of Type I anomalies should include exploration and excision of the mass and its tract down to the EAC at its bony junction (**Fig. 19.3**). Management of Type II anomalies entails excision via parotidectomy incision and complete excision of the tract. Conservative parotidectomy with identification of the facial nerve is required in most cases. Limited cystectomies will result in recurrence and the incidence of facial nerve injury is higher if the nerve is not identified.[4] Facial nerve monitors are often used during these operations, but a thorough knowledge of the relationship of the tracts with the facial nerve is essential. If the sinus tract involves the cartilaginous EAC, it should be marsupialized with an ellipse of cartilage removed.

Second BAs

The external skin opening should be excised in an elliptical fashion. Methods to aid in identifying the tract have included injection of methylene blue, insertion of probes and catheters, or paraffin injection. Careful dissection of the tract should be carried as far superiorly as possible and ligated. Tract length is variable and long tracts may require several "stepladder" incisions (**Fig. 19.4**). In many cases, sinuses extend to the level of the carotid bifurcation and even into the tonsillar fossa.[2] In rare circumstances it may be necessary to perform a tonsillectomy to identify the internal oropharyngeal opening. The tract can be cannulated from the mouth and the tract pulled through from the neck for a complete surgical excision. Potential surgical complications include persistence of the cyst, pharyngocutaneous fistula formation, and cranial nerve (glossopharyngeal or hypoglossal) and vascular injury.

Third and Fourth BAs

Third and fourth BAs are excised with a cervical neck incision similar to that for second BA. Treatment should include complete excision of the lesion as well as a left thyroid lobectomy, if indicated. After multiple neck infections or surgical procedures, these lesions may be densely adherent to the carotid sheath. There is debate on the best method of addressing pyriform sinus tracts.[9] Some suggest initial cannulation with a lacrimal probe or Fogarty catheter under direct laryngoscopy. Once identified, the tract is followed proximally and completely excised with a purse-string closure (**Fig. 19.5**). Dissection may continue all the way up to the pyriform sinus. Potential surgical complications include pharyngocutaneous fistula formation and nerve (superior and recurrent laryngeal) and vascular injury.

Various endoscopic cauterization techniques have been described as an alternative to open surgery. Endoscopic cauterization is performed under suspension laryngoscopy with identification of the fistulous opening in the pyriform sinus. Chen et al reported success with endoscopic electrocauterization alone, using a urologic instrument (5 French Flexible Bugbee Cautery Electrode, EET-107B, Greenwald Surgical Company, Inc., Lake Station, IN).[10] Other obliterative methods such as chemical cauterization with 40% trichloroacetic acid and injection of fibrin glue into the pyriform sinus apex have also been described.[11] These methods are performed in conjunction with drainage of the neck abscess, when present.

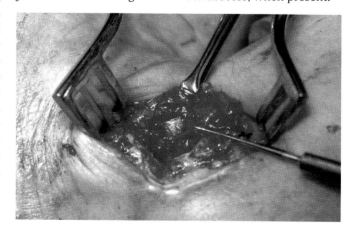

Figure 19.5 Localization of pyriform apex fistula in the neck using a Fogarty balloon.

Table 19.2 deSerres Classification of Lymphatic Malformations

Stage I	Unilateral infrahyoid disease
Stage II	Unilateral suprahyoid disease
Stage III	Unilateral suprahyoid and infrahyoid disease
Stage IV	Bilateral suprahyoid disease
Stage V	Bilateral suprahyoid and infrahyoid disease

Note: This classification system correlates increasing stage with clinical complications including: need for airway intervention, speech and feeding difficulties, preoperative infection requiring antibiotics, cosmesis, dental malocclusion, and persistent or recurrent disease.

Adapted from: Wiegand S, Eivazi B, Zimmermann AP, Sesterhenn AM, Werner JA. Sclerotherapy of lymphangiomas of the head and neck. *Head Neck* 2011;33(11):1649–1655.

LMs

Embryology and Anatomy

LMs are generally considered benign congenital neoplasms of the lymphatic system. Histopathologically, LMs have been classified into simple lymphangiomas, cavernous lymphangiomas, and cystic hygromas.[12] This classification system is based on thickness of the adventitia and size of the vascular spaces. An alternative system categorizes LMs into three relatively distinct morphologic types: macrocystic, microcystic, or mixed lesions.[13] The macrocystic type is composed of large cysts ≥2 mL filled with lymphatic fluid. The microcystic type comprise dysplastic lymphatic tissue with a variable fibrofatty component, small cysts <2 mL or ectatic channels. In the mixed form, a solid soft-tissue mass is associated with a cystic component.

The most commonly accepted staging system, used for prognosis, was developed by deSerres based on laterality and relationship to the hyoid bone (**Table 19.2**).[14] deSerres recognized that suprahyoid lesions are more difficult to excise completely than infrahyoid lesions.

Clinical Presentation and Diagnosis

LMs occur frequently in the head and neck, with the neck often considered the most likely location.[14] Malformations are present at birth, although they may have delayed clinical presentations. Males and females are equally affected. They most commonly present as a painless, soft, compressible mass in the anterior or posterior cervical triangle. Floor of mouth, hypopharyngeal, or laryngeal malformations can cause airway compromise, as well as speech and feeding difficulties. Facial and parotid lesions can be disfiguring. Orbital lesions may affect vision and neck lesions can cause torticollis. Cervicofacial LMs can result in long-term mandibular deformity and dental malocclusion. Inferior thoracocervical LMs can cause mediastinal widening or great vessel displacement, often without aerodynamic compromise.

Cervicofacial LMs are diagnosed by history and physical examination. Lesions grow commensurate with the child and are often transilluminate. Sudden enlargement results from intralesional hemorrhage or infection causing an inflammatory response. Thin-walled lesions permit bleeding into vessels, resulting in a reddish hue of the overlying skin. With large head and neck LMs, a comprehensive airway evaluation should include fiberoptic laryngoscopy to identify any involvement of the larynx or hypopharynx.

Imaging

Ultrasound may demonstrate hypoechogenic, multilocular cysts with septae of variable thickness. It is of limited use for identifying mediastinal extension or retropharyngeal LMs. Prenatal diagnosis of LMs is increasingly common. Ultrasound in the first or second trimester may diagnose nuchal LMs, but these lesions generally resolve. In utero LMs are associated with aneuploidy syndromes such as Turner or Down syndrome.[15]

MRI with gadolinium is the best study for evaluating LMs and differentiating them from low-flow venous lesions. LMs are hypo- or isodense on T1-weighted images and hyperintense on T2-weighted images.[13] Septations are clearly demarcated and margins are often distinguishable from adjacent tissue (**Fig. 19.6**). Recent infection or hemorrhage into the cyst appears as a heterogeneous fluid–fluid level. Chest radiographs can identify thoracic extension.

Management/Treatment

Treatment options vary based on LM size, location, and associated symptoms. The risks of surgery are considered as well as the potential for complete excision. Airway management is essential in all patients with potential airway compromise, but especially in infants with large cervicofacial lesions extending to the oral floor and tongue base. Tracheostomy is

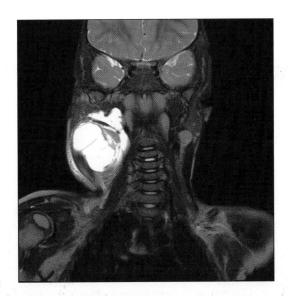

Figure 19.6 Coronal gadolinium-enhanced magnetic resonance image of right neck lymphatic malformation.

considered if there are airway concerns related to mass effect, acute enlargement, or inflammatory reaction to treatment. An ex utero intrapartum treatment (EXIT) for airway management is scheduled if there is concern for respiratory compromise.[16]

Potential for recurrent infection, airway compromise, feeding and speech difficulties, and cosmetic concerns makes these lesions challenging. A multidisciplinary approach should assess treatment plans that may include surgery, sclerotherapy, or observation.

Observation

The goal of treatment is improvement or preservation of functional and aesthetic integrity. Small, asymptomatic (nondisfiguring, nonobstructing) LMs are often not treated. Nonetheless, spontaneous regression is rare and occurs in less than 5% of cases.[17]

Treatment may be delayed (i.e., 6 to 12 months of age), in the absence of airway obstruction. However, resection should be scheduled before the child develops self-image and memory (at about age 3). Multiple procedures beyond the neonatal period are typically necessary in these patients to obviate the need for tracheostomy.

Surgical Excision

The general dictum is that LMs do not involute and surgery is the treatment of choice. The most important factor is to perform complete surgical excision without significant morbidity. Safe and complete removal depends on the extent, location, and wall thickness. Lesions can infiltrate surrounding tissues making excision difficult without sacrifice of neurovascular structures. In reality, many LMs are treated repeatedly with multiple or combined modalities. Surgery is particularly appropriate for focal lesions (Stages I and II) that involve the anterior tongue, neck, parotid, or mediastinum (**Fig. 19.7A, B**). Surgery may be indicated for microcystic

lesions because sclerotherapy is generally less effective. Incomplete excision carries a high risk of recurrence (50 to 100%).[14,17] Typically, recurrences are evident soon after surgery, but some LMs can recur even after a long period of quiescence.

Extensive LMs of the oral cavity are particularly difficult to resect. Postoperative feeding and speech morbidity can result from neuromuscular damage. The facial nerve is at risk in lesions with parotid, buccal, and submandibular involvement, with the marginal mandibular branch most commonly injured.[14] Hypoglossal nerve injury results from resection of floor of mouth masses while the accessory nerve is at risk in posterior cervical lesions. Frey syndrome (gustatory sweating) and Horner syndrome (ptosis, miosis, and anhidrosis) can occur after excision of parotid masses or malformations with carotid sheath involvement, respectively.

Sclerotherapy

Percutaneous sclerotherapy is most effective for unilocular macrocystic lesions and some microcystic lesions. OK-432 (picibanil), a lyophilized low-virulence strain of group A *Streptococcus pyogenes*, has been used effectively with few side effects in children with macrocystic LMs.[13,18] Although the exact mechanism of this action is unknown, it causes an intense inflammatory reaction followed by fibrosis and shrinkage. Doxycycline is an effective sclerosing agent that does not cause neural toxicity. Other sclerosants include 50% dextrose, sodium tetradecyl foam, bleomycin, ethanol, and interferon alfa-2a. Each of these agents has unique potential complications. Sclerosing technique involves aspiration to confirm the lymphatic character of the lesion, followed by instillation into the cyst under ultrasound or fluoroscopic guidance. Adverse reactions are mostly temporary and limited to pain, erythema, edema, and fever associated with an inflammatory response. When injected into the

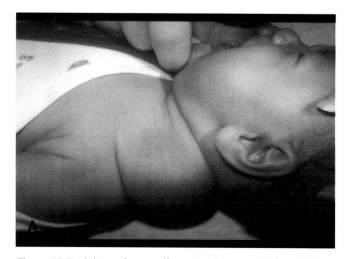
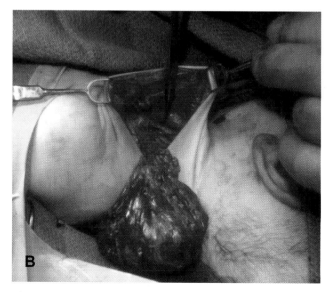

Figure 19.7   (A) Lymphatic malformation (preoperative) and (B) intraoperative resection.

neck, there is a risk of airway compromise from swelling, and need for emergent tracheostomy has been described.[13] Sclerotherapy does not seem to complicate subsequent surgery for residual LMs.[18]

Laser Therapy

The carbon dioxide (CO_2) laser is an invisible laser (10,600 nm), which is preferentially absorbed by water. It can reduce the size of superficial mucosal lymphatic lesions. Intra-oral lesions may be treated with a handheld laser while hypopharyngeal and laryngeal lesions require suspension microlaryngoscopy.[19] CO_2 laser debulking does not completely excise tissue in patients with obstructing airway lesions. Nd:YAG and pulsed dye laser are useful in treating the superficial components of LMs and can improve cosmesis. As these lasers do not address the deep component, recurrence is inevitable.

Radiofrequency Ablation

Bipolar radiofrequency plasma ablation (coblation) can be an effective means of treating or diminishing microcystic LMs of the oral cavity.[20] Coblation destroys lesion tissues at low temperature (40 to 70°C) with minimal damage to adjacent structures. Submucosal tongue lesions are typically treated under general anesthesia with suspension microlaryngoscopy.

TGDC

Embryology and Anatomy

Early in gestation, the thyroid gland begins to form from the median thyroid anlage at the foramen cecum. The gland descends anteroinferiorly over the hyoid to its destination in the lower midline of the neck. During this process, the median thyroid anlage elongates, forming the thyroglossal duct. Persistence of ductal elements leads to the formation of cysts.

Clinical Presentation and Diagnosis

TGDCs are the most frequent congenital neck mass requiring excision (**Fig. 19.8**). They present as a soft compressible painless neck mass in the region of the hyoid bone at or around midline.[21] Most patients present in the first 5 years of life, although they may present in adulthood. Classically, the mass moves cranially with swallowing and tongue protrusion because of its association with the hyoid bone.

Some patients may present with a draining midline fistula that occurs after infection. Lingual thyroglossal duct cysts are rare variants that present in the central tongue base. Left untreated, these patients may present with life-threatening airway obstruction.

Imaging

The extent of preoperative testing in children with TGDC has evolved over the past several decades. Patients with

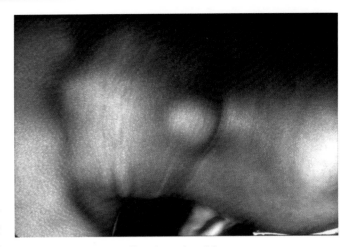
Figure 19.8 A large midline thyroglossal duct cyst.

suspected TGDC should undergo preoperative ultrasound to establish the presence of a normal thyroid gland in the normal location, effectively ruling out the possibility of ectopic thyroid as the etiology of the mass. Ultrasound of TGDC demonstrates a hypoechoic or anechoic, thin-walled cyst with prominent enhancement. Debris may suggest hemorrhage or infection. When the thyroid gland is absent on ultrasound, a radionuclide scan may be useful.

Management/Treatment

Surgical Excision

TGDCs are removed to prevent subsequent infection. The Sistrunk procedure, reported about 90 years ago, entails complete excision of the cyst, tract and fistula, and the central portion of the hyoid bone (**Fig. 19.9**). The thyroid cartilage is identified and the hyoid is skeletonized and suprahyoid muscles are released to remove a central portion of bone.

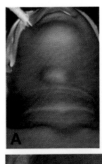
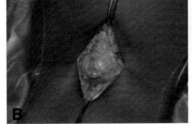
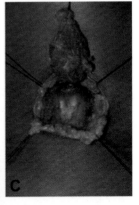

Figure 19.9 The classic Sistrunk procedure involves the en bloc resection of cyst tract, central body of hyoid followed to foramen cecum. (A) After procedure; (B) after tract; and (C) after cecum.

Dissection proceeds proximally, coring tissue around the tract through the base of tongue muscles to the foramen cecum including this in the specimen. The tract is ligated at the tongue base and the specimen is removed en bloc. The pyramidal lobe may be included in the surgical specimen to prevent recurrence.[22]

Various modifications of the classic surgical technique have been described to reduce the recurrence risk. Perkins et al describe a "suture-guided transhyoid pharyngotomy" technique for recurrent TGDC, which involves removal of a tissue block from the foramen cecum under direct visualization.[23]

Hemangiomas

Embryology and Anatomy

Infantile hemangiomas (IHs) are the most common tumor of infancy (affecting about 5% of infants) and the most common airway neoplasm in children. They are proliferating embryonal tumors that may stem from placental tissue. Localized hemangiomas originate from a central point, while segmental hemangiomas follow developmental segments. These lesions have a three-phase natural history: proliferation, plateau, and involution.

Clinical Presentation and Diagnosis

Most hemangiomas are not seen at birth but present in the first month of life and continue to proliferate until 24 months of age. The rate of growth during the proliferative phase is unpredictable. Spontaneous regression typically occurs after 18 to 24 months of age. The most common sites in the head and neck are the scalp, neck, and face. On physical examination, these lesions are generally soft, painless, and compressible.

Airway hemangiomas can be life-threatening. Signs and symptoms include stridor, croup-like cough, respiratory distress, and oral intolerance. Patients with airway symptoms and those with cutaneous hemangiomas in the V3 beard distribution should undergo airway evaluation including flexible nasopharyngoscopy, and perhaps direct laryngoscopy and bronchoscopy.[24] PHACE syndrome (posterior fossa malformations, head and neck hemangiomas, arterial anomalies, cardiac defects, eye abnormalities) has a significant association with cervical hemangiomas in the V3 distribution.[25]

Imaging

Imaging of preschool age children with extensive neck and airway hemangiomas may require sedation and endotracheal intubation. CT scan of the neck with contrast provides good tissue detail. MRI or magnetic resonance angiography is helpful in defining the extent of the lesion and its vascularity. The diagnostic findings of hemangiomas on T2-weighted MRI are multiple septated lobules of high signal intensity resembling a "bunch of grapes" (**Fig. 19.10**).[25] Thrombosis

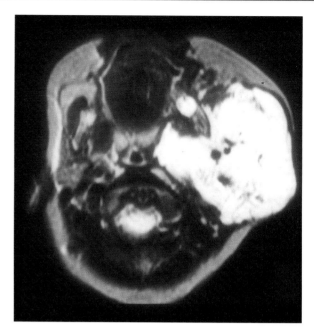

Figure 19.10   Magnetic resonance image of large neck (parotid) hemangioma.

appears as circular areas of low signal intensity similar to phleboliths.

Management/Treatment

Surgical Excision

Subtotal removal using the microdebrider or laser can debulk obstructive lesions but may not obviate the need for medical treatment (**Fig. 19.11**).[26] Open resection of airway hemangiomas with laryngotracheoplasty is an effective method of treatment for larger focal airway hemangiomas.[27] For lesions extending beyond the airway into the neck, surgical options are more limited and less efficacious.

Corticosteroids

Traditionally, corticosteroids have been the mainstay of medical treatment for hemangiomas. Although effective,

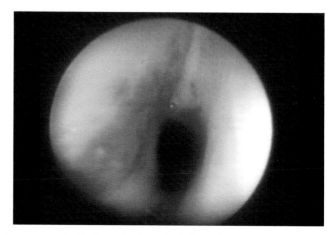

Figure 19.11   Endoscopic view of subglottic hemangioma.

long-term systemic steroids cause side effects (especially in the growing child) that include immunosuppression, cushingoid facies, and muscle weakness. Intralesional injected steroids may be effective and reduce the risk of systemic side effects.

Beta-Blockers

Propranolol, a nonspecific β-adrenergic receptor blocker, is a new and effective treatment for hemangiomas. In a study conducted by Truong et al, use of propranolol results in improvement of airway obstruction, avoidance of surgical intervention, and decreased duration of corticosteroid use.[28] Clinical response to propranolol is typically noted in the first 1 to 3 weeks following treatment initiation. Potential side effects such as hypotension, bradycardia, and hypoglycemia warrant careful patient monitoring. Treatment progress is based on clinical examination and serial endoscopy or repeat imaging. When there is no response to therapy, biopsy with GLUT-1 immunohistochemical staining can be considered to confirm diagnosis.[28]

A protocol was developed at our institution (The Children's Hospital of Philadelphia) for the initial management of complicated airway hemangiomas with propranolol (**Table 19.3**). Treatment duration varies between institutions and depends on patient factors such as age, initial response, and reaction to discontinuation of therapy. The anticipation is that therapy will continue for about 3 to 6 months, or until the child reaches 6 to 12 months of age. Acebutolol, a selective β₁-receptor blocker, has been investigated for subglottic hemangiomas with some positive results in a small number of patients.[29] Unlike propranolol, acebutolol is cardioselective, has a less frequent dosing schedule (twice a day vs. thrice a day dosing), and has less effect on resting heart rate.

Dermoids

Embryology and Anatomy

Dermoid cysts represent up to 25% of midline congenital neck masses.[30] These lesions occur throughout the head and neck,

Table 19.3 Propranolol Protocol for Airway Hemangiomas (Abbreviated)

Premedication screening
- Baseline evaluation is performed including history and physical examination, electrocardiogram, and if indicated, echocardiogram or cardiac MRI/A to screen for structural cardiac abnormalities associated with decreased cardiac output.
- Consultation with Cardiology team at the discretion of the admitting team. In most cases, screening history and physical examination with specific attention to contraindications (e.g., active reactive airway disease, hypoglycemia, prematurity <32 wk, bradycardia or hypotension, and other medications that would contraindicate concomitant use of β-blockers) is sufficient.
- Consultation of other services based on anatomic location of lesion or organ dysfunction.
- For those with suspected PHACE syndrome, evaluation should include:
  - Cardiology consultation and echocardiogram with attention to right and transverse aortic arch.
  - MRI/A of the head and neck to r/o ischemic intracranial vascular anomalies.
  - Ophthalmology consultation to evaluate for structural eye anomalies.
  - Screening thyroid function testing and rT3 measurement.

Preadmission protocol
- Determination if child should be admitted to ICU or inpatient hospital floor
  - ICU admission for infants <2 mo (chronological or corrected gestational age) or those with unstable health conditions.

Inpatient admission protocol
- On inpatient ward, baseline vitals are obtained, then q2h × 2 doses following initial dose and subsequent dose escalations, then standard q4h.
- ICU patients are monitored continuously.

Dosing protocol
- Day 1: Initiation as oral dose at 0.5 mg/kg/d divided q8h ×3 doses
- Day 2: Oral dose at 1 mg/kg/d divided q8h × 3 doses
- Day 3: Oral dose at 2 mg/kg/d divided q8h × 3 doses
- Blood glucose measurements as well as hold criterion are specified in full protocol.
- If suboptimal or partial results, doses may be escalated to 3–5 mg/kg/d in 0.5–1 mg increments as tolerated. Caution is necessary in patients with bronchospastic disease, diabetes, hepatic or renal impairment, and Wolf-Parkinson-White syndrome.
- Once the target dose is achieved, ambulatory heart rate and blood pressure monitoring is recommended weekly or biweekly for 1 mo and then monthly while on treatment. Closer follow-up may be necessary if oral steroids are being tapered while still on β-blocker.

MRI/A, magnetic resonance imaging/angiography; wk, weeks; PHACE syndrome, posterior fossa malformations, head and neck hemangiomas, arterial anomalies, cardiac defects, eye abnormalities; ICU, intensive care unit; mo, months; q2h, every 2 hours; q4h, every 4 hours; d, day; q8h, every 8 hours.

typically along the lines of embryonic fusion. The histology and anatomic distribution of dermoid lesions suggests they may result from entrapment of epithelial elements along embryonic lines of fusion (**Fig. 19.12**).

Clinical Presentation and Diagnosis

Dermoid cysts typically present before age 3 as painless cervical subcutaneous masses in the anterior neck that move with overlying skin manipulation. Infection is rare, but superficial cysts can rupture and present with granulomatous inflammation. Diagnostic confusion arises when dermoids are located near the hyoid.

Management/Treatment

Surgical excision of the mass is curative. However, some have recommended techniques for performing the Sistrunk procedure when a midline neck mass shares characteristics of dermoid and TGDC.[31]

Cervical Teratomas

Embryology and Anatomy

Teratomas are rare embryonal neoplasms that arise when totipotent germ cells escape developmental control and form tissue masses derived from all three cell layers (endoderm, mesoderm, and ectoderm). Head and neck teratomas represent only 2 to 6% of all teratomas.[30,32]

Clinical Presentation and Diagnosis

The most common sites of head and neck teratomas are cervical and nasopharyngeal.[32] Teratomas may become symptomatic in utero causing polyhydramnios from esophageal obstruction. Diagnosis is often made on prenatal ultrasound, but >50% of these teratomas are diagnosed at birth.[32,33] The α-fetoprotein (AFP) assay is a useful adjunct in establishing a prenatal diagnosis.

Imaging

Ultrasound demonstrates a mixed solid and cystic mass originating most commonly from the anterolateral aspect of the neck with calcifications. MRI provides key anatomic details about the mass and adjacent airway. It can distinguish a predominately cystic teratoma from a cystic lymphatic malformation. Prenatal ultrafast MRI has the advantage of high-contrast resolution, which is unaffected by fetal motion.[33]

Management/Treatment

When prenatal diagnosis of cervical teratoma is made and

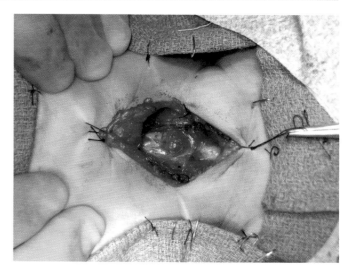

Figure 19.12   Surgical resection of midline neck dermoid.

airway compromise is suspected, an EXIT procedure is planned. Delivery via cesarean section is preferred because the size of the neck mass may preclude vaginal delivery.[16] Sometimes aspiration of a large cystic teratoma is necessary to deliver the head and neck. If initial attempt at direct laryngoscopy or rigid bronchoscopy fails to establish an airway, a tracheostomy is performed. Rare situations of cardiovascular instability or difficult tracheostomy require tumor removal or debulking at the time of delivery while on uteroplacental bypass.[16]

Surgical excision should be performed electively in the first weeks of life because these lesions occupy critical spaces and tend to grow rapidly. The goal is to remove all tumor tissue without sacrificing vital structures. A clean cleavage plane is usually found between the tumor and the structures of the neck because these lesions tend to be encapsulated or psuedoencapsulated.[31,32] Unfortunately, some teratomas are densely adherent to nearby tissues. The risk to anatomic structures depends on location. Postoperatively, serial AFP levels should be obtained to screen for recurrence. Malignant degeneration can occur. Presence of metastasis at birth has also been reported.

Late sequelae including pharyngocutaneous fistula, vocal cord paralysis/paresis, tracheomalacia, hypoparathyroidism, and bleeding have been described.[33] A multidisciplinary team of obstetricians, anesthesiologists, pediatric surgeons, pediatric otolaryngologists, and neonatologists may be required for optimal management of this condition. Some fetuses with large teratomas or severe hydrops may not be viable and termination or open fetal surgery is an option.

References

1. Schroeder JW Jr, Mohyuddin N, Maddalozzo J. Branchial anomalies in the pediatric population. Otolaryngol Head Neck Surg 2007;137(2):289–295

2. Ford GR, Balakrishnan A, Evans JN, Bailey CM. Branchial cleft and pouch anomalies. J Laryngol Otol 1992;106(2):137–143

3. Triglia JM, Nicollas R, Ducroz V, Koltai PJ, Garabedian EN. First branchial cleft anomalies: a study of 39 cases and a review of the literature. Arch Otolaryngol Head Neck Surg 1998;124(3):291–295

4. D'Souza AR, Uppal HS, De R, Zeitoun H. Updating concepts of first branchial cleft defects: a literature review. Int J Pediatr Otorhinolaryngol 2002;62(2):103–109

5. Work WP. Newer concepts of first branchial cleft defects. Laryngoscope 1972;82(9):1581–1593

6. Celis I, Bijnens E, Peene P, Cleeren P. The use of preoperative fistulography in patients with a second branchial cleft anomaly. Eur Radiol 1998;8(7):1179–1180

7. Pereira KD, Davies JN. Piriform sinus tracts in children. Arch Otolaryngol Head Neck Surg 2006;132(10):1119–1121

8. Shrime M, Kacker A, Bent J, Ward RF. Fourth branchial complex anomalies: a case series. Int J Pediatr Otorhinolaryngol 2003;67(11):1227–1233

9. Nicoucar K, Giger R, Jaecklin T, Pope HG Jr, Dulguerov P. Management of congenital third branchial arch anomalies: a systematic review. Otolaryngol Head Neck Surg 2010;142(1):21–28, e2

10. Chen EY, Inglis AF, Ou H, et al. Endoscopic electrocauterization of pyriform fossa sinus tracts as definitive treatment. Int J Pediatr Otorhinolaryngol 2009;73(8):1151–1156

11. Stenquist M, Juhlin C, Aström G, Friberg U. Fourth branchial pouch sinus with recurrent deep cervical abscesses successfully treated with trichloroacetic acid cauterization. Acta Otolaryngol 2003;123(7):879–882

12. Sobol SM, Bailey SB. Evaluation and surgical management of tumors of the neck: benign tumors. In: Thawley SE, Panje WR, Batsakis JG, Lindberg RD, eds. Comprehensive Management of Head and Neck Tumors. Philadelphia, PA: WB Saunders 1999;(65):1416–1449

13. Giguère CM, Bauman NM, Sato Y, et al. Treatment of lymphangiomas with OK-432 (Picibanil) sclerotherapy: a prospective multi-institutional trial. Arch Otolaryngol Head Neck Surg 2002;128(10):1137–1144

14. de Serres LM, Sie KC, Richardson MA. Lymphatic malformations of the head and neck. A proposal for staging. Arch Otolaryngol Head Neck Surg 1995;121(5):577–582

15. Gedikbasi A, Gul A, Sargin A, Ceylan Y. Cystic hygroma and lymphangioma: associated findings, perinatal outcome and prognostic factors in live-born infants. Arch Gynecol Obstet 2007;276(5):491–498

16. Bauman NM, Giguere CM, Manaligod JM, Sato Y, Burke DK, Smith RJH. Management of lymphatic malformations: if, when and how. Oper Tech Otolaryngol Head Neck Surg 2002;13:85–92

17. Riechelmann H, Muehlfay G, Keck T, Mattfeldt T, Rettinger G. Total, subtotal, and partial surgical removal of cervicofacial lymphangiomas. Arch Otolaryngol Head Neck Surg 1999;125(6):643–648

18. Wiegand S, Eivazi B, Zimmermann AP, Sesterhenn AM, Werner JA. Sclerotherapy of lymphangiomas of the head and neck. Head Neck 2011;33(11):1649–1655

19. Burns AJ, Navarro JA. Role of laser therapy in pediatric patients. Plast Reconstr Surg 2009;124(Suppl 1):82e–92e

20. Grimmer JF, Mulliken JB, Burrows PE, Rahbar R. Radiofrequency ablation of microcystic lymphatic malformation in the oral cavity. Arch Otolaryngol Head Neck Surg 2006;132(11):1251–1256

21. Allard RH. The thyroglossal cyst. Head Neck Surg 1982;5(2):134–146

22. Foley DS, Fallat ME. Thyroglossal duct and other congenital midline cervical anomalies. Semin Pediatr Surg 2006;15(2):70–75

23. Perkins JA, Inglis AF, Sie KC, Manning SC. Recurrent thyroglossal duct cysts: a 23-year experience and a new method for management. Ann Otol Rhinol Laryngol 2006;115(11):850–856

24. O TM, Alexander RE, Lando T, et al. Segmental hemangiomas of the upper airway. Laryngoscope 2009;119(11):2242–2247

25. Vilanova JC, Barceló J, Villalón M. MR and MR angiography characterization of soft tissue vascular malformations. Curr Probl Diagn Radiol 2004;33(4):161–170

26. Pransky SM, Canto C. Management of subglottic hemangioma. Curr Opin Otolaryngol Head Neck Surg 2004;12(6):509–512

27. Wiatrak BJ, Reilly JS, Seid AB, Pransky SM, Castillo JV. Open surgical excision of subglottic hemangioma in children. Int J Pediatr Otorhinolaryngol 1996;34(1–2):191–206

28. Truong MT, Perkins JA, Messner AH, Chang KW. Propranolol for the treatment of airway hemangiomas: a case series and treatment algorithm. Int J Pediatr Otorhinolaryngol 2010;74(9):1043–1048

29. Blanchet C, Nicollas R, Bigorre M, Amedro P, Mondain M. Management of infantile subglottic hemangioma: acebutolol or propranolol? Int J Pediatr Otorhinolaryngol 2010;74(8):959–961

30. Azizkhan RGGM, Haase GM, Applebaum H, et al. Diagnosis, management, and outcome of cervicofacial teratomas in neonates: a Children's Cancer Group study. J Pediatr Surg 1995;30(2):312–316

31. Soucy P, Penning J. The clinical relevance of certain observations on the histology of the thyroglossal tract. J Pediatr Surg 1984;19(5):506–509

32. De Backer A, Madern GC, van de Ven CP, Tibboel D, Hazebroek FW. Strategy for management of newborns with cervical teratoma. J Perinat Med 2004;32(6):500–508

33. Breysem L, Bosmans H, Dymarkowski S, et al. The value of fast MR imaging as an adjunct to ultrasound in prenatal diagnosis. Eur Radiol 2003;13(7):1538–1548

20 Malignant Pediatric Neck Tumors

Kenneth R. Whittemore Jr. and Michael J. Cunningham

The majority of neck masses in the pediatric age group are of infectious, inflammatory, or congenital origin. Although comparatively less frequent, malignant cervical neoplasms occur and can be a significant cause of pediatric morbidity and mortality. This chapter focuses on the presentation, evaluation, and management of the more common pediatric neck malignancies.

Cervical malignancies arise primarily from structures in the neck, extend secondarily from adjacent regions such as the mediastinum or skull base, or represent from metastases from distant sites. As a result, the potential diagnoses of a firm neck mass in a child or adolescent can be quite broad. The patient's age, location of the mass, clinical history, associated physical examination findings, and evaluative work-up all help narrow this differential diagnosis.

Evaluation

A child presenting with a mass in the neck requires a thorough medical examination. The risk of malignancy is increased by positive family history, a history of radiation exposure, immunodeficiency or immunosuppression, or the presence of certain syndromes and genetic disorders. The age of the child is also predicative of the likelihood of particular malignancies.[1]

Given that cervical malignancies may be primary, secondary, or metastatic, both a thorough head and neck and systemic examination are necessary. The cervicofacial examination should include the skin seeking pigmented lesions, a complete cranial nerve review, and a detailed assessment of the upper aerodigestive tract including the nasopharynx, hypopharynx, and larynx. Depending on the age, cooperativeness, and health of the child, the latter examination may require a diagnostic laryngoscopy with or without a bronchoscopy and esophagoscopy.

Imaging is often necessary in the evaluation of pediatric neck masses and the type of imaging depends on the location and character of the mass, age of the patient, presence of hardware such as braces, and medical conditions such as renal insufficiency or potential airway obstruction with sedation. Ultrasonography has several advantages. It involves no radiation, can be performed even in children of all ages without sedation, and allows determination of mass location, consistency, and vascular flow characteristics. Ultrasound is also ideal for guiding fine-needle aspiration biopsies. Greater anatomical detail is often required for both diagnostic and therapeutic decision-making; such is provided by either computed tomography (CT) or magnetic resonance imaging (MRI). CT imaging is useful for masses adjacent to osseous or cartilaginous structures seeking evidence of erosion. CT imaging can be coordinated with a guided biopsy. In the case of a potential thyroid malignancy, contrast enhancement should be avoided as it precludes the subsequent use of radioactive iodine. MRI provides the greatest degree of soft tissue detail. Gadolinium enhancement determines vascularity, and magnetic resonance angiography may provide even greater detail. The anatomical detail and lack of radiation are major advantages of MRI. The presence of hardware can preclude its performance, and the need for anesthesia in younger children is a disadvantage. Additional imaging studies such as positron emission tomography (PET) and bone scans may be considered, particularly when metastatic disease is likely or the cervical lesion itself is a potential metastasis. Nonimaging evaluative studies of potential utility include a complete blood count with a manual differential, chemistry panel, lactate dehydrogenase level, liver function tests, renal function indices, and urinalysis. Metastatic assessment may require chest films, lumbar puncture, and bone marrow biopsy. Early consultation with an oncologist can be helpful in guiding the staging work-up, suggesting specific genetic marker screening, and speaking with the family both before and after a diagnosis is made. A tissue biopsy is nearly always required for diagnosis. On occasion in older children and adolescents, and with specific lesions such as suspected thyroid malignancies, ultrasound or CT-guided fine-needle aspiration biopsy may suffice. More frequently, operative incisional or excisional biopsy is necessary. The method of obtaining the tissue depends on several factors including the size, anatomical location and vascularity of the lesion, its potential resectability, and the probability that the primary treatment of the lesion will be surgical or nonsurgical.

Differential Diagnosis

The differential diagnosis of a firm neck mass in the pediatric population is broad given the variety of tissue types present within and adjacent to the neck, as well as the potential for regional and systemic metastases.[2] This chapter will focus on the more common entities including Hodgkin lymphoma and non-Hodgkin lymphomas, rhabdomyosarcoma and neuroblastoma.

Hodgkin Lymphoma

Hodgkin lymphoma (HL) is a malignant neoplasm of the lymphoreticular system with a bimodal distribution, one peak of which occurs in adolescence and the second in young adulthood. In contrast to NHL, HL is uncommon in preadolescent children and rarely occurs in children younger than 5 years of age.[3] Although no definitive causal factors are known, there is an association between Epstein-Barr virus (EBV) infection and HL.

HL is distinguished pathologically by the diagnostic presence of Reed-Sternberg (RS) cells admixed within the appropriate pleomorphic cellular background. The historical HL classification system—the Rye classification system—recognizes four subtypes based upon this cellular background: lymphocyte predominant, lymphocyte depletion, nodular sclerosis, and mixed cellularity.[4] The lymphocyte predominant category is characterized by an abundance of mature lymphocytes with only occasional RS cells. Such nodular lymphocyte predominant Hodgkin lymphoma (NLPHL) can also be distinguished from the other subtypes of HL by immunohistochemical staining techniques. The Revised European-American Lymphoma classification system accounts for this differentiation, dividing HL into two broad categories: classic HL and NLPHL.[5] Further rationale for this classification system is documentation that NLPHL has different virologic features and is clinically less aggressive than classic HL.

HL arises within lymph nodes in more than 90% of childhood, adolescent, and young adult cases. The typical patient with HL has asymmetric firm, rubbery, and nontender lymphadenopathy. The cervical, supraclavicular, and mediastinal lymph nodes are the most frequently involved. Obstruction of the superior vena cava or tracheobronchial tree may occur as a complication of mediastinal lymphadenopathy. Extranodal involvement does occur with disease progression; the spleen, liver, lung, bone, and bone marrow are common organ systems affected. At presentation, 25 to 30% of HL patients manifest nonspecific systemic symptoms such as unexplained fever, night sweats, weight loss, weakness, anorexia, and pruritis.[3]

The diagnosis of HL is made by lymph node biopsy. Once the diagnosis is established, it is essential to define the full extent of disease before instituting specific treatment. The Ann Arbor staging system (**Table 20.1**) is used to stratify risk for HL patients. This staging system is based on the premise that HL arises in a unifocal lymph node site, spreads via lymphatics to contiguous lymph node groups, and involves extralymphatic sites, including the spleen, principally by hematogenous dissemination. The system recognizes that patients with localized extralymphatic spread—denoted by the letter E—do as well as comparable patients of the same stage without such disease extension. Systemic symptoms are considered significant in HL staging and are designated A when absent and B when present.[6]

The treatment of HL varies according to stage and is typically multimodal. Stage IA and IIA disease is usually treated with a combination of low-dose multiagent chemotherapy and radiation therapy to the involved field. Intermediate risk patients include those with Stage IIIA disease or Stages I or II disease with B symptoms, bulky disease, or spleen involvement. These patients require an increased number of chemotherapy cycles and either increased dose or volume of radiation therapy. For patients with high-risk advanced Stage IIIB and IV diseases, multiagent chemotherapy alone or in combination with radiation therapy is used. The recent management of HL distinguishes between children who have obtained full growth and those who are still growing in an attempt to limit the high doses and extended fields of radiation therapy that cause considerable long-term morbidity for children and young adolescents. Similarly, chemotherapeutic regimens have been changed to reduce the risks

Table 20.1 Ann Arbor Staging Classification of Hodgkin Lymphoma

Stage	Definition
I	Involvement of a single lymph node region (I) or of a single extralymphatic organ or site (I_E).
II	Involvement of two or more lymph node regions on the same side of the diaphragm (II) or localized involvement of extralymphatic organ or site and of one or more lymph node regions on the same side of the diaphragm (II_E). An optional recommendation is that the numbers of node regions involved be indicated by a subscript numerals (e.g., II_3).
III	Involvement of lymph node regions on both sides of the diaphragm (III), which may also be accompanied by localized involvement of extralymphatic organ or site (III_E) or by involvement of the spleen (III_S), or both (III_{SE}).
IV	Diffuse or disseminated involvement of one or more extralymphatic organs or tissues with or without associated lymph node enlargement. The reason for classifying the patient as Stage IV should be identified further by defining site by symbols.

[a]Each stage is subdivided into A and B categories indicating the absence or presence, respectively, of documented unexplained fever, night sweats, or weight loss (>10% of body weight in the past 6 months).

Adapted from: Cunningham MJ, Myers EN, Bluestone CD. Malignant tumors of the head and neck in children: a twenty-year review. *Int J Pediatr Otorhinolaryngol* 1987;13(3):279–292 of sterility, pulmonary toxicity, and secondary malignancies. HL patients who relapse may be candidates for autologous stem cell transplantation.

With current treatments, more than 90% of all HL patients, regardless of stage, initially achieve a complete remission. Prolonged remission and cure is achieved in approximately 90% of patients with early Stage I and II disease and in 35 to 60% of patients with advanced Stage III and IV disease. Patients with lymphocyte predominant lesions have the most favorable survival statistics.[3,7]

Non-Hodgkin Lymphoma

Non-Hodgkin lymphoma (NHL) designates a heterogeneous group of solid primary neoplasms of the lymphoreticular system. In children, NHL most commonly occurs between the ages of 2 and 12 years and, as in HL, demonstrates a male predilection. Both congenital and acquired immunodeficiency disorders predispose to the development of NHL.[8]

Immunologic staining techniques allow separation of NHL into categories of B-cell, T-cell, and histiocytic origin. The B- and T-cell lymphomas are further subdivided based on their morphologic appearance, degree of lymphocytic transformation, and responsiveness to therapy.[9] The classification schema of NHL is dynamic due to constant advances in immunophenotyping.

The clinical features of NHL reflect the site of origin of the primary tumor and the extent of local and systemic disease. Asymptomatic cervical lymphadenopathy is the most common initial presentation; inguinal, axillary, and generalized nodal presentations are comparatively less frequent. Although nodal growth may be rapid, insidious presentations are more typical.

Extranodal NHL occurs frequently in children.[10] Extranodal head and neck sites include the oropharynx and naso-

pharynx, the nose and paranasal sinuses, the orbit, and the maxilla and mandible. The signs and symptoms attributable to extranodal cervicofacial NHL are quite variable and site specific; these may include nasal blockage and other manifestations of upper airway obstruction, dysphagia, orbital or facial swelling, and cranial nerve deficits. Oronasopharyngeal NHL may mimic benign adenotonsillar hypertrophy; biopsy via adenoidectomy or tonsillectomy may be warranted if there is asymmetry, discoloration, or evidence of systemic symptoms.

The St. Jude's classification system (**Table 20.2**) is the staging system most commonly used for NHL. This system attempts to account for both the characteristic extranodal presentations and the tendency toward hematogenous dissemination, bone marrow infiltration, and central nervous system (CNS) involvement in childhood NHL.[11] The clinical staging of NHL of the head and neck requires a comprehensive history and physical examination, serologic testing such as a complete blood count and lactate dehydrogenase level, chest radiograph, skeletal survey or bone scan, bone marrow biopsy, and cerebrospinal fluid analysis in addition to appropriate head and neck imaging by means of CT and MRI. Abdominal CT with contrast or ultrasound may be used to assess for mesenteric lymph node involvement. More recently, gallium-67 scanning and PET with ^{18}F-fluoro-2-deoxy-D-glucose have been used for disease staging and for following treatment response.

The diagnosis of NHL requires biopsy; typically excisional biopsy for nodal disease or incisional biopsy for extranodal disease. Surgery plays little additional role in NHL treatment with the exception of surgical debulking in selected cases of aerodigestive tract compression or when reduction of tumor load may lower the risk of development of tumor lysis syndrome. The latter is particularly true for Burkitt lymphoma.

Stage I NHL is infrequently diagnosed in the pediatric age

Table 20.2   St. Jude's Classification System of Non-Hodgkin Lymphoma

Stage	Criteria for Extent of Disease
I	A single tumor (extranodal) or single anatomic area (nodal), with the exclusion of mediastinum or abdomen.
II	• A single tumor (extranodal) with regional node involvement. • Two or more nodal areas on the same side of the diaphragm. • Two single (extranodal) tumors with or without regional node involvement on the same side of the diaphragm. • A primary gastrointestinal tract tumor, usually in the ileocecal area, with or without involvement of associated mesenteric nodes only.
III	• Two single tumors (extranodal) on opposite sides of the diaphragm. • Two or more nodal areas above and below the diaphragm. • All the primary intrathoracic tumors (mediastinal, pleural, thymic). • All extensive primary intra-abdominal disease. • All paraspinal or epidural tumors, regardless of other tumor site(s).
IV	Any of the above with initial central nervous system and/or bone marrow involvement.

Adapted from: Murphy SB. Childhood non-Hodgkin lymphoma. *N Engl L Med* 1978;299:1446–1448.

group; the exception to this rule is follicular lymphoma. The vast majority of children with NHL have advanced Stage II, III, or IV disease at presentation. The principal treatment for nearly all stages of pediatric head and neck NHL is systemic chemotherapy; the rapid doubling time of high-grade NHL makes it very chemoresponsive.[12]

Both early and late therapeutic complications are common. Early complications generally result from the rapid lysis of tumor cells and bone marrow suppression. The most significant long-term complications relate to the development of secondary malignancies.

Prognosis is principally associated with disease stage and response to initial therapy. The current overall 5-year disease-free survival rate for NHL of the head and neck approximates 70 to 76%. The event-free survival rate for NHL, irrespective of site of origin, is 85 to 95% for stage I and II disease, and 50 to 85% for stage III and IV disease, depending on immunohistopathologic subtype.[10,13]

Rhabdomyosarcoma

Rhabdomyosarcoma (RMS) is the most common soft tissue malignancy in children with an incidence of about 6 in 1,000,000 in the pediatric population. Anderson et al reported that 50% of cases occur in children younger than 6 years of age, and a cervicofacial presentation is common, accounting for 40% cases.[14]

RMS is of primitive muscle cell origin and is considered one of the small blue-cell tumors. Positive staining for muscle-specific proteins such as vimentin, muscle actin, desmin, myoglobin, and myo-D1 is diagnostic.[15] RMS is classified into four histopathologic subtypes—embryonal, alveolar, undifferentiated, and botryoid (meaning grape-like)—with relative percentages at presentation of 55, 20, 20, and 5%, respectively.[16]

RMS generally presents as a rapidly growing, painless, cervicofacial mass. Symptomatic manifestations reflect the site of origin; these may include dysphonia, dysphagia, dyspnea, trismus, cranial nerve deficits, brachial plexus neuropathy, and Horner syndrome. RMS may also manifest at systemic sites with presenting symptoms dependent upon the organ system involved. Metastatic spread may occur through direct extension, via the lymphatic system, and hematogenously to distal organs. The risk of CNS involvement is particularly high if the primary tumor is in a parameningeal location.

The treatment of RMS is guided by the primary site of involvement and stage of disease. The Intergroup Rhabdomyosarcoma Study Group (IRSG) established a staging system (**Table 20.3**) based on extent of disease (localized, regional, or systemic) and if excision of local or regional disease can be accomplished.[17,18] Extent of disease is determined by the bounds of the primary tumor, regional lymphatic spread, and the presence of metastatic disease. Various studies may be ordered to aid in assessing the stage

of disease. A complete blood count may show anemia if there is bone marrow invasion; liver enzyme elevation can indicate hepatic metastases. Contrast-enhanced CT or MRI will aid in determining the extent of the primary tumor, specifically if there is extension beyond the muscle group of origin. Imaging of the chest, abdomen, and brain may also be required to complete the metastatic work-up. Both CNS imaging and lumbar puncture are necessary if the primary tumor is in a parameningeal location.

Complete excision of the primary tumor is indicated when removal imposes no major functional disability and permits either the elimination of postoperative radiation therapy or a reduction in radiation dose. When only partial tumor resection is possible, initial surgery is often limited to biopsy. A study comparing the role of surgical biopsy versus debulking in patients with IRSG III disease showed no difference in outcome.[19]

The role of a "second-look" surgical procedure following primary therapy is controversial. In the IRSG III study, patients with group III disease, confirmed to be partial responders to multimodality therapy based on a "second-look" surgical procedure, benefited from additional chemotherapy.[20] Postoperative radiation therapy in patients with group III nonalveolar RMS may benefit from the use of follow-up radiotherapy even when a "second-look" procedure shows a complete response.[21] Another study looking at the prognostic significance of RMS at the end of primary therapy suggests that there is no improvement in disease recurrence or mortality whether the patients were complete responders or partial or nonresponders, suggesting that in this group of patients aggressive follow-up therapy may not be necessary.[22] These study results suggest that a second-look procedure may be helpful to determine if further radiotherapy or chemotherapy may be beneficial depending on the stage and histology of the disease.

Chemotherapy is typically administered postoperatively to patients with small resectable lesions and preoperatively to patients with larger lesions to decrease tumor volume before local treatment. Such local treatment may require a combination of surgical resection and radiation. Radiation therapy is also indicated for patients with group II, III, or IV tumors. Children with a clinically positive neck benefit from neck dissection and postoperative radiotherapy.

Prognosis is dependent on histopathologic subtype, genetic predisposition, and stage of disease. Alveolar and undifferentiated RMS have a poorer survival rate compared with embryonal and botryoid RMS.[23] Chromosomal abnormalities such as the PAX3-FKHR fusion associated with the translocation t(2;13) (q35;q14) have a negative prognostic implication.[24] Spontaneous occurrence of RMS has been associated with a mutation of the *PTCH* gene (abnormality in 9q22.3 locus), implying that environmental exposure may play a role.[25,26]

The IRSG was formed in 1972 to systematically study patients with RMS regarding treatment, prognosis, and

Table 20.3   Staging of rhabdomyosarcoma according to the Intergroup Rhabdomyosarcoma Study

Group I	Localized disease with tumor completely resected and regional nodes not affected. Confined to muscle or organ of origin. No contiguous involvement or infiltration outside the muscle or organ of origin.
Group II	Localized disease with microscopic residual disease, or regional disease with neither microscopic nor residual disease. Grossly resected tumor with microscopic residual disease (nodes negative). Regional tumor completely resected (nodes positive or negative). Regional disease with involved nodes grossly resected but with evidence of microscopic residual disease.
Group III	Incomplete resection or biopsy with gross residual disease.
Group IV	Metastatic disease present at onset.

staging.[27] The IRSG summary studies are designated as RMS-I, -II, -III, -IV. These designations need to be distinguished from the group staging of patients with RMS.

The 5-year survival rate in IRSG-III for select groups is as follows: group I favorable histology (93%); group I unfavorable histology and group II (54 to 81%); group III (74%); and group IV (27 to 31%).[20] Individuals who are free of recurrence 2 years after treatment are probably cured.[28] The time to relapse appears to have prognostic significance that is independent of histology or tumor site: children in whom recurrence was at less than 6 months, between 6 and 12 months, and after 12 months had 4-year survival rates of 12, 21, and 41%, respectively.[29]

The overall 5-year survival rate for patients with nonmetastatic RMS approximates 80%; this rate decreases to 30% in patients with metastatic disease.[30] The IRSG-IV protocol addresses distant metastases with trials of various chemotherapeutic agents before the introduction of standard chemotherapy and radiation therapy.[31] IRSG-V is in progress and groups patients based on their risk of recurrence and is looking at the best combination of therapies based on these groupings.[27]

Neuroblastoma

Neuroblastoma is a malignancy that most commonly arises in patients under the age of 5 years. It is slightly more common in boys, with an overall incidence of about 1 in 100,000. Cervicofacial neuroblastoma may represent either primary or metastatic disease. Approximately 2 to 4% of primary neuroblastoma arises in the cervical region.

Mutations in the *ALK* and *PHOX2B* genes have been identified in patients with neuroblastoma. The PHOX2B mutation is also associated with congenital central hypoventilation syndrome and Hirschsprung disease; a family history of either of these diseases or neuroblastoma warrants genetic screening.[32,33] Only 1 to 2% of children with neuroblastoma have this familial form which is autosomal dominant with incomplete penetrance.

Neuroblastoma arises from neural crest cells of the sympathetic nervous system. It falls into the category of small, round, blue-cell tumors that also include desmoplastic small cell tumor, Ewing sarcoma, acute leukemia, primitive neuroectodermal tumor, RMS, and Wilms tumor. The cells are round with a high nuclear to cytoplasmic ratio, may form rosettes, and have necrotic areas. Positive immunohistochemical staining for neuron-specific enolase distinguishes neuroblastoma from the other small, round, blue-cell tumors.

Primary cervical neuroblastoma usually arises in children in the first few years of life. The lesion typically occurs in the lateral neck and is often firm. Both the specific location of the mass and any present neurological deficits may predict what structures are affected by the lesion. Numbness or weakness of the upper limbs indicates involvement of the brachial plexus. Horner syndrome and/or heterochromia are reflective of sympathetic chain involvement.[34] Dysphagia, dysphonia, or dyspnea may be found secondary to compression of the aerodigestive tract or by involvement of cranial nerves IX through XII.

Cervical neuroblastoma most commonly represents metastatic disease from a distant systemic site. As the adrenal medulla is a frequent primary site, palpation of the abdomen is needed to evaluate for a mass. Spinal tenderness may be indicative of disease in a vertebral body. Dissemination of disease through the vascular system occurs in 25% of children below 1 year of age and in 68% of children older than 1 year of age; common hematogenous metastatic sites include bone marrow, skin, and liver.[35,36]

The diagnosis of neuroblastoma requires adequate tissue for histopathologic examination; an open biopsy is often necessary. The evaluation of a child with suspected or confirmed neuroblastoma should additionally include the following: 24-hour urinalysis for the catecholamine by-products homovanillic acid and vanillylmandelic acid; imaging of the neck, abdomen, and chest with contrast-enhanced CT or MRI; bone scanning to detect osseous metastases; and meta-iodobenzylguanidine (MIBG) scintiscan

Table 20.4 International Neuroblastoma Staging System Classification

Stage 1	Localized tumor with complete gross excision, with or without microscopic residual disease; representative ipsilateral lymph nodes negative for tumor microscopically (nodes attached to and removed with the primary tumor may be positive).
Stage 2A	Localized tumor with incomplete gross excision; representative ipsilateral nonadherent lymph nodes negative for tumor microscopically.
Stage 2B	Localized tumor with or without complete gross excision, with ipsilateral nonadherent lymph nodes positive for tumor. Enlarged contralateral lymph nodes must be negative microscopically.
Stage 3	Unresectable unilateral tumor infiltrating across the midline, with or without regional lymph node involvement; or localized unilateral tumor with contralateral regional lymph node involvement; or midline tumor with bilateral extension by infiltration (unresectable) or by lymph node involvement.
Stage 4	Any primary tumor with dissemination to distant lymph nodes, bone, bone marrow, liver, skin, and/or other organs (except as defined for Stage 4S).
Stage 4S	Localized primary tumor (as defined for Stages 1, 2A, or 2B), with dissemination limited to skin, liver, and/or bone marrow (limited to infants <1 year of age).

to identify tumors particularly in nonosseous sites, as MIBG is taken up by sympathetic tissue.

A risk-stratification protocol categorizes neuroblastoma patients into 4 broad groups based on 13 parameters. Several of the more important parameters include age, tumor histology, stage of disease (**Table 20.4**), tumor ploidy, and the presence or absence of the molecular genetic marker N-myc.[37] Tumors that are determined to be triploidy tend to not metastasize and have a better prognosis than those tumors that are diploid. The presence of N-myc amplification is less common in localized disease compared with more disseminated disease, and the higher the amplification of N-myc in a tumor, the poorer the patient's prognosis.

Primary cervical neuroblastoma may be treated with surgical removal alone if completely resectable. Partly resectable primary or metastatic cervical neuroblastoma requires chemotherapy and/or radiation therapy in accordance with the following parameters. Surgery alone with minimal morbidity is recommended for low-risk, isolated disease. Intermediate risk disease involves surgery and moderately intensive chemotherapy. High-risk disease requires intensive chemotherapy, surgery, and external beam radiotherapy to

primary tumor and resistant metastatic sites, myeloablative chemotherapy with autologous hematopoietic stem cell rescue, and possible immunotherapy.[38] Five-year event-free survival rates based on these risk groups are as follows: very low risk (>85%), low risk (>75 to ≤85%), intermediate risk (≥50 to ≤75%), and high risk (<50%).[37]

Conclusion

Children diagnosed with a head and neck malignancy require multiple services for optimal care. In addition to the management provided by various surgical and medical pediatric specialists, there is a need for social and psychological support of the child, parents, and other family members. Child psychiatry, social work, child-life specialists, chaplin services, and parental support groups will complement the medical and surgical care of both the child and the family through this difficult time. In addition, one must also keep in mind that this is a lifelong commitment, as the survivors of childhood malignancies require long-term follow-up due to potential therapeutic complications and the risk of secondary malignancies.

References

1. Cunningham MJ, Myers EN, Bluestone CD. Malignant tumors of the head and neck in children: a twenty-year review. Int J Pediatr Otorhinolaryngol 1987;13(3):279–292
2. Albright JT, Topham AK, Reilly JS. Pediatric head and neck malignancies: US incidence and trends over 2 decades. Arch Otolaryngol Head Neck Surg 2002;128(6):655–659
3. Hudson MM, Donaldson SS. Hodgkin's disease. Pediatr Clin North Am 1997;44(4):891–906
4. Lukes RJ, Craver LF, Hall TC, Rappaport H, Ruben P. Report of the Nomenclature Committee. Cancer Res 1966;26:1311–1383
5. Harris NL, Jaffe ES, Stein H, et al. A revised European-American

classification of lymphoid neoplasms: a proposal from the International Lymphoma Study Group. Blood 1994;84(5):1361–1392
6. Carbone PP, Kaplan HS, Musshoff K, Smithers DW, Tubiana M. Report of the Committee on Hodgkin's Disease Staging Classification. Cancer Res 1971;31(11):1860–1861
7. Pötter R. Paediatric Hodgkin's disease. Eur J Cancer 1999;35(10): 1466–1474, discussion 1474–1476
8. Sandlund JT, Downing JR, Crist WM. Non-Hodgkin's lymphoma in childhood. N Engl J Med 1996;334(19):1238–1248
9. National Cancer Institute sponsored study of classifications of

non-Hodgkin lymphomas: summary and description of a working formulation for clinical usage. The Non-Hodgkin Lymphoma Pathologic Classification Project. Cancer 1982;49:2112–2135

10. La Quaglia MP. Non-Hodgkin's lymphoma of the head and neck in childhood. Semin Pediatr Surg 1994;3(3):207–215

11. Murphy SB. Classification, staging and end results of treatment of childhood non-Hodgkin's lymphomas: dissimilarities from lymphomas in adults. Semin Oncol 1980;7(3):332–339

12. Whalen TV, La Quaglia MP. The lymphomas: an update for surgeons. Semin Pediatr Surg 1997;6(1):50–55

13. Murphy SB. Childhood non-Hodgkin's lymphoma. N Engl J Med 1978;299(26):1446–1448

14. Anderson GJ, Tom LW, Womer RB, Handler SD, Wetmore RF, Potsic WP. Rhabdomyosarcoma of the head and neck in children. Arch Otolaryngol Head Neck Surg 1990;116(4):428–431

15. Pilch BZ. Head and Neck Surgical Pathology. Philadelphia, PA: Lippincott Williams and Wilkins; 2001:422–424

16. Pappo AS, Shapiro DN, Crist WM, Maurer HM. Biology and therapy of pediatric rhabdomyosarcoma. J Clin Oncol 1995;13(8):2123–2139

17. Barnes L. Tumors and tumor-like lesions of the soft tissues. In: Barnes L, ed. Surgical Pathology of the Head and Neck. New York, NY: Marcel Dekker; 1985:725–880

18. Maurer HM, Moon T, Donaldson M, et al. The intergroup rhabdomyosarcoma study: a preliminary report. Cancer 1977; 40(5):2015–2026

19. Cecchetto G, Bisogno G, De Corti F, et al; Italian Cooperative Group. Biopsy or debulking surgery as initial surgery for locally advanced rhabdomyosarcomas in children?: the experience of the Italian Cooperative Group studies. Cancer 2007;110(11):2561–2567

20. Crist W, Gehan EA, Ragab AH, et al. The third intergroup rhabdomyosarcoma study. J Clin Oncol 1995;13(3):610–630

21. Cecchetto G, Carretto E, Bisogno G, et al. Complete second look operation and radiotherapy in locally advanced non-alveolar rhabdomyosarcoma in children: A report from the AIEOP soft tissue sarcoma committee. Pediatr Blood Cancer 2008;51(5):593–597

22. Rodeberg DA, Stoner JA, Hayes-Jordan A, et al. Prognostic significance of tumor response at the end of therapy in group III rhabdomyosarcoma: a report from the children's oncology group. J Clin Oncol 2009;27(22):3705–3711

23. Hays DM, Newton W Jr., Soule EH, et al. Mortality among children with rhabdomyosarcomas of the alveolar histologic subtype. J Pediatr Surg 1983;18(4):412–417

24. Anderson J, Gordon T, McManus A, et al; UK Children's Cancer Study Group (UKCCSG) and the UK Cancer Cytogenetics Group. Detection of the *PAX3-FKHR* fusion gene in paediatric rhabdomyosarcoma: a reproducible predictor of outcome? Br J Cancer 2001;85(6):831–835

25. Calzada-Wack J, Schnitzbauer U, Walch A, et al. Analysis of the PTCH coding region in human rhabdomyosarcoma. Hum Mutat 2002;20(3):233–234

26. Tostar U, Malm CJ, Meis-Kindblom JM, Kindblom LG, Toftgård R, Undén AB. Deregulation of the hedgehog signalling pathway: a possible role for the PTCH and SUFU genes in human rhabdomyoma and rhabdomyosarcoma development. J Pathol 2006; 208(1):17–25

27. Raney RB, Maurer HM, Anderson JR, et al. The Intergroup Rhabdomyosarcoma Study Group (IRSG): major lessons from the IRS-I through IRS-IV studies as background for the current IRS-V treatment protocols. Sarcoma 2001;5(1):9–15

28. Raney RB Jr., Crist WM, Maurer HM, Foulkes MA. Prognosis of children with soft tissue sarcoma who relapse after achieving a complete response. A report from the Intergroup Rhabdomyosarcoma Study I. Cancer 1983;52(1):44–50

29. Mattke AC, Bailey EJ, Schuck A, et al. Does the time-point of relapse influence outcome in pediatric rhabdomyosarcomas? Pediatr Blood Cancer 2009;52(7):772–776

30. Punyko JA, Mertens AC, Baker KS, Ness KK, Robison LL, Gurney JG. Long-term survival probabilities for childhood rhabdomyosarcoma. A population-based evaluation. Cancer 2005;103(7):1475–1483

31. Raney RB Jr., Tefft M, Maurer HM, et al. Disease patterns and survival rate in children with metastatic soft-tissue sarcoma. A report from the Intergroup Rhabdomyosarcoma Study (IRS)-I. Cancer 1988;62(7):1257–1266

32. Mosse YP, Laudenslager M, Khazi D, et al. Germline PHOX2B mutation in hereditary neuroblastoma. Am J Hum Genet 2004;75(4):727–730

33. Trochet D, Bourdeaut F, Janoueix-Lerosey I, et al. Germline mutations of the paired-like homeobox 2B (*PHOX2B*) gene in neuroblastoma. Am J Hum Genet 2004;74(4):761–764

34. Jaffe N, Cassady R, Petersen R, Traggis D. Heterochromia and Horner syndrome associated with cervical and mediastinal neuroblastoma. J Pediatr 1975;87(1):75–77

35. Brodeur GM, Castleberry RP, Pizzo PA. Principles and Practice of Pediatric Oncology: Neuroblastoma. Philadelphia, PA:JB Lippincott;1997:771

36. Castleberry RP. Predicting outcome in neuroblastoma. N Engl J Med 1999;340(25):1992–1993

37. Cohn SL, Pearson AD, London WB, et al; INRG Task Force. The International Neuroblastoma Risk Group (INRG) classification system: an INRG Task Force report. J Clin Oncol 2009;27(2):289–297

38. Maris JM. Recent advances in neuroblastoma. N Engl J Med 2010;362(23):2202–2211

Index